Breast Cancer: Gene Regulation and Metastasis

Breast Cancer: Gene Regulation and Metastasis

Edited by **Sandra Lekin**

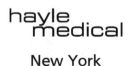

New York

Published by Hayle Medical,
30 West, 37th Street, Suite 612,
New York, NY 10018, USA
www.haylemedical.com

Breast Cancer: Gene Regulation and Metastasis
Edited by Sandra Lekin

© 2015 Hayle Medical

International Standard Book Number: 978-1-63241-066-5 (Hardback)

Contents

Preface

The main aim of this book is to educate learners and enhance their research focus by presenting diverse topics covering this vast field. This is an advanced book which compiles significant studies by distinguished experts in the area of analysis. This book addresses successive solutions to the challenges arising in the area of application, along with it; the book provides scope for future developments.

Commonly known to occur in women, breast cancer can also occur in men. Cancer is the principal reason of death in the majority of countries and it results in enormous financial, societal and mental burden. Breast cancer is the most diagnosed kind of cancer and the foremost reason of death due to cancer amongst women. This book deals with various aspects of breast cancer. It discusses topics related to gene regulation and metastasis of breast cancer. It intends to help students and experts in gaining more knowledge regarding the topic.

It was a great honour to edit this book, though there were challenges, as it involved a lot of communication and networking between me and the editorial team. However, the end result was this all-inclusive book covering diverse themes in the field.

Finally, it is important to acknowledge the efforts of the contributors for their excellent chapters, through which a wide variety of issues have been addressed. I would also like to thank my colleagues for their valuable feedback during the making of this book.

Editor

Part 1

Breast Cancer Gene Regulation

Histone Modification and Breast Cancer

Xue-Gang Luo, Shu Guo, Yu Guo and Chun-Ling Zhang
Tianjin University of Science and Technology
P. R. China

1. Introduction

In eukaryotic cells, DNA is maintained in a highly ordered and condensed form via its association with small, basic histone proteins. The fundamental subunit of chromatin, the nucleosome, is composed of an octamer of four core histones, an H3/H4 tetramer and two H2A/H2B dimers, around which 146 bp of DNA are wrapped. Dynamic modulation of chromatin structure, that is, chromatin remodeling, is a key component in the regulation of gene expression, apoptosis, DNA replication and repair and chromosome condensation and segregation. Enzymes that eovalently modify histones control many cellular processes by affecting gene expression. These modifications of core histones mainly include of methylation, acetylation, phosphorylation, ubiquitination/sumoylation, ADP-ribosylation, deamination, and proline isomerisation (Ito, 2007; Bartova et al., 2008). The abnormal regulation of these processes is intimately associated with human diseases, including cancer.

Breast cancer, the leading cause of death from cancer in women, is a heterogeneous disease ranging from premalignant hyperproliferation to invasive and metastatic carcinomas (Jemal et al., 2011). The disease progression is poorly understood but is likely due to the accumulation of genetic mutations leading to widespread changes in gene expression. Accumulating evidence has suggested that abnormal alteration of histone modification plays roles in the process of breast cancer. This chapter will summarize the relationship between histone modification and the molecular mechanism of breast cancer, and the therapy strategies focused on histone modification for breast cancer will also be discussed.

2. Histone modification and breast cancer

2.1 Chromatin structure and histone modifications

Chromatin is the physiological template of eukaryotic genome. Its fundamental unit, the nucleosome core particle, contains ~200 bp of DNA, organized by an octamer of small, basic proteins. The protein components are histones (two copies of each highly conserved core histone protein – H2A, H2B, H3 and H4). They form an interior core; the DNA lies on the surface of the particle. Nucleosomes are an invariant component of euchromatin and heterochromatin in the interphase nucleus, and of mitotic chromosomes. The nucleosome core particle represents the first level of organization, with a packing ratio of ~6. The second level of organization is the coiling of the series of nucleosomes into a helical array to form the fiber with ~30 nm diameter, which is found in both interphase chromatin and mitotic chromosomes. This brings the packing ratio of DNA to ~40 in chromatin. The fiber-like structure requires additional proteins, which has not been well defined. The final packing ratio is determined by the third level of organization, the packaging of the 30 nm fiber itself. This gives a total packing ratio of ~ 1000 in euchromatin, cyclically interchangeable with packing into mitotic chromosomes to reach an overall ratio of ~10,000. Heterochromatin generally has a packing ratio -10,000 in both interphase and mitosis (Fig 1) (Lewin, 2004).

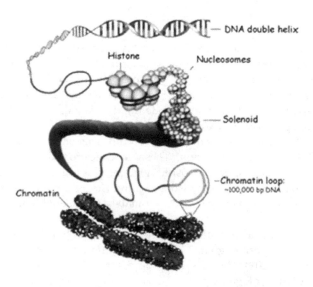

Fig. 1. Chromatin structure in eukaryotic cells

Local chromatin architecture is now generally recognized as an important factor in the regulation of gene expression. This architecture of chromatin is strongly regulated by post-translational modifications of the N-terminal tails of the histones. Core histones are subjected to a wide range of covalent modifications including methylation, acetylation, phosphorylation, ubiquitination, sumoylation, ADP ribosylation, deamination, prolineisomerization (Fig 2) (Jovanovic et al., 2010). These modifications lead to a combinatorial histone code that demarcates chromatin regions for transcription activation or repression. Although the histone code is not fully investigated, specific marks such as lysine acetylation (H3K9ac, H3K18ac, and H4K12ac), lysine trimethylation (H3K4me3), and arginine dimethylation (H4R3me2) are generally associated with transcriptionally active gene promoters, whereas some other modifications such as lysine methylation (H3K9me2, H3K9me3 and H4K20me3) are associated with transcriptional repression. Global loss of acetylation (K16) and trimethylation (K20) of histone H4 have been shown to be characteristic of human cancer (Elsheikh et al., 2009).

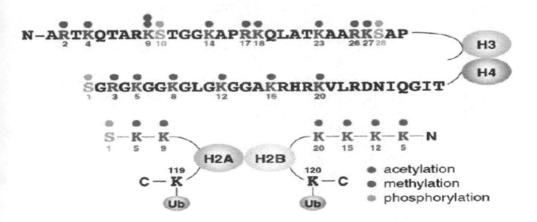

Fig. 2. Major sites of histone modifications

2.2 Histone modifications in breast cancer
2.2.1 Histone acetylation in breast cancer
Histone acetylation is a dynamic process directed by histone acetyltransferases (HATs) and histone deacetylases (HDACs). Normally, Transcription factors recruit coactivators with HAT activity to regulatory DNA sites, whereas transcriptional repressors recruit corepressors with HDAC activity (Sun et al., 2001). A summary of known HAT proteins is presented in Table 1 (Sterner et al., 2000; Yang, 2004; Kimura et al., 2005).

Many HATs have also be showed to be involved in breast cancer. Among of them, p300/CBP and NCOAs are the most important and well-characterised HAT proteins associated with breast cancer.

2.2.1.1 p300/CBP

p300 and its close homolog CBP (CREB-binding protein) are often referred to as a single entity. p300 and CBP share several conserved domains: (1) the bromodomain (Br), which is frequently found in mammalian HATs; (2) three cysteine-histidine (CH)-rich domains (CH1, CH2 and CH3); (3) a KIX domain; and (4) an ADA2-homology domain, which shows extensive similarity to Ada2p, a yeast transcriptional co-activator. The N- and C-terminal domains of p300/CBP can act as transactivation domains, and the CH1, CH3 and the KIX domains are likely to be important in mediating protein-protein interactions, and a number of cellular and viral proteins bind to these regions. The acetyl-transferase domain is located in the central region of the protein, and the Br domain could function in recognising different acetylated motifs (Fig 3A, B) (Chan et al., 2001). p300/CBP contribute to acetylation of H3-K56 and promotes the subsequent assembly of newly-synthesized DNA into chromatin (Das et al., 2009). It is a non-DNA-binding transcriptional coactivator which stimulates transcription of target genes by interacting, either directly or through cofactors, with numerous promoter-binding transcription factors such as CREB, nuclear hormone receptors, and oncoprotein-related activators such as c-Fos, c-Jun, c-Myb and AML1 (Fig 3C) (Kitabayashi et al., 1998; Sterner et al., 2000).

Family	Members	Histone specificity	Basic functions
P300/CBP		H2A/H2B/H3/H4	Global transcriptional coactivator
Nuclear receptor coactivators (p160, SRC)		H3/H4	Nuclear receptor coactivators (transcriptional response to hormone signals)
	NCOA1 (SRC-1)		
	NCOA2 (SRC-2)		
	NCOA3 (SRC-3)		
GNAT			
	Hat1	H4	Histone deposition, chromatin assembly and gene silencing
	Gcn5	H3/H4	Transcriptional coactivator
	PCAF	H3/H4	Transcriptional coactivator
MYST			
	Tip60	H2A/H3/H4	Transcriptional co-regulator, DNA repair and apoptosis
	MOZ	H3	Transcriptional coactivator
	MORF	H2A/H3/H4	Transcriptional coactivator (strong homology to MOZ)
	HBO1	H3/H4	DNA replication, transcriptional corepressor
TAF$_{II}$250		H3/H4	TBP-associated factor, transcription initiation, kinase and ubiquitin ligase
TFIIIC		H3/H4	RNA polymerase III transcription initiation
	TFIIIC220		
	TFIIIC110		
	TFIIIC90		
ATF-2		H4/H2B	Transcriptional activator
CIITA		H4	Transcriptional coactivator
CDY		H4	Histone-to-protamine transition during spermatogenesis

Table 1. Summary of major human HATs

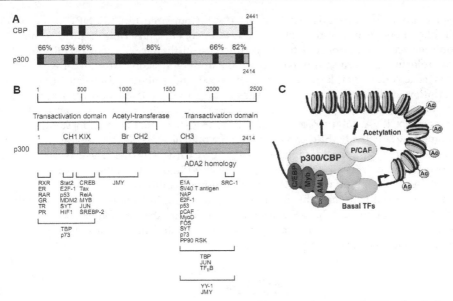

Fig. 3. Organisation of p300/CBP proteins. (A) Comparison of p300 and CBP. The dark regions indicate the areas of highest homology; (B) The functional domains in p300; (C) One of the potential model for the action of p300/CBP in the transcriptional regulation (Kitabayashi et al., 1998; Sterner et al., 2000).

p300/CBP is a ubiquitously expressed, global transcriptional coactivator that is involved in most important cellular programs, such as cell cycle control, differentiation, and apoptosis. Mice nullizygous for p300 or double heterozygous for p300 and CBP showed defects in neurulation and heart development, and then exhibited embryonic lethality, and mutations in p300 and CBP are associated with certain human disease processes (Giles et al., 1998; Yao et al., 1998; Giordano et al., 1999). A role for p300 in tumor suppression has been proposed by the fact that disturbance of p300 function by viral oncoproteins is essential for the transformation of rodent primary cells and, consistent with this hypothesis, mutations of p300 have been identified in certain types of human cancers, including breast carcinomas (Gayther et al., 2000).

It showed that both the localization of p300 and the recruitment to aggresomes differ between breast cancers and normal mammary glands. The expression level of p300 in breast cancer epithelia is higher than that in normal mammary gland. Cytoplasmic localization of p300 was also observed in tumor epithelia whereas nuclear localization was found in normal mammary glands in both animal models and in non-malignant adjacent areas of human breast cancer specimens. Proteasomal inhibition induced p300 redistribution to aggresomes in tumor but not in normal mammary gland-derived cells (Fermento et al., 2010).

The regulation of gene expression by nuclear receptors (NRs) controls the phenotypic properties and diverse biologies of target cells. In breast cancer cells, estrogen receptor alpha (ERα) is a master regulator of transcriptional stimulation and repression (Frasor et al., 2003). Upon E2 treatment, gene transcription is widely impacted, creating highly complex regulatory networks whose ultimate goal is the stimulation or suppression of specific biological processes. p300/CBP can function as a transcriptional cofactor of ERs and other nuclear hormone receptors (Hanstein et al., 1996). Compared to CBP, NRIP1 and NCOAs, which play more gene-specific roles in the ER-dependent transcription, p300 seemed to be the only cofactor that appeared to be recruited at all the target genes of ER and plays a central role in both transcriptional activation and repression. After E2 treatment, ERα recruits coactivator complexes including of p300 and initiates transient stimulation of transcription via binds to ERα binding sites of target genes. If it could offer a more stable nucleation site for coactivator proteins (i.e. SRC-3), leading to histone acetylation and engagement of RNA polymerase II (Pol II), the transcriptional activation status would be maintained. Alternatively, ERα can cause transcriptional repression by recruiting, via p300, CtBP1-containing repressor complexes which lead to RNA polymerase II dismissal and histone deacetylation (Fig 4) (Stossi et al., 2009). In addition, the breast cancer susceptibility gene BRCA1 can strongly inhibits the transcriptional activity of ERα in human breast and prostate cancer cell lines, and this event is correlates with its down-regulation of p300 (but not CBP) (Fan et al., 2002). p300 also plays roles in the regulation of CYP19 I.3/II (aromatase), the key enzyme in estrogen biosynthesis and an important target in breast cancer (Subbaramaiah et al., 2008).

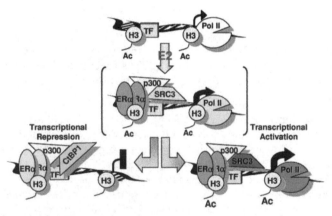

Fig. 4. Proposed model for ERα-mediated activation or repression of target genes via p300 (Stossi et al., 2009).

Another important role of p300 in breast cancer is the regulation of p53, a famous tumor suppressor. p53 can be acetylated by p300 in response to DNA damage to regulate its DNA-binding and transcriptional functions (Yuan et al., 1999). What's more, the N terminus of p300/CBP exhibits the ubiquitin ligase E3/E4 activity and is required for physiologic p53 polyubiquitination and degradation. Depletion of CBP or p300 could enhance the stabilization of p53 (Grossman et al., 2003; Shi et al., 2009).

Furthermore, p300/CBP has also been identified as a coactivator of HIF1α (hypoxia-inducible factor 1 alpha), and thus plays a role in the stimulation of hypoxia-induced genes (such as VEGF, GLUT1, etc) and development of glycolysis, which is the most important metabolic marker of cancer (Ruas et al., 2005).

2.2.1.2 Nuclear receptor coactivators

The Nuclear receptor coactivator family (NCOA), also named as p160 or steroid receptor coactivator, contains three homologous members: NCOA1 (SRC-1), NCOA2 (SRC-2, GRIP1 or TIF2) and NOCA3 (SRC-3, p/CIP, RAC3, ACTR, AIB1 or TRAM-1). These three members have an overall sequence similarity of 50–55% and sequence identity of 43–48%. They contain three structural domains. The N-terminal basic helix-loop-helix-Per/ARNT/ Sim (bHLH-PAS) domain is the most conserved region and is required for interact with several transcription factors (such as myogenin, MEF-2C and TEF, but not be obligator for NRs) and then enhance the transcription (Onate et al., 1995; Belandia et al., 2000). The central region contains three LXXLL (L, leucine; X, any amino acid) motifs, which form an amphipathic α-helix and are responsible for interacting with NRs (Heery et al., 1997; Darimont et al., 1998). The C-terminus contains two intrinsic transcriptional activation domains (AD1 and AD2). The AD1 region binds p300/CBP (but not interact with NRs), and this recruitment of p300/CBP to the chromatin is essential for NCOA-mediated transcriptional activation (Yao et al., 1996). The AD2 domain interacts with histone methyltransferases, coactivator-associated arginine methyltransferase 1 (CARM1) and protein arginine methyltransferases (PRMT1) (Koh et al., 2001). Based on such molecular features, NCOAs interact with ligand-bound nuclear receptors and recruit histone acetyltransferases and methyltransferases to specific enhancer/promotor regions, which in turn results in chromatin remodeling, assembly of general transcription factors and recruitment of RNA Polymerase II for transcriptional activation (Fig 5) (Zhang et al., 2004; Xu et al., 2009). Furthermore, The C-termini of NCOAs itself also contain HAT activity domains (Chen et al., 1997; Spencer et al., 1997), and the poly Q encoding sequence in the C-terminal of NCOA3 gene is genetically unstable and is an easy target for somatic mutations in cancer cells (Wong et al., 2006).

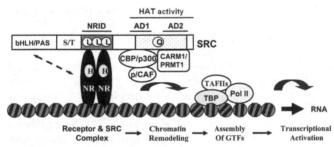

Fig. 5. Molecular structure of NCOAs and their functional mechanisms in steroid hormone-induced gene expression. Abbreviations: H, hormone; NRID, NR interaction domain; TBP, the TATA binding protein; TAFIIs, TBP-associated general transcription factors (GTFs).

Except of NRs, NCOAs also serve as coactivators for many other transcription factors associated with breast cancer, such as HIF1, NF-κB, E2F1, p53, RB and MRTFs (Zhang et al., 2004; Xu et al., 2009). By regulating a broad range of gene expression controlled by NRs and non-NR transcription factors, NCOAs regulate diverse events in the development of breast cancer. Either NCOA1 or NCOA2 deficiency can reduce ductal side branching and alveologenesis in the mammary gland (Xu et al., 1998; Mukherjee et al., 2006), and NCOA3−/− mice show growth retardation, delayed puberty, reduced female reproductive function and blunted mammary gland development (Xu et al., 2000).

In normal human breast, the levels of the three NCOA proteins in epithelial cells are usually low or undetectable (Hudelist et al., 2003). NCOA1 is overexpressed in 19% to 29% of breast cancers and plays important roles in cell proliferation, lymph node metastasis, disease recurrence and poor disease-free survival (DFS) (Fleming et al., 2004). Therefore, elevated

NCOA1 has been regarded as an independent predictor of breast cancer recurrence following therapy (Redmond et al., 2009). Although the evidence were not very sufficient, NCOA2 overexpression might also promote proliferation and invasion of breast cancer cells (Kishimoto et al., 2005). The amplification (in less than 10%) and elevated expression (in over 30%) of NCOA3 were be detected in breast cancer, and its overexpression in breast cancer usually correlates with the expression of ERBB2 , matrix metalloproteinase 2 (MMP2), MMP9 and PEA3 and with larger tumor size, higher tumor grade, and/or poor DFS (Anzick et al., 1997; Hudelist et al., 2003; Harigopal et al., 2009; Xu et al., 2009). What's more, elevated NCOA3 is able to promote estrogen-independent cell proliferation depends on the function of E2F1 and the association between NCOA3 and E2F1, but not ER (Louie et al., 2004).

In addition, NCOAs play important roles in the chemotherapy resistance of breast cancer. Increased expression levels of the ER-NCOA3 complex were found in tamoxifen-resistant cells, and such overexpression of NCOA3 could enhance the agonist activity of tamoxifen and therefore, reduces its antitumor activity in patients with breast cancer (Smith et al., 1997; Zhao et al., 2009).

2.2.1.3 HDACs

The 18 HDACs identified so far can be categorized into four classes: class I (HDAC1-3, HDAC8), class II (HDAC4-7, 9-10), class III (Sirtuin1-7) and class IV (HDAC11). Class I, II, and IV HDACs share homology in both sequence and structure and all require a zinc ion for catalytic activity. In contrast, class III HDACs shares no similarities in their sequence or structure with class I, II, or IV HDACs and requires nicotinamide adenine dinucleotide (NAD+) for catalytic activity (Ellis et al., 2009; Mottet et al., 2010). HDACs remove the acetyl groups from histone lysine tails and are thought to facilitate transcriptional repression by decreasing the level of histone acetylation. Like HATs, HDACs also have non-histone targets (Bolden et al., 2006; Wang et al., 2007).

Several HDACs have been found to be involved in breast cancer. In ER-positive breast cancer MCF-7 cells, expression of HDAC6 was increased after being treated by estradiol, and the elevated HDAC6 could deacetylate alpha-tubulin and increase cell motility. While the ER antagonist tamoxifen (TAM) or ICI 182,780 could prevent estradiol-induced HDAC6 upregulation, and then reduce cell motility. The *in vivo* assays showed that the patients with high levels of HDAC6 mRNA tended to be more responsive to endocrine treatment than those with low levels, indicating that the levels of HDAC6 expression might be used as both as a marker of endocrine responsiveness and also as a prognostic indicator in breast cancer (Zhang et al., 2004; Saji et al., 2005). Besides, HDAC1, Sirtuin3 (SIRT3), SIRT7 are all overexpressed in breast cancer (Zhang et al., 2005; Michan et al., 2007; Saunders et al., 2007). HDAC4 overexpression and mutations have also been found in breast cancer samples (Sjoblom et al., 2006).

2.2.2 Histone methylation in breast cancer

Histones can be mono-, di-, or tri-methylated at lysine or arginine residues by histone methyltransferases (HMTs). Many HMTs, including both lysine-specific HMTs (eg. SMYD3) and arginine-specific HMTs (eg. PRMT1 and CARM1), have been shown to act as ER coactivators and be involved in breast cancer.

2.2.2.1 Histone lysine methyltransferase (HKMTs)

Histone lysine methylation occurs on histone H3 at ε-amino group of lysines 4, 9, 14, 27, 36, and 79 and on histone H4 at lysines 20 and 59 (Strahl et al., 2000; Lee et al., 2005). In general, methylation at H3K4 or H3K36, mono- methylations of H3K27, H3K9, H4K20, H3K79, and H2BK5 is associated with transcriptional activation, whereas trimethylations of H3K27, H3K9 H3K79, and H4K20 are linked to transcriptional repression (Rea et al., 2000; Kouzarides, 2007; Wang et al., 2007). Many HKMTs have been isolated and characterized (Tab 2). Up to now, except of Dot1, all the HKMTs contains a conserved SET [Su(var), Enhancer of zeste, trithorax] domain that is responsible for catalysis and binding of cofactor S-adenosyl-l- methionine (AdoMet), and many of them has been shown to play roles in the breast cancer.

NSD3 is amplified in human breast cancer cell lines and primary tumors and identified at the breakpoint of t(8;11)(p11.2;p15), resulting in a fusion of the NUP98 and NSD genes (Angrand et al., 2001; Rosati et al., 2002).

SMYD3 is a novel SET-domain-containing lysine histone methyltransferase which has been regarded as an important factor in carcinogenesis. Formed a complex with RNA polymerase II through an interaction with the RNA helicase HELZ, SMYD3 specifically methylates H3K4 and activates the transcription of a set of downstream genes (including of Nkx2.8, hTERT, WNT10B, VEGFR1, c-Met, etc) containing a "5' - CCCTCC - 3'" or "5' - GGAGGG - 3" sequence in the promoter region (Fig 6) (Hamamoto et al., 2004; Hamamoto et al., 2006; Kunizaki et al., 2007; Zou et al., 2009). It seems that the N-terminal region of SMYD3 plays an important role for the regulation of its methyltransferase activity, and the cleavage of 34 amino acids in the N-terminal region or interaction with heat shock protein 90 alpha (HSP90α) may enhance the histone methyltransferase (HMTase) activity compared to the full-length protein (Silva et al., 2008). Enhanced expression of SMYD3 is essential for the growth of many cancer cells (such as breast cancer, colorectal carcinoma, hepatocellular carcinoma, etc), and it also could stimulate cell adhesion and migration, whereas suppression of SMYD3 by RNAi or other reagents induces apoptosis and inhibits cell proliferation and migration (Hamamoto et al., 2004; Hamamoto et al., 2006; Luo et al., 2007; Wang et al., 2008; Luo et al., 2009; Zou et al., 2009; Luo et al., 2010). SMYD3 may be an important coactivator of estrogen receptor (ER) in the estrogen signal pathway. It can directly interact with the ligand binding domain of ER, in turn augments ER target gene expression via histone H3-K4 methylation (Kim 2009).

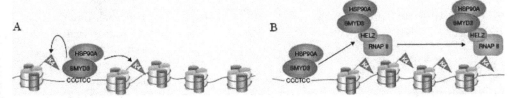

Fig. 6. SMYD3-mediated histone H3-K4 methylation and transcriptional regulation. (Sims et al., 2004)

EZH2 overexpression has been found in breast cancer, its elevation is associated with poor prognosis. It seems that EZH2 might be associated with the regulation of pRB–E2F pathway and genes involved in homologous recombination pathway of DNA repair (Zeidler et al., 2005). However, the detailed mechanism of EZH2 in cancer is not yet clear. Another study has shown that EZH2 is also overexpressed in preneoplastic breast lesions and morphologically normal breast epithelium adjacent to the pre-invasive and invasive lesions, indicating that it might be a marker of epithelium at higher risk for neoplastic transformation (Ding et al., 2006).

Family	Members	Histone specificity	Basic functions
SET domain-containing proteins			
SUV39	SUV39H1, SUV39H2, SULT1E1, G9A, CLLL8	H3K9	Transcriptional repression
SET1	MLL1, MLL2, MLL3	H3K4	Transcriptional activation
SET2	NSD1	H3K36, H4K20	Transcriptional activation
	NDS2	H4K20	Transcriptional activation
	NSD3	H3K4, H3K27	Mainly be transcriptional repression
	SETD2	H3K36	Transcriptional activation
SMYD	SMYD1	H3K4	Transcriptional repression
	SMYD2	H3K36	Transcriptional activation
	SMYD3	H3K4	Mainly be transcriptional activation
	SMYD4	Unclear	Transcriptional repression
	SMYD5	Unclear	Unclear
EZ	EZH2	H3K27	Transcriptional repression
SUV4~20	SUV4~20H1, SUV4~20H2	H4K20	Heterochromatin
PRDM2		H3K9	Transcriptional activation
Others	SET7/9	H3K4	Transcriptional activation
	SETD8	H4K20	Transcriptional repression
	SETDB1	H3K9	Transcriptional repression
	EHMT1	H3K9, H3K27	Transcriptional repression
Non-SET domain-containing proteins			
Dot1	Dot1L	H3K79	Transcriptional repression

Table 2. Summary of major human HKMTs (Pan et al., 2010)

PRDM2 (RIZ1) was originally identified as a pRb-binding protein, and its inactivation and underexpression via mutations or promoter hypermethylation had been found in a number of tumors including breast, colon, liver and lung cancers, as well as neuroblastoma, melanoma and osteosarcomas (Kim et al., 2003; Wang et al., 2007). Overexpression of PRDM2 induces G2/M cell-cycle arrest and apoptosis in tumor cell lines, while PRDM2-/- mice are prone to developing B cell lymphoma and stomach cancer (Steele-Perkins et al., 2001; Gibbons, 2005).

2.2.2.2 Histone arginine methyltransferase (HRMTs)

The protein arginine methyltransferase (PRMT) family is the major HRMTs up to now. The PRMTs are classified into four groups depending on the type of methylarginine they generate: Type I PRMTs (PRMT1, PRMT2, PRMT3, PRMT4, PRMT6 and PRMT8) catalyze the formation of ω-NG, monomethylarginines (MMA) and ω-NG, NG-asymmetric dimethylarginines (aDMA); Type II PRMTs (PRMT5, PRMT7 and PRMT9) catalyze the formation of MMA and ω-NG, N'G-symmetric dimethylarginines (sDMA); Type III PRMTs (remained unclear) catalyze only the monomethylation of arginine residues in proteins; Type IV PRMTs (only be found in *Saccharomyces cerevisiae* up to date) catalyze the methylation at delta (Δ) nitrogen atom of arginine residues (Niewmierzycka et al., 1999; Boisvert et al., 2005; Bachand, 2007).

Compared to HKMTs, The evidence for the involvement of HRMTs in human cancers is not as solid. However, underexpression of PRMT1 has been observed in breast cancer (Scorilas et al., 2000). PRMT4, also known as coactivator-associated arginine methyltransferase-1 (CARM1), is a coactivator for nuclear receptors and is oversexpressed in prostate and breast cancers (El et al., 2006). PRMT4 plays an important role in estrogen-induced cell cycle progression in the MCF-7 breast cancer cell line. Upon estrogen stimulation, the E2F1 promoter is subject to PRMT4-dependent dimethylation on H3R17, and this recruitment of PRMT4 by ERα are dependent on the presence of the NCOA3 (Frietze et al., 2008).

2.2.2.3 Histone demethylase

It used to be considered that histone methylation was a permanent and irreversible histone modification. However, in recent decade, many enzymes have been identified with the ability to demethylate methylated histone lysine/arginine residues via amine oxidation, hydroxylation or deimination (Cloos et al., 2008). The histone demethylases could be divided into three distinct classes. The first class (petidylarginine deiminase 4, PADI4) converts a methyl-lysine to citrulline. The second class (lysine-specific demethylase 1, LSD1) reverses histone H3K4 and H3K9 modifications by an oxidative demethylation reaction. The third class of demethylases is the family of Jumonji C (JmjC)-domain containing histone demethylases (JHDMs). Contrast to LSD1, JHDMs can demethylate all three methylated states (mono- di- and tri-methylated lysine). Up to now, JHDMs have been found to demethylate H3K36 (JHDM1), H3K9 (JHDM2A) and H3K9/K27 (JHDM3 and JMJD2A-D) (Klose et al., 2006; Miremadi et al., 2007).

Histone demethylase JARID1B (PLU-1) is shown to be overexpressed in breast cancers but low expressed in normal adult tissues, and it is essential for the proliferation of the MCF-7 breast cancer cell line and for the tumor growth of mammary carcinoma cells in nude mice. Several target genes of JARID1B have also been identified to be associated with breast cancer proliferation, such as 14–3–3σ, BRCA1, CAV1, and HOXA5 (Lu et al., 1999; Yamane et al., 2007). LSD1 might be a coactivator in the ER signalling (Garcia-Bassets et al., 2007). JMJD1C expression is decreased in breast cancer tissues compared with normal breast tissues, indicating that it might be a tumor suppressor (Wolf et al., 2007).

2.2.3 Histone phosphorylation in breast cancer

Phosphorylation is also thought to have a role in chromatin remodeling and in the initiation of gene transcription, and therefore be associated with the development of human cancer (Espino et al., 2006; Wang et al., 2007). Phosphorylation of H3 on S10 and S28 is important not only during mitotic chromosome condensation but also in transcriptional activation of immediate early genes. The number of H3 pS10 foci was increased, and these TPA-induced foci were positioned next to actively transcribed regions in the nucleus after TPA stimulating of MCF-7 breast cancer cells. Presumably, these nuclear sites represent the nuclear location of genes that are induced or in a competent state. Thus, growth factors stimulating the Ras/MAPK and increasing H3 pS10 at transcriptionally active loci may contribute to aberrant gene expression and breast cancer progression (Espino et al., 2006).

2.2.4 The other histone modifications in breast cancer

Besides the acetylation, methylation and phosphorylation, there are some other modification occurred in the histone. These epigenetic changes include ubiquitination/sumoylation, ADP-ribosylation, deamination, and proline isomerisation. Although the knowledge of their functions and mechanisms is still little, some studies have showed that they are also associated with breast cancer and other human cancers.

The regulation of gene expression by phosphorylated and undersumoylated PRs is a novel form of hormone independent PR action that is predicted to contribute to breast cancer cell growth and survival (Daniel et al., 2009). Recent studies revealed that E3 ubiquitin ligases play important roles in breast carcinogenesis. ubiquitin-mediated protein degradation plays an important role in many cancer-related cellular processes. E3s play critical roles because they control the substrate specificity. Accumulating evidence suggests that genetic and expression alteration of E3s contributes to breast carcinogenesis (Chen et al., 2006).

histone sumoylation as a component of the group of modifications that appear to govern chromatin structure and function to mediate transcriptional repression and gene silencing (Shiio et al., 2003). A better understanding of the epigenetic mechanisms that cause transcriptional repression has allowed researchers to find new agents that are very effective in inducing apoptosis , differentiation, and/or cell growth arrest in human breast cancer, lung cancer, thoracic cancer, leukemia, and colon cancer cell lines (Giacinti et al., 2006).

2.3 Histone modification inhibitors and breast cancer

As discussed above, histone modification could be used as a novel target for the research of anticancer drugs. So far, several histone modification inhibitors have been developed. HDAC inhibitors are the most studied type of histone modification inhibitor up to now (Tab 3).

It showed that combination of the HDAC inhibitor vorinostat with paclitaxel and bevacizumab could induce a partial or complete response in more than 50% of patients with metastatic breast cancer (Wong, 2009; Jovanovic et al., 2010). In addition, the HDAC inhibitors have different role in ER+ and ER- breast cancer cells. In ER+ cells, HDAC inhibitors reduce the transcriptional level of ER and its response genes, while they reestablish ER expression in ER- cell lines. But the HDAC inhibitor could potentiate and restore the efficacy of anti-estrogen therapy in preclinical models in either ER+ or ER- breast cancer cells. This has led to the initiation of several clinical trials combining HDAC inhibitors with anti-estrogen therapy (Thomas et al., 2009). LAQ824 is a novel inhibitor of HDAC that shows antineoplastic activity and can activate genes that produce cell cycle arrest. Combination of the LAQ824 and a DNMT inhibitor (decitabine) showed a synergistic (re-)activation of silenced tumor-suppressor genes in human MDA-MB-231 and MCF-7 breast carcinoma cells (Hurtubise et al., 2006).

Class	In vivo preclinical activity	Clinical phase
Carboxylates (short-chain fatty acids)		
PA	Leukemia, glioblastoma	I/II
PB	Prostate, endometrial	I/II
VA	Brain, melanoma	I/II
AN-9	NSCLC, leukemia	I/II
Hydroxamic acids		
SAHA	Lung, prostate, melanoma	I/II
m-Carboxycinnamic acid bishydroxamic acid	Neuroblastoma	
Suberic bishydroxamic acid	Melanoma, sarcoma	
Pyroxamide		I
TSA	Cervical, hepatoma,	
Oxamflatin	Melanoma	
NVP-LAQ824	Colon, multiple myeloma	I
Electrophillic ketones (epoxides)		
TPX		
AOE		

Class	In vivo preclinical activity	Clinical phase
Depudecin		
Cyclic peptides		
Apicidin	Melanoma, leukemia	
FK-228, FR901228	Melanoma, colon, sarcoma, fibrosarcoma, lung, gastric	I/II
Benzamides		
MS-275	Leukemia, colorectal, gastric, pancreatic, lung, ovarian	I/II
CI-994	Colorectal, pancreatic, mammary, prostate, sarcoma, leukemia	I
Other hybrid compounds		
CHAPs	Melanoma, lung, stomach, breast	
Scriptaid		
Tubacin		
JNJ16241199		
A-161906		
6-(3-Chlorophenylureido)caproic hydroxamic acid		
PXD101	Breast, prostate, ovarian, colon, NSCLC	

Table 3. Summary of major HDAC inhibitors (Acharya et al., 2005; Laird, 2005).

3. Conclusion

In summary, Histone modifications provide crucial regulatory functions in the process of gene transcription, and they play very important roles in the proliferation, metastasis, chemotherapy and other aspects of breast cancer, as well as many other human cancers. The reversibility of histone modification makes it could be regarded as one valuable target for the development of novel anticancer strategies. The understanding of all these epigenetics changes and their contribution to breast cancer might take great progress in the field of diagnosis, prognosis and therapy of breast cancer.

4. Acknowledgment

This work was financially supported by the National Basic Research Program of China (973 Program) (NO. 2009CB825504), the National Natural Science Fundation of China (NO. 31000343), the High School Science & Technology Development Fundation of Tianjin (NO.20090602) and the Scientific Research Launch Fund for Introduction of Talents into Tianjin University of Science & Technology (No. 20080414).

5. References

Acharya, M. R., A. Sparreboom, J. Venitz and W. D. Figg (2005). "Rational development of histone deacetylase inhibitors as anticancer agents: a review." Mol Pharmacol 68 (4): 917-32.

Angrand, P. O., F. Apiou, A. F. Stewart, B. Dutrillaux, R. Losson and P. Chambon (2001). "NSD3, a new SET domain-containing gene, maps to 8p12 and is amplified in human breast cancer cell lines." Genomics 74 (1): 79-88.

Anzick, S. L., J. Kononen, R. L. Walker, D. O. Azorsa, M. M. Tanner, X. Y. Guan, G. Sauter, O. P. Kallioniemi, J. M. Trent and P. S. Meltzer (1997). "AIB1, a steroid receptor coactivator amplified in breast and ovarian cancer." Science 277 (5328): 965-8.

Bachand, F. (2007). "Protein arginine methyltransferases: from unicellular eukaryotes to humans." Eukaryot Cell 6 (6): 889-98.

Bartova, E., J. Krejci, A. Harnicarova, G. Galiova and S. Kozubek (2008). "Histone modifications and nuclear architecture: a review." J Histochem Cytochem 56 (8): 711-21.

Belandia, B. and M. G. Parker (2000). "Functional interaction between the p160 coactivator proteins and the transcriptional enhancer factor family of transcription factors." J Biol Chem 275 (40): 30801-5.

Boisvert, F. M., C. A. Chenard and S. Richard (2005). "Protein interfaces in signaling regulated by arginine methylation." Sci STKE 2005 (271): re2.

Bolden, J. E., M. J. Peart and R. W. Johnstone (2006). "Anticancer activities of histone deacetylase inhibitors." Nat Rev Drug Discov 5 (9): 769-84.

Chan, H. M. and N. B. La Thangue (2001). "p300/CBP proteins: HATs for transcriptional bridges and scaffolds." J Cell Sci 114 (Pt 13): 2363-73.

Chen, C., A. K. Seth and A. E. Aplin (2006). "Genetic and expression aberrations of E3 ubiquitin ligases in human breast cancer." Mol Cancer Res 4 (10): 695-707.

Chen, H., R. J. Lin, R. L. Schiltz, D. Chakravarti, A. Nash, L. Nagy, M. L. Privalsky, Y. Nakatani and R. M. Evans (1997). "Nuclear receptor coactivator ACTR is a novel histone acetyltransferase and forms a multimeric activation complex with P/CAF and CBP/p300." Cell 90 (3): 569-80.

Cloos, P. A., J. Christensen, K. Agger and K. Helin (2008). "Erasing the methyl mark: histone demethylases at the center of cellular differentiation and disease." Genes Dev 22 (9): 1115-40.

Daniel, A. R. and C. A. Lange (2009). "Protein kinases mediate ligand-independent derepression of sumoylated progesterone receptors in breast cancer cells." Proc Natl Acad Sci U S A 106 (34): 14287-92.

Darimont, B. D., R. L. Wagner, J. W. Apriletti, M. R. Stallcup, P. J. Kushner, J. D. Baxter, R. J. Fletterick and K. R. Yamamoto (1998). "Structure and specificity of nuclear receptor-coactivator interactions." Genes Dev 12 (21): 3343-56.

Das, C., M. S. Lucia, K. C. Hansen and J. K. Tyler (2009). "CBP/p300-mediated acetylation of histone H3 on lysine 56." Nature 459 (7243): 113-7.

Ding, L., C. Erdmann, A. M. Chinnaiyan, S. D. Merajver and C. G. Kleer (2006). "Identification of EZH2 as a molecular marker for a precancerous state in morphologically normal breast tissues." Cancer Res 66 (8): 4095-9.

El, M. S., E. Fabbrizio, C. Rodriguez, P. Chuchana, L. Fauquier, D. Cheng, C. Theillet, L. Vandel, M. T. Bedford and C. Sardet (2006). "Coactivator-associated arginine methyltransferase 1 (CARM1) is a positive regulator of the Cyclin E1 gene." Proc Natl Acad Sci U S A 103 (36): 13351-6.

Ellis, L., P. W. Atadja and R. W. Johnstone (2009). "Epigenetics in cancer: targeting chromatin modifications." Mol Cancer Ther 8 (6): 1409-20.

Elsheikh, S. E., A. R. Green, E. A. Rakha, D. G. Powe, R. A. Ahmed, H. M. Collins, D. Soria, J. M. Garibaldi, C. E. Paish, A. A. Ammar, M. J. Grainge, G. R. Ball, M. K. Abdelghany, L. Martinez-Pomares, D. M. Heery and I. O. Ellis (2009). "Global histone modifications in breast cancer correlate with tumor phenotypes, prognostic factors, and patient outcome." Cancer Res 69 (9): 3802-9.

Espino, P. S., L. Li, S. He, J. Yu and J. R. Davie (2006). "Chromatin modification of the trefoil factor 1 gene in human breast cancer cells by the Ras/mitogen-activated protein kinase pathway." Cancer Res 66 (9): 4610-6.

Fan, S., Y. X. Ma, C. Wang, R. Q. Yuan, Q. Meng, J. A. Wang, M. Erdos, I. D. Goldberg, P. Webb, P. J. Kushner, R. G. Pestell and E. M. Rosen (2002). "p300 Modulates the BRCA1 inhibition of estrogen receptor activity." Cancer Res 62 (1): 141-51.

Fermento, M. E., N. A. Gandini, C. A. Lang, J. E. Perez, H. V. Maturi, A. C. Curino and M. M. Facchinetti (2010). "Intracellular distribution of p300 and its differential recruitment to aggresomes in breast cancer." Exp Mol Pathol 88 (2): 256-64.

Fleming, F. J., E. Myers, G. Kelly, T. B. Crotty, E. W. McDermott, N. J. O'Higgins, A. D. Hill and L. S. Young (2004). "Expression of SRC-1, AIB1, and PEA3 in HER2 mediated endocrine resistant breast cancer; a predictive role for SRC-1." J Clin Pathol 57 (10): 1069-74.

Frasor, J., J. M. Danes, B. Komm, K. C. Chang, C. R. Lyttle and B. S. Katzenellenbogen (2003). "Profiling of estrogen up- and down-regulated gene expression in human breast cancer cells: insights into gene networks and pathways underlying estrogenic control of proliferation and cell phenotype." Endocrinology 144 (10): 4562-74.

Frietze, S., M. Lupien, P. A. Silver and M. Brown (2008). "CARM1 regulates estrogen-stimulated breast cancer growth through up-regulation of E2F1." Cancer Res 68 (1): 301-6.

Garcia-Bassets, I., Y. S. Kwon, F. Telese, G. G. Prefontaine, K. R. Hutt, C. S. Cheng, B. G. Ju, K. A. Ohgi, J. Wang, L. Escoubet-Lozach, D. W. Rose, C. K. Glass, X. D. Fu and M. G. Rosenfeld (2007). "Histone methylation-dependent mechanisms impose ligand dependency for gene activation by nuclear receptors." Cell 128 (3): 505-18.

Gayther, S. A., S. J. Batley, L. Linger, A. Bannister, K. Thorpe, S. F. Chin, Y. Daigo, P. Russell, A. Wilson, H. M. Sowter, J. D. Delhanty, B. A. Ponder, T. Kouzarides and C. Caldas (2000). "Mutations truncating the EP300 acetylase in human cancers." Nat Genet 24 (3): 300-3.

Giacinti, L., P. P. Claudio, M. Lopez and A. Giordano (2006). "Epigenetic information and estrogen receptor alpha expression in breast cancer." Oncologist 11 (1): 1-8.

Gibbons, R. J. (2005). "Histone modifying and chromatin remodelling enzymes in cancer and dysplastic syndromes." Hum Mol Genet 14 Spec No 1: R85-92.

Giles, R. H., D. J. Peters and M. H. Breuning (1998). "Conjunction dysfunction: CBP/p300 in human disease." Trends Genet 14 (5): 178-83.

Giordano, A. and M. L. Avantaggiati (1999). "p300 and CBP: partners for life and death." J Cell Physiol 181 (2): 218-30.

Grossman, S. R., M. E. Deato, C. Brignone, H. M. Chan, A. L. Kung, H. Tagami, Y. Nakatani and D. M. Livingston (2003). "Polyubiquitination of p53 by a ubiquitin ligase activity of p300." Science 300 (5617): 342-4.

Hamamoto, R., F. P. Silva, M. Tsuge, T. Nishidate, T. Katagiri, Y. Nakamura and Y. Furukawa (2006). "Enhanced SMYD3 expression is essential for the growth of breast cancer cells." Cancer Sci 97 (2): 113-8.

Hamamoto, R., Y. Furukawa, M. Morita, Y. Iimura, F. P. Silva, M. Li, R. Yagyu and Y. Nakamura (2004). "SMYD3 encodes a histone methyltransferase involved in the proliferation of cancer cells." Nat Cell Biol 6 (8): 731-40.

Hanstein, B., R. Eckner, J. DiRenzo, S. Halachmi, H. Liu, B. Searcy, R. Kurokawa and M. Brown (1996). "p300 is a component of an estrogen receptor coactivator complex." Proc Natl Acad Sci U S A 93 (21): 11540-5.

Harigopal, M., J. Heymann, S. Ghosh, V. Anagnostou, R. L. Camp and D. L. Rimm (2009). "Estrogen receptor co-activator (AIB1) protein expression by automated quantitative analysis (AQUA) in a breast cancer tissue microarray and association with patient outcome." Breast Cancer Res Treat 115 (1): 77-85.

Heery, D. M., E. Kalkhoven, S. Hoare and M. G. Parker (1997). "A signature motif in transcriptional co-activators mediates binding to nuclear receptors." Nature 387 (6634): 733-6.

Hudelist, G., K. Czerwenka, E. Kubista, E. Marton, K. Pischinger and C. F. Singer (2003). "Expression of sex steroid receptors and their co-factors in normal and malignant breast tissue: AIB1 is a carcinoma-specific co-activator." Breast Cancer Res Treat 78 (2): 193-204.

Hurtubise, A. and R. L. Momparler (2006). "Effect of histone deacetylase inhibitor LAQ824 on antineoplastic action of 5-Aza-2'-deoxycytidine (decitabine) on human breast carcinoma cells." Cancer Chemother Pharmacol 58 (5): 618-25.

Ito, T. (2007). "Role of histone modification in chromatin dynamics." J Biochem 141 (5): 609-14.

Jemal, A., F. Bray, M. M. Center, J. Ferlay, E. Ward and D. Forman (2011). "Global cancer statistics." CA Cancer J Clin 61 (2): 69-90.

Jovanovic, J., J. A. Ronneberg, J. Tost and V. Kristensen (2010). "The epigenetics of breast cancer." Mol Oncol 4 (3): 242-54.

Kim, K. C., L. Geng and S. Huang (2003). "Inactivation of a histone methyltransferase by mutations in human cancers." Cancer Res 63 (22): 7619-23.

Kimura, A., K. Matsubara and M. Horikoshi (2005). "A decade of histone acetylation: marking eukaryotic chromosomes with specific codes." J Biochem 138 (6): 647-62.

Kishimoto, H., Z. Wang, P. Bhat-Nakshatri, D. Chang, R. Clarke and H. Nakshatri (2005). "The p160 family coactivators regulate breast cancer cell proliferation and invasion through autocrine/paracrine activity of SDF-1alpha/CXCL12." Carcinogenesis 26 (10): 1706-15.

Kitabayashi, I., A. Yokoyama, K. Shimizu and M. Ohki (1998). "Interaction and functional cooperation of the leukemia-associated factors AML1 and p300 in myeloid cell differentiation." EMBO J 17 (11): 2994-3004.

Klose, R. J., E. M. Kallin and Y. Zhang (2006). "JmjC-domain-containing proteins   and histone demethylation." Nat Rev Genet 7 (9): 715-27.

Koh, S. S., D. Chen, Y. H. Lee and M. R. Stallcup (2001). "Synergistic enhancement of nuclear receptor function by p160 coactivators and two coactivators with protein methyltransferase activities." J Biol Chem 276 (2): 1089-98.

Kouzarides, T. (2007). "Chromatin modifications and their function." Cell 128 (4): 693-705.

Kunizaki, M., R. Hamamoto, F. P. Silva, K. Yamaguchi, T. Nagayasu, M. Shibuya, Y. Nakamura and Y. Furukawa (2007). "The lysine 831 of vascular endothelial growth factor receptor 1 is a novel target of methylation by SMYD3." Cancer Res 67 (22): 10759-65.

Laird, P. W. (2005). "Cancer epigenetics." Hum Mol Genet 14 Spec No 1: R65-76.

Lee, D. Y., C. Teyssier, B. D. Strahl and M. R. Stallcup (2005). "Role of protein methylation in regulation of transcription." Endocr Rev 26 (2): 147-70.

Lewin, B. (2004). Genes VIII. Upper Saddle River, NJ, Pearson Prentice Hall.

Louie, M. C., J. X. Zou, A. Rabinovich and H. W. Chen (2004). "ACTR/AIB1 functions as an E2F1 coactivator to promote breast cancer cell proliferation and antiestrogen resistance." Mol Cell Biol 24 (12): 5157-71.

Lu, P. J., K. Sundquist, D. Baeckstrom, R. Poulsom, A. Hanby, S. Meier-Ewert, T. Jones, M. Mitchell, P. Pitha-Rowe, P. Freemont and J. Taylor-Papadimitriou (1999). "A novel gene (PLU-1) containing highly conserved putative DNA/chromatin binding motifs is specifically up-regulated in breast cancer." J Biol Chem 274 (22): 15633-45.

Luo, X. G., J. N. Zou, S. Z. Wang, T. C. Zhang and T. Xi (2010). "Novobiocin decreases SMYD3 expression and inhibits the migration of MDA-MB-231 human breast cancer cells." IUBMB Life 62 (3): 194-9.

Luo, X. G., T. Xi, S. Guo, Z. P. Liu, N. Wang, Y. Jiang and T. C. Zhang (2009). "Effects of SMYD3 overexpression on transformation, serum dependence, and apoptosis sensitivity in NIH3T3 cells." IUBMB Life 61 (6): 679-84.

Luo, X. G., Y. Ding, Q. F. Zhou, L. Ye, S. Z. Wang and T. Xi (2007). "SET and MYND domain-containing protein 3 decreases sensitivity to dexamethasone and stimulates cell adhesion and migration in NIH3T3 cells." J Biosci Bioeng 103 (5): 444-50.

Michan, S. and D. Sinclair (2007). "Sirtuins in mammals: insights into their biological function." Biochem J 404 (1): 1-13.

Miremadi, A., M. Z. Oestergaard, P. D. Pharoah and C. Caldas (2007). "Cancer genetics of epigenetic genes." Hum Mol Genet 16 Spec No 1: R28-49.

Mottet, D. and V. Castronovo (2010). "Histone deacetylases: anti-angiogenic targets in cancer therapy." Curr Cancer Drug Targets 10 (8): 898-913.

Mukherjee, A., S. M. Soyal, R. Fernandez-Valdivia, M. Gehin, P. Chambon, F. J. Demayo, J. P. Lydon and B. W. O'Malley (2006). "Steroid receptor coactivator 2 is critical for progesterone-dependent uterine function and mammary morphogenesis in the mouse." Mol Cell Biol 26 (17): 6571-83.

Niewmierzycka, A. and S. Clarke (1999). "S-Adenosylmethionine-dependent methylation in Saccharomyces cerevisiae. Identification of a novel protein arginine methyltransferase." J Biol Chem 274 (2): 814-24.

Onate, S. A., S. Y. Tsai, M. J. Tsai and B. W. O'Malley (1995). "Sequence and characterization of a coactivator for the steroid hormone receptor superfamily." Science 270 (5240): 1354-7.

Pan, H., X. G. Luo, S. Guo and Z. P. Liu (2010). "[Histone methylation and its relationship with cancer]." Sheng Li Ke Xue Jin Zhan 41 (1): 22-6.

Rea, S., F. Eisenhaber, D. O'Carroll, B. D. Strahl, Z. W. Sun, M. Schmid, S. Opravil, K. Mechtler, C. P. Ponting, C. D. Allis and T. Jenuwein (2000). "Regulation of chromatin structure by site-specific histone H3 methyltransferases." Nature 406 (6796): 593-9.

Redmond, A. M., F. T. Bane, A. T. Stafford, M. McIlroy, M. F. Dillon, T. B. Crotty, A. D. Hill and L. S. Young (2009). "Coassociation of estrogen receptor and p160 proteins predicts resistance to endocrine treatment; SRC-1 is an independent predictor of breast cancer recurrence." Clin Cancer Res 15 (6): 2098-106.

Rosati, R., R. La Starza, A. Veronese, A. Aventin, C. Schwienbacher, T. Vallespi, M. Negrini, M. F. Martelli and C. Mecucci (2002). "NUP98 is fused to the NSD3 gene in acute myeloid leukemia associated with t(8;11)(p11.2;p15)." Blood 99 (10): 3857-60.

Ruas, J. L., L. Poellinger and T. Pereira (2005). "Role of CBP in regulating HIF-1-mediated activation of transcription." J Cell Sci 118 (Pt 2): 301-11.

Saji, S., M. Kawakami, S. Hayashi, N. Yoshida, M. Hirose, S. Horiguchi, A. Itoh, N. Funata, S. L. Schreiber, M. Yoshida and M. Toi (2005). "Significance of HDAC6 regulation via estrogen signaling for cell motility and prognosis in estrogen receptor-positive breast cancer." Oncogene 24 (28): 4531-9.

Saunders, L. R. and E. Verdin (2007). "Sirtuins: critical regulators at the crossroads between cancer and aging." Oncogene 26 (37): 5489-504.

Scorilas, A., M. H. Black, M. Talieri and E. P. Diamandis (2000). "Genomic organization, physical mapping, and expression analysis of the human protein arginine methyltransferase 1 gene." Biochem Biophys Res Commun 278 (2): 349-59.

Shi, D., M. S. Pop, R. Kulikov, I. M. Love, A. L. Kung and S. R. Grossman (2009). "CBP and p300 are cytoplasmic E4 polyubiquitin ligases for p53." Proc Natl Acad Sci U S A 106 (38): 16275-80.

Shiio, Y. and R. N. Eisenman (2003). "Histone sumoylation is associated with transcriptional repression." Proc Natl Acad Sci U S A 100 (23): 13225-30.

Silva, F. P., R. Hamamoto, M. Kunizaki, M. Tsuge, Y. Nakamura and Y. Furukawa (2008). "Enhanced methyltransferase activity of SMYD3 by the cleavage of its N-terminal region in human cancer cells." Oncogene 27 (19): 2686-92.

Sims, R. R. and D. Reinberg (2004). "From chromatin to cancer: a new histone lysine methyltransferase enters the mix." Nat Cell Biol 6 (8): 685-7.

Sjoblom, T., S. Jones, L. D. Wood, D. W. Parsons, J. Lin, T. D. Barber, D. Mandelker, R. J. Leary, J. Ptak, N. Silliman, S. Szabo, P. Buckhaults, C. Farrell, P. Meeh, S. D. Markowitz, J. Willis, D. Dawson, J. K. Willson, A. F. Gazdar, J. Hartigan, L. Wu, C. Liu, G. Parmigiani, B. H. Park, K. E. Bachman, N. Papadopoulos, B. Vogelstein, K. W. Kinzler and V. E. Velculescu (2006). "The consensus coding sequences of human breast and colorectal cancers." Science 314 (5797): 268-74.

Smith, C. L., Z. Nawaz and B. W. O'Malley (1997). "Coactivator and corepressor regulation of the agonist/antagonist activity of the mixed antiestrogen, 4-hydroxytamoxifen." Mol Endocrinol 11 (6): 657-66.

Spencer, T. E., G. Jenster, M. M. Burcin, C. D. Allis, J. Zhou, C. A. Mizzen, N. J. McKenna, S. A. Onate, S. Y. Tsai, M. J. Tsai and B. W. O'Malley (1997). "Steroid receptor coactivator-1 is a histone acetyltransferase." Nature 389 (6647): 194-8.

Steele-Perkins, G., W. Fang, X. H. Yang, M. Van Gele, T. Carling, J. Gu, I. M. Buyse, J. A. Fletcher, J. Liu, R. Bronson, R. B. Chadwick, A. de la Chapelle, X. Zhang, F. Speleman and S. Huang (2001). "Tumor formation and inactivation of RIZ1, an Rb-binding member of a nuclear protein-methyltransferase superfamily." Genes Dev 15 (17): 2250-62.

Sterner, D. E. and S. L. Berger (2000). "Acetylation of histones and transcription-related factors." Microbiol Mol Biol Rev 64 (2): 435-59.

Stossi, F., Z. Madak-Erdogan and B. S. Katzenellenbogen (2009). "Estrogen receptor alpha represses transcription of early target genes via p300 and CtBP1." Mol Cell Biol 29 (7): 1749-59.

Strahl, B. D. and C. D. Allis (2000). "The language of covalent histone modifications." Nature 403 (6765): 41-5.

Subbaramaiah, K., C. Hudis, S. H. Chang, T. Hla and A. J. Dannenberg (2008). "EP2 and EP4 receptors regulate aromatase expression in human adipocytes and breast cancer cells. Evidence of a BRCA1 and p300 exchange." J Biol Chem 283 (6): 3433-44.

Sun, J. M., H. Y. Chen and J. R. Davie (2001). "Effect of estradiol on histone acetylation dynamics in human breast cancer cells." J Biol Chem 276 (52): 49435-42.

Thomas, S. and P. N. Munster (2009). "Histone deacetylase inhibitor induced modulation of anti-estrogen therapy." Cancer Lett 280 (2): 184-91.

Wang, G. G., C. D. Allis and P. Chi (2007). "Chromatin remodeling and cancer, Part I: Covalent histone modifications." Trends Mol Med 13 (9): 363-72.

Wang, S. Z., X. G. Luo, J. Shen, J. N. Zou, Y. H. Lu and T. Xi (2008). "Knockdown of SMYD3 by RNA interference inhibits cervical carcinoma cell growth and invasion in vitro." BMB Rep 41 (4): 294-9.

Wolf, S. S., V. K. Patchev and M. Obendorf (2007). "A novel variant of the putative demethylase gene, s-JMJD1C, is a coactivator of the AR." Arch Biochem Biophys 460 (1): 56-66.

Wong, L. J., P. Dai, J. F. Lu, M. A. Lou, R. Clarke and V. Nazarov (2006). "AIB1 gene amplification and the instability of polyQ encoding sequence in breast cancer cell lines." BMC Cancer 6: 111.

Wong, S. T. (2009). "Emerging treatment combinations: integrating therapy into clinical practice." Am J Health Syst Pharm 66 (23 Suppl 6): S9-S14.

Xu, J., L. Liao, G. Ning, H. Yoshida-Komiya, C. Deng and B. W. O'Malley (2000). "The steroid receptor coactivator SRC-3 (p/CIP/RAC3/AIB1/ACTR/TRAM-1) is required for normal growth, puberty, female reproductive function, and mammary gland development." Proc Natl Acad Sci U S A 97 (12): 6379-84.

Xu, J., R. C. Wu and B. W. O'Malley (2009). "Normal and cancer-related functions of the p160 steroid receptor co-activator (SRC) family." Nat Rev Cancer 9 (9): 615-30.

Xu, J., Y. Qiu, F. J. DeMayo, S. Y. Tsai, M. J. Tsai and B. W. O'Malley (1998). "Partial hormone resistance in mice with disruption of the steroid receptor coactivator-1 (SRC-1) gene." Science 279 (5358): 1922-5.

Yamane, K., K. Tateishi, R. J. Klose, J. Fang, L. A. Fabrizio, H. Erdjument-Bromage, J. Taylor-Papadimitriou, P. Tempst and Y. Zhang (2007). "PLU-1 is an H3K4 demethylase involved in transcriptional repression and breast cancer cell proliferation." Mol Cell 25 (6): 801-12.

Yang, X. J. (2004). "The diverse superfamily of lysine acetyltransferases and their roles in leukemia and other diseases." Nucleic Acids Res 32 (3): 959-76.

Yao, T. P., G. Ku, N. Zhou, R. Scully and D. M. Livingston (1996). "The nuclear hormone receptor coactivator SRC-1 is a specific target of p300." Proc Natl Acad Sci U S A 93 (20): 10626-31.

Yao, T. P., S. P. Oh, M. Fuchs, N. D. Zhou, L. E. Ch'Ng, D. Newsome, R. T. Bronson, E. Li, D. M. Livingston and R. Eckner (1998). "Gene dosage-dependent embryonic development and proliferation defects in mice lacking the transcriptional integrator p300." Cell 93 (3): 361-72.

Yuan, Z. M., Y. Huang, T. Ishiko, S. Nakada, T. Utsugisawa, H. Shioya, Y. Utsugisawa, K. Yokoyama, R. Weichselbaum, Y. Shi and D. Kufe (1999). "Role for p300 in stabilization of p53 in the response to DNA damage." J Biol Chem 274 (4): 1883-6.

Zeidler, M., S. Varambally, Q. Cao, A. M. Chinnaiyan, D. O. Ferguson, S. D. Merajver and C. G. Kleer (2005). "The Polycomb group protein EZH2 impairs DNA repair in breast epithelial cells." Neoplasia 7 (11): 1011-9.

Zhang, H., X. Yi, X. Sun, N. Yin, B. Shi, H. Wu, D. Wang, G. Wu and Y. Shang (2004). "Differential gene regulation by the SRC family of coactivators." Genes Dev 18 (14): 1753-65.

Zhang, Z., H. Yamashita, T. Toyama, H. Sugiura, Y. Ando, K. Mita, M. Hamaguchi, Y. Hara, S. Kobayashi and H. Iwase (2005). "Quantitation of HDAC1 mRNA expression in invasive carcinoma of the breast*." Breast Cancer Res Treat 94 (1): 11-6.

Zhang, Z., H. Yamashita, T. Toyama, H. Sugiura, Y. Omoto, Y. Ando, K. Mita, M. Hamaguchi, S. Hayashi and H. Iwase (2004). "HDAC6 expression is correlated with better survival in breast cancer." Clin Cancer Res 10 (20): 6962-8.

Zhao, W., Q. Zhang, X. Kang, S. Jin and C. Lou (2009). "AIB1 is required for the acquisition of epithelial growth factor receptor-mediated tamoxifen resistance in breast cancer cells." Biochem Biophys Res Commun 380 (3): 699-704.

Zou, J. N., S. Z. Wang, J. S. Yang, X. G. Luo, J. H. Xie and T. Xi (2009). "Knockdown of SMYD3 by RNA interference down-regulates c-Met expression and inhibits cells migration and invasion induced by HGF." Cancer Lett 280 (1): 78-85.

Epigenetics and Breast Cancer

Majed Saleh Alokail
Department of Biochemistry, College of Science
King Saud University
Saudi Arabia

1. Introduction

The term epigenetic was introduced by Conard Waddington in 1942 as a concept of environmental influence in inducing phenotype modification. His work on developmental plasticity states that the environmental influences during development could induce alternative phenotypes from one genotype, one of the clearest examples is polyphenisms in insects. He showed that exposing the pupae of wild type Drosophila melanogaster to heat shock treatment, results in altered wing vein patterns (Waddington, 1952;Waddington, 1959a). Breeding individuals who have been exposed to these environmentally induced changes led to a stable population exhibiting the phenotype without the environmental stimulus. As a result of Waddington's observations of the dynamic interaction between genes and variation in the environment during the plastic phase of development, he described phenotype induction as genetic canalization. Canalization describes the robustness of phenotypes in response to perturbation (Waddington, 1959b;Waddington, 1961;Waddington & Robertson, 1966).

The epigenome controls the genome in both normal and abnormal cellular processes and events (Szyf et al., 2008;Vaissiere et al., 2008). Epigenetic system includes DNA methylation and histone modification and non-coding RNAs, which work cooperatively to control gene expression. As a result, epigenetic mechanisms are essential for normal development and maintenance of tissue-specific gene expression patterns in mammals. Disruption of epigenetic processes can lead to altered gene function and malignant cellular transformation. Global changes in the epigenetic landscape are a hallmark of cancer (Hanahan & Weinberg, 2000). Methylation of cytosine bases in DNA provides a layer of epigenetic control in many eukaryotes that has important implications for normal biology and disease. DNA methylation is a crucial epigenetic modification of the genome that is involved in regulating many cellular processes. These include embryonic development, transcription, chromatin structure, X-chromosome inactivation, genomic imprinting, and chromosome stability.

Additionally, in 1975, DNA methylation was related to the process of X chromosome inactivation in females (Riggs, 1975). Since then, it has been used as a marker for gene silencing and extensively studied as an important mechanism of epigenetic control (Jaenisch & Bird, 2003). For instance, methylation of CpG islands within the imprinted gene promoters ensures transcriptional silencing of the associated parental allele (Nafee et al., 2008). Consistent with these important roles, a growing number of human diseases including cancer have been found to be associated with aberrant DNA methylation. Therefore we will summarize the, in this chapter the current knowledge on mechanisms of epigenetic and its potential application in breast cancers.

2. DNA methylation

DNA methylation is a well conserved process that occurs in eukaryotes and prokaryotes (Klose & Bird, 2006). DNA methylation refers to the covalent addition of a methyl group to carbon number five in the nitrogenous base cytosine at the DNA strand (Fuks, 2005;Szyf et al., 2008). However, methylation does not occur in every cytosine, but only those adjacent to guanine are targets for the methylation by the methyltransferases enzymes. The CpG may occur in multiple repeats which are known as CpG islands (Fuks, 2005). These regions are often associated with the promoter regions of genes. Almost half of the genes in our genome have CpG rich promoter regions. In the whole genome, about 80% of the CpG dinucleutides not associated with CpG islands are heavily methylated (Robertson & Jones, 2000). In contrast the CpG islands associated with gene promoters are usually unmethylated (Singal & Ginder, 1999). There are a number of factors that may maintain the undermethylated state of CpG islands, such as sequence feature, SP1 binding sites, specific acting enhancer elements, as well as specific histone methylation mark H3K4me3, which prevents the binding of de novo methylation complexes (Straussman et al., 2009). Methylation of the CpG islands in the promoter region silences gene expression, and the absence of methylation is associated with active transcription. Thus unmethylated CpG islands are associated with the promoters of transcriptionally active genes, such as housekeeping genes and many regulated genes, such as genes showing tissue specific expression (Bird, 1986;Song et al., 2005).

CpG dinucleotides are under-represented in the genome except for small clusters, referred to as CpG islands, located in or near the promoter of greater than 70% of all genes (Balch et al, 2007; Brena et al, 2006; Hellebrekers et al, 2007). Promoter methylation is known to participate in reorganizing chromatin structure and also plays a role in transcriptional inactivation. It is believed that the chromatin surrounding an active promoter containing an unmethylated CpG island is "open" and allows for the access of transcription factors and other coactivators. An inactive promoter containing methylated CpG dinucleotides is associated with a "closed" chromatin configuration and results in transcription factors unable to access the promoter (Dworkin et al., 2009).

2.1 DNA methylation and breast cancer

There are well understood genetic alterations associated with breast carcinogenesis, including specific gene amplifications, deletions, point mutations, chromosome rearrangements, and aneuploidy. In addition to these highly characterized mutations, epigenetic alterations resulting in aberrant gene expression are key contributor to breast tumorigenesis (Campan et al., 2006; Giacinti et al., 2006; Mirza et al., 2007; Sharma et al., 2005; Sui et al., 2007; Vincent-Salomon et al., 2007; Visvanathan et al., 2006; Zhou et al., 2006. Decreased methylation of repetitive sequences in the satellite DNA of the pericentric region of chromosomes is associated with increased chromosomal rearrangements, mitotic recombination, and aneuploidy (Eden et al., 2003,Karpf and Matsui, 2005). Intragenomic endoparasitic DNA, such as L1 (long interspersed nuclear elements) (Schulz, 2006) and Alu (recombinogenic sequence) repeats, are silenced in somatic cells and become reactivated in human cancer (Berdasco & Esteller, 2010). Furthermore, aberrations in DNA methylation patterns of the CpG islands in the promoter regions of tumor-suppressor genes are accepted as being a common feature of human cancer (Esteller, 2008). CpG island promoter hypermethylation affects genes from a wide range of cellular pathways, such as cell cycle, DNA repair, toxic catabolism, cell adherence, apoptosis, and angiogenesis, among others (Esteller, 2008), and may occur at various stages in the development of cancer. (Berdasco & Esteller, 2010).

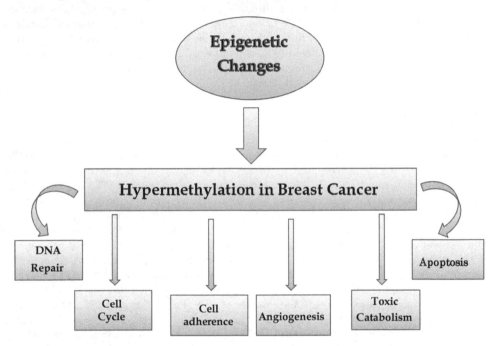

Fig. 1. Hypothetical model that explain how CpG island promoter hypermethylation. Multiple genes are hypermethylated in breast cancer compared to non-cancerous tissue which are affected genes from a wide range of cellular pathways induced by epigenetic changes.

Therefore, DNA methylation not only participates in cancer but has been found to regulate the histone modifications involved in tumor formation. The presence of certain histone modifications such as H4 R3 me2 is a marker of prostate cancer and increased expression of HDAC6 in breast cancer (Kurdistani, 2007). In addition the prognosis of certain malignancies can be affected by epigenetic status (Sakuma et al., 2007) . In normal cells, repetitive genomic sequences (e.g., centromeric satellite α-DNA and juxtacentromeric satellite DNA) are heavily methylated (Esteller, 2007; Jones & Baylin, 2002). The maintenance of methylation in this repetitive DNA could be important for the protection of chromosomal integrity by preventing chromosomal rearrangements, translocations and gene disruption through the reactivation of transposable elements (Eden et al., 2003; Ehrlich, 2002; Jones & Baylin, 2002). Besides hypermethylation of gene-associated CpG islands, hypomethylation of repetitive genomic DNA has also been identified as a specific feature in human cancers (Feinberg & Vogelstein, 1983; Narayan et al., 1998; Jones & Baylin, 2002). Although less well studied than DNA hypermethylation, several lines of investigation indicate that the global DNA hypomethylation identified in cancer cells might contribute to structural changes in chromosomes, loss of imprinting (LOI), micro satellite and chromosome instability through aberrant DNA recombination, aberrant activation of proto-oncogene expression and increased mutagenesis (Chen et al.,1998; Eden et al., 2003; Kaneda & Feinberg, 2005; Jones & Baylin, 2002). Global genomic hypomethylation in breast cancer has been known to correlate with some clinical features such as disease stage, tumor size and histological grade (Soares et al., 1999). Some proto-oncogenes implicated in proliferation and metastasis (e.g., synuclein γ and urokinase genes) or drug resistance to endocrine therapy (e.g., N-cadherin, ID4, annexin A4, β-catenin and WNT11 genes) have been found to be upregulated in breast cancer through the hypomethylation of their promoters (Fan et al., 2006; Gupta et al., 2003; Pakneshan et al., 2004).

3. DNA methyltransferases

The methylation process is catalyzed by the DNA methyltransferases. There are currently four known DNMTs; DNMT1, 2, 3A and 3B (Okano et al., 1998). DNMT3A and DNMT3B are the de novo methyltransferases while DNMT1 maintains the methylation patterns during DNA replication (mitosis) (Bestor, 2000). The actual function of DNMT2 is not clear. It has been shown that DNMT2 possesses weak methyltransferase activity, and its deletion in the embryonic cells caused no detectible effect on global methylation (Okano et al., 1998). DNMT1 has a 5-30 fold preference for hemimethylated DNA (Goyal et al., 2006;Yoder et al., 1997). As well as to the epigenetic silencing of particular genes, DNMT1 supports the long term silencing of non-coding DNA, including most of the repetitive elements (Brannan & Bartolomei, 1999;Fuks, 2005;Jaenisch & Bird, 2003;Jones & Takai, 2001). DNMT1 exist as a component of the DNA replication complex, and thus methylates the newly synthesized DNA strand in correspondence to the template strand (Vertino et al., 2002). DNMT1 has different isoforms, the somatic tissue isoform DNMT1S, the oocyte specific isoform DNMT1o and the spermatocyte isoform DNMT1p. DNMT1o is responsible for maintaining maternal imprints during cleavage (Howell et al., 2001). In addition to that, over expression of DNMT1 has been reported in human tumours and many contribute to the global methylation abnormalities seen in cancer cells although increased expression of the DNMTs likely to be only partially responsible for the observed methylation abnormalities since not all tumours overexpress these enzymes (Robertson & Jones, 2000).

On the other hand, de novo DNA methylation is catalyzed by DNMT3a, DNMT3b and DNMT3L (Okano et al.,1999; Chedin et al., 2002). DNMT3L lacks the ability to bind to SAM, and is responsible for increasing the binding of DNMT3a to SAM (Chedin et al., 2002; Aapola et al., 2000). DNMT2, a small 391-amino-acid protein, is reported to possess weak DNA methyltransferase activity, but its biological function is not yet elucidated (Dong et al, 2001). Very recent studies have shown that Dicer-mediated microRNA biogenesis is involved in modulation of DNA methylation by indirectly regulating the expression of DNMT3 genes (Sinkkonen et al., 2008; Benetti et al., 2008). Dicer belongs to the RNase III family enzymes and is implicated in processing the biosynthesis of small interfering RNAs (siRNAs) and microRNAs (miRNAs) (Kim et al., 2005). In dicer$^{-/-}$ cells, the microRNAs of the miR-290 cluster are depleted and expression levels of their target Rbl2 protein (retinoblastoma-like protein) are increased, leading to downregulation of DNMT3 gene expression through Rbl2-

mediated transcriptional repression, and in turn causing the DNA methylation defect (global hypomethylation) (Sinkkonen et al., 2008; Benetti et al., 2008). Regarding the role of DNMTs in breast tumorigenesis, it has been reported that DNMT3b mRNA is overexpressed in breast cancer, a finding that correlates well with the hypermethylator phenotype and poor prognosis in breast tumors (Girault et al., 2003; Roll et al.,2008).

4. Histone conformation

Histones are five basic nuclear proteins that form the core of the nuclesome. The histone octamer contains two molecules each of histones H2A, H2B, H3 and H4. Histone H1 the linker histone is located outside the core and involve in the packing of DNA (Kornberg & Lorch, 1999). DNA wraps around the octamer in two turns of 146 base pairs (Luger et al., 1997), and the adjacent nucleosomes are connected and wrapped on each other by H1. Consequently histone modifications play a major role in regulating gene expression and extend the information potential of the DNA which explains the growing interest of the 'Histone Code' (Jenuwein & Allis, 2001;Zhang & Reinberg, 2001a). Modifications to amino acids on the N-terminal tails of histones protruding from the nucleosome core can induce both an open or closed chromatin structure and these affect the ability of transcription factors to access promoter regions to activate transcription. The covalent modification can be acetylation, methylation, phosphorylation and ubiquitination. Methylation of some residues is associated with both transcriptional repression, such as methylation of histone 3 lysine 9 (H3 K9) (Nakayama et al., 2001a)and others with transcriptional activation, such as methylation of histone 3 lysine 4 (H3 K4) (Strahl et al., 1999). Histone methylation is performed by histone methltransferase (HMTs) which can transfer up to three methyl groups to lysine residues within the tails of the histones with different effects on gene activity. Acetylation which occurs at lysine residue is associated with transcriptional activation (Turner, 2000). This modification is performed by histone acetylases (HATs) and removed by the histone deacetylases (HDACs).

Other important regulators of chromatin conformation include the polycomb group (PcG) and trithorax group (trxG) proteins, which have key role in developmental gene regulation (Schuettengruber et al., 2007). They are recruited to response elements near proximal promoters to direct histone modifications, which induce both an active chromatin structure (trxG) and an inactive chromatin structure (PcG). Trithorax group proteins methylate H3 K4 to induce an active chromatin configuration (Schuettengruber et al., 2007), while PcG proteins direct the methylation of H3 K27 to induce a repressive chromatin configuration. The effect of PcG protein are however reversible, as removal of PcG during development leads to gene activation. PcG protein have been found to be implicated in regulation of developmental transcription factors, genomic imprinting and X chromosome inactivation (Heard, 2005).

Acetylation of histones has been extensively studied as one of the key regulatory mechanisms of gene expression (Grant, 2001). Histone acetylation was found to affect RNA transcription as early as the 1960s (Allfrey et al., 1964). The highly conserved lysine residue at the N-terminal of H3 at position 9, 14, 18 and 23, and H4 lysine 5,8,12 and 16, are frequently targeted for modification (Roth et al., 2001). Acetylations of the lysine residues neutralize the positive charge of the histone tails. And therefore, decrease their affinity for DNA which results in open chromatin conformation allowing the transcriptional machinery to reach its target (Hong et al., 1993). Additionally, many histone acetylases (HATs) (Brownell & Allis, 1996; Parthun et al., 1996) and histone deacetylases (HDACs) (Taunton et al., 1996) have been described previously.

The acetyltransferases catalyse the addition of the acetyl group from acetyl coenzyme A (acetyl-CoA) to the epsilon-amino group of specific lysine residues (it-Si-Ali et al., 1998;Kim et al., 2000), where deacetylases reverse the reaction (Kuo & Allis, 1998). There are eighteen HDAC enzymes in mammalian cells which are divided into two families: a) zinc metalloenzymes that catalyses the hydrolysis of acetylated specific residues on histone tails and include class I, II and 1V HDACs, and b) NAD-dependent Sir2 deactylases which are considerd as class III HDACs (Glaser, 2007;Vigushin et al., 2001).

Class I is a group of four enzymes known as HDAC1, 2, 3 and 8 and this class is associated with gene regulation. They are expressed ubiquitously and they function exclusively in the nucleus (Brehm et al., 1998;Glaser, 2007). Class II is subdivided into class IIA, which includes HDAC 4, 5, 7 and 9 and class IIB that includes HDAC 6 and 10. Class II enzymes shuttle between cytoplasm and nucleus, and they involve mainly in cell differentiation and are highly expressed in certain tissues such as heart, skeletal muscle and brain (de Ruijter et al., 2003;Glaser, 2007;Grozinger et al., 1999;Vigushin et al., 2001). Class III includes the NAD-dependent deacetylases which is a group of seven enzymes that are involved in maintaining the chromatin stability. They can remove the acetyl groups from histones as will as other proteins (Kyrylenko et al., 2003). Class IV contains one member which is HDAC 11. It is closely related to class I thus some reviewers consider it as a member of that class. The function of HDAC 11 has not been characterized yet (Crabb et al., 2008;de Ruijter et al., 2003).

5. DNA methylation and histone modification

Besides to the promoter methylation, chromatin modification may also contribute to silencing genes in cancer cells. Post-translational modifications to histone proteins occur after translation primarily in the NH2 terminal tail of histones and include acetylation, methylation, phosphorylation, or ubiquitination (Dworkin et al., 2009). Three decade ago Razin and Cedar (1977) have reported the presence of tight correlation between DNA and chromatin structure (Razin & Cedar, 1977). It was believed the relationship is a unidirectional relationship i.e the state of DNA methylation defines chromatin structure; methylated DNA results in closed chromatin configuration while unmethylated DNA results in open chromatin configuration. This hypothesis was supported by research finding that showed that methylated DNA binding proteins recruits chromatin modification enzymes to methylated genes such as MeCP2 (Meehan et al., 1992;Nan et al., 1997). There is increasing evidence showing that changes in chromatin structure would alter DNA methylation patterns. Furthermore, the targeting of DNA methylation enzymes to genes promoters is guided by chromatin modifying enzymes. The fact that is chromatin configuration is dynamic and that is chromatin modifying enzymes activated by cellular signaling pathways. This provides a link between the extracellular environment and the state of DNA methylation (Szyf, 2007). One of the evidence of the link between chromatin modiling and DNA methylation in humans and mice mutation of the SWI-SNF proteins which are involved in chromatin remidling, result in defect in DNA methylation (Szyf, 2007). A number of histone methyltransferases, such as G9a, SUV39H1 and EZH2, a member of the multiprotein polycomb complex PRC2 can regulate DNA methylation by either recruiting or regulating the stability of DNMTs. DNMTs in turn can recruit HDACs and MBPs to achieve chromatin condensation and gene silencing (Sharma et al., 2010). This relationship between the epigenetic machinery makes the epigenetic mechanisms of genome expression a tightly regulated process.

As a result of that, cancer was thought to be exclusively a consequence of genetic changes in key tumor-suppressor genes and oncogenes that regulate cell proliferation, DNA repair, cell differentiation, and other homeostatic functions. During the last decade, the study of epigenetic mechanisms in cancer, such as DNA methylation, histone modification, nucleosome positioning, and micro RNA expression, has provided extensive information about the mechanisms that contribute to the neoplastic phenotype through the regulation of expression of genes critical to transformation pathways. Regarding DNA methylation, the low level of CpG methylation in tumors compared with that in their normal-tissue counterparts was one of the first epigenetic alterations to be found in human cancer (Feinberg & Vogelstein, 1983;Goelz et al., 1985) this let us to think that the cancer cells have a specific epigenome. hypomethylation in cancer cells is associated with a number of adverse products, including chromosome instability, activation of transposable elements, and loss of genomic imprinting (Berdasco & Esteller, 2010).

6. Micro RNA and epigenetic

As well documented, about 80 % of human transcribed RNA is not translated into protein. This RNA was thought to be either functionless (Mattick, 2001), or transcriptional noise (Dennis, 2002). From this population, micro RNAs (miRNA) have an established epigenetic role with the potential to be implicated in programming. micro RNA (miRNA) are small untranslated RNAs generally 21-25 mucleotides in length (Bartel, 2004), they regulate gene expression by affecting the stability or the translation efficiency of target mRNA. They bind their complementary mRNA and thus dsRNA is formed, this recognized as foreign RNA and cleaved to be degraded. Matching between the miRNAs and mRNA doesn't have to be perfect as even incomplete binding can block translation (Mattick & Makunin, 2005). Nearly 30% of genes expression is probably regulated by miRNA via the interaction between miRNAs and their target mRNA. Individual miRNA may regulate 200 targets by partial base pairing to mRNA, sugessting that one miRNA may control numerous biological or pathological signaling pathway by affecting the expressions and functions of their targets. It has been reported that miRNA has a role in the development process (He & Hannon, 2004), including a role in the process of stem cell differentiation (Houbaviy et al., 2003). Also it has been shown in cancer studies of miRNA that DNA methylation and histone modification control the expression of these small RNAs. This was achieved by studying the effect of DNA demethylating agents and hisdtone deacetylases inhibitors on the expression of miRNA expression particularly the miR-127 which is embedded in CpG island (Saito & Jones, 2006;Saito et al., 2006).

7. Genomic imprinting

Genomic imprinting is a developmental phenomenon that describes a unique form of gene regulation that leads to only one parental allele being expressed depending on its parental origin (Delaval & Feil, 2004;Surani, 1991). Insulin-like growth factor 2 (IGF2) and its receptor IGF2R are two of the first reported genes subjected to imprinting regulation (Barlow et al., 1991;DeChiara et al., 1991). In mouse genome there are 600 predicted imprinted genes (Luedi et al., 2005). These identified imprinted genes have a major common feature in that they are associated with at least one regulatory DNA element, often referred to as imprinted control region (ICR). The ICR region is essential in regulating the parental origin-specific expression via interaction with specific transcription factors (Kim et al., 2007;Yang et al., 2003). Differential DNA methylation of the parental ICRs is one of the most common features associated with imprinted genes (Kim et al., 2003;Liang et al., 2000;Mancini-Dinardo et al., 2003). Typical disorders associated with imprinted genes include Prader-Willi and Angelman syndromes, Beckwith-Wiedemann syndrome and multiple forms of neoplasia (Weksberg et al., 2003;Zeschnigk et al., 1997). In addition to that, X inactivation is a mechanism that functionally equalizes the difference of X-linked genes between XX females and XY males by silencing one of the two X chromosomes in females. Dosage compensation is a widely known method of silencing the X chromosome in females. This is achieved epigenetically through a cascade of CpG methylation superimposed by global histone deacetylation (Avner & Heard, 2001;Lyon, 1999;Monk, 2002;Pfeifer et al., 1990).

8. PcG and cancer epigenetics

Other epigenetic modifiers have been identified, including the Polycomb group (PcG) proteins and small non-coding RNAs. PcG repressors serve as a docking platform for DNA methyltransferases and target a gene for permanent silencing by methylation of hisone H3 on lysine 27 (H3K27). Reversal of permanent silencing is only overcome by de-differentiation processes in the germline. Small non-coding RNA molecules, such as microRNAs, regulate gene expression by targeting RNA degradation (Luczak & Jagodzinski, 2006). These RNAs have also been found to also target gene promoters and result in transcriptional gene silencing (Balch et al., 2007; Han et al., 2007).

Increasing evidence from cancer epigenomic studies suggests a critical role for PcG factors in abnormal epigenetic silencing of tumor suppressor genes in cancer cells (Baylin & Ohm, 2006;Jones & Baylin, 2007;Lund & van Lohuizen, 2004;Valk-Lingbeek et al., 2004;Ting et al., 2006). There are at least four different PcG complexes identified in mammalian, including the maintenance complex, PRC1, composed of RING, HPC, HPH, and BMI1, and three different initiation complexes, PRC2 through PRC4, which are formed by enhancer of zeste homolog 2 (EZH2), suppressor of zeste 12 (SUZ12), and different isoforms of embryonic ectoderm development (EED) (Baylin & Ohm, 2006;Ting et al., 2006;Kuzmichev et al., 2004;Kuzmichev et al., 2005). In particular, PRC4 exists in embryonic, stem, progenitor and cancer cells and associates with a class III HDAC called SIRT1 ((Baylin & Ohm, 2006;Ting et al., 2006). The crucial function of PRC complexes in H3K27 methylation is mediated by EZH2, a histone lysine methyltransferase, that catalyzes this lysine methylation (Cao et al., 2002;Cao & Zhang, 2004;Martin & Zhang, 2005). Methylation of H3K27 possibly stabilizes the binding of PcG complexes to this histone mark to facilitate long-term gene silencing (Fischle et al., 2003;Martin & Zhang, 2005). Importantly, H3K27me is often present at the promoters of the DNA hypermethylated and silenced cancer genes investigated thus far (McGarvey et al., 2006), indicating that PcG proteins play an essential role in aberrant gene silencing in cancer cells. A recent study also showed that PcG-targeted genes in normal cells are closely associated with de novo DNA methylation in cancer cells, suggesting that PcG may preprogram its targeted genes as targets of subsequent DNA methylation in cancer cells (Keshet et al., 2006;Schlesinger et al., 2007).

In addition, several studies have shown that expression of PcG proteins such as EZH2, SUZ12 and BMI1 is aberrantly elevated in breast cancer and other cancers (Dimri et al., 2002;Kleer et al., 2003), suggesting deregulation of components of nucleosomal remodeling complexes can also be a mechanism resulting in gene silencing in cancer cells. In the case of another repressive histone mark, H3K9me2 (me3), this lysine methylation is catalyzed by several histone lysine methyltransferases, including SUV39H, SETDB1, G9a and GLP among others (Schultz et al., 2002;Lehnertz et al., 2003;Tachibana et al., 2005). Although the defined role of H3K9 methylation in epigenetic gene silencing remains elusive, one possible mechanism is that this mark can serve as a binding site for heterochromatin protein HP1, which has an intrinsic ability to recruit DNA methyltransferases to the silenced genes (Fuks et al., 2003;Lachner et al., 2001).

To establish DNA methylation in a subset of genes, polycomb protein EZH2 must associate with DNMTs (Esteller, 2007). It is thought that polycomb proteins could collaborate with DNMTs by recruiting them to silenced promoters to establish long-term silencing (Matarazzo et al., 2007). Leu et al (2004) investigated whether the removal of ERα signaling could cause changes in DNA methylation and chromatin structure of ERα target promoters. They used RNAi to transiently disable ERα in breast cancer cells and found that polycomb repressors and histone deacetylases assemble in the promoter of an ERα target gene. Accumulation of DNA methylation in these silenced targets like the PR promoter region then occurs and can be stably transmitted to cell progeny for long-term silencing. Both ERα expression and DNA demethylation appear to be required to restore PR expression. They also observed a trend that more ERα negative tumors had more methylated loci than ERα positive tumors (Leu et al., 2004). This indicates that dysregulation of normal signaling in cancer cells may result in stable silencing of downstream targets maintained by epigenetic machinery (Dworkin et al., 2009).

The epigenetic mechanisms for gene silencing involve the interplay between DNA methylation, histone modifications and nucleosomal remodeling. The families of methyl-CpG binding proteins (MBD and Kaiso families) have been identified to play a key role in this interplay. The molecular functions of methyl-CpG binding proteins are dependent on their ability to recognize and bind methylated DNA (Clouaire & Stancheva, 2008;Meehan et al., 1989; ing et al., 2006). Accumulating evidence suggests that methyl-CpG binding proteins can associate directly or indirectly with DNMTs, HDACs and HMTs and cooperate with them to modify chromatin structure and suppress initiation of gene transcription (Fuks et al., 2003;Jones et al., 1998;Kimura & Shiota, 2003;Sarraf & Stancheva, 2004). The associated partners of methyl-CpG binding proteins have also been found to include many nucleosomal remodeling complexes such as NuRD, CoREST, NCoR/SMRT, Sin3A, SUV39H and SWI/SNF (Fujita et al., 2003;Harikrishnan et al., 2005;Le Guezennec et al., 2006;Yoon et al., 2003;Wade et al., 1999;Zhang et al., 1999). The significant role of methyl-CpG binding proteins in cancer epigenetics is supported by the findings that they are localized to DNA hypermethylated and aberrantly silenced cancer genes (Bakker et al., 2002; Lopez-Serra et al., 2006; Nguyen et al., 2001).

Thus, it has been postulated that methyl-CpG binding proteins initially recognize and bind to methylated DNA, and then bring down nucleosomal remodeling complexes to modify chromatin to the repressive compact heterochromatin structure, which causes gene silencing. Inversely, the results from some other studies show that chromatin remodeling activities can further facilitate binding of methyl-CpG binding proteins to methylated DNA sites (Feng & Zhang, 2001;Harikrishnan, et al., 2005), suggesting interaction between methyl-CpG binding proteins and nucleosomal remodeling complexes results in mutual stimulation of each others' activity. Taken together, methyl-CpG binding proteins represent an important class of chromosomal proteins that associate with multiple protein partners to modify surrounding chromatin and silence transcription, providing a functional link between DNA methylation and chromatin modification and remodeling (Lo & Sukumar, 2008).

Again, cancer generally has been viewed as a disease that is driven by progressive genetic abnormalities, involving chromosomal abnormalities, mutations in oncogenes and tumor suppressor genes (Hanahan & Weinberg, 2000;Vogelstein & Kinzler 2004). Nevertheless, it has been shown that breast cancer, similar to other types of cancer, is also a disease that is driven by epigenetic alterations, which do not affect the primary DNA sequence (Widschwendter & Jones, 2002;Polyak, 2007). The result of these alterations is aberrant transcriptional regulation that leads to a modify in expression patterns of genes implicated in survival, differentiation and cellular proliferation (Baylin & Ohm, 2006;Esteller, 2007;Widschwendter & Jones, 2002). In transformed cells, epigenetic alterations occur at the chromosomal level. These involve changes in DNA methylation, histone modifications, altered expression and function of factors implicated in regulating assembly and remodeling of nucleosomes (Baylin & Ohm, 2006;Esteller, 2007;Jones & Baylin, 2002;Jones & Baylin, 2007;Ting et al., 2006). Alterations in DNA methylation include global hypomethyation and focal hypermethylation.

Global hypomethylation has been found to increase with age and is linked to genomic instability and activation of oncogene expression (Eden et al., 2003;Feinberg & Tycko, 2004;Richardson, 2002). Epigenetic inactivation due to aberrant promoter methylation is a key process in breast tumorigenesis. DNA Methylation silencing of tumor suppressor genes, aberrant expression of DNMT1 or demethylation of oncogenes can lead to the conversion of a normal cell to a malignant cell. In addition chromosomal instability and inactivation of the DNA repair system has both the genetic and epigenetic backgrounds (Esteller & Herman, 2002;Szyf, 2008). Epigenetic silencing of tumour suppressor genes is an early event in breast carcinogenesis and reversion of gene silencing by epigenetic reprogramming can provide clues to the mechanisms responsible for tumour initiation and progression. Hypermethylation of the mismatch repair gene MLH1 is associated with tumors exhibiting microsatellite instability, and hypermethylation of the breast cancer gene BRCA1 is found in 10%- 15% of women with non-familial breast cancer (Jones & Baylin, 2002).

9. Epigenetic modifications and breast cancer

Epigenetic modifications are believed to be early events in cancer development (Leu et al., 2004) and breast cancer is a disease characterized by both genetic and epigenetic alterations. It is thought that once epigenetic alterations are established in premalignant tissues, the extent of modifications will accumulate as the disease progresses (Dworkin et al., 2009). Varying theories have been proposed on how this field defect arises. One theory is based on the self-metastasis model and the idea that the primary tumor is composed of multiple self-metastases that form around a seed from the tumor to itself (Norton, 2005). A second theory has been seen in gastric cancers and is based on cell methylation profiles influencing H. pylori infection which leads to additional methylation of promoters in gastric mucosal cells and accompanying increases in risk for gastric cancer (Maekita et al., 2006). Another theory has supportive evidence in breast cancer and is based on the idea that early epigenetic changes are associated with a large area of pre-malignant changes, and the "epicenter" appears to accumulate additional epigenetic changes (Yan et al., 2006).

Allelic losses of 3p, including a critical region at 3p21.3, are frequently detected in many cancers including breast cancer. The Ras-associated domain family member 1 gene (RASSF1) maps to the region of frequent loss. It is comprised of eight exons and through different promoter usage and alternative splicing generates seven unique transcripts, RASSF1A-G.

RASSF1A is transcribed from a CpG island promoter region, and is one of the most frequently hypermethylated genes thus far described in human cancer. The CpG island of RASSF1A is hypermethylated in 60–77% of breast cancers (Lewis et al., 2005;Vincent-Salomon et al., 2007) resulting in gene silencing in cancer cell lines and primary tissues. Its diverse functions include regulation of apoptosis, growth regulation, and microtubule dynamics during mitotic progression. Specifically, RASSF1A is a Ras effector and induces apoptosis through its interactions with pro-apoptotic kinase MST1. When cells lacking RASSF1A expression are treated with a DNA methyltransferase, such as 5-aza-2'-deoxycytidine, expression can be reactivated (Pfeifer & Dammann, 2005). Mouse knockout studies show that RASSF1A$^{-/-}$ mice are prone to spontaneous development of lung adenomas, lymphomas and breast adenocarcinomas. These mice are prone to early spontaneous tumorigenesis and show a severe tumor susceptibility phenotype compared to that of littermate wild-type mice (Pfeifer & Dammann, 2005).

Furthermore, it has been reported that the DNA methylation assay might be used for risk assessment and prognosis of breast cancer. Lewis et al. studied five frequently methylated genes, including RASSF1A, APC, H-cadherin, RARβ, and cyclin D2, and found a higher methylation frequency of both RASSF1A and APC genes in unaffected women at high risk for breast cancer compared with those at low or intermediate risk based on the Gail model analysis. This suggests that promoter hypermethylation of these genes is associated with epidemiologic markers of increased breast cancer risk (Lewis et al., 2005). This finding needs confirmation that such alterations do indeed occur earlier than abnormal histological findings, and by follow-up studies to examine whether these changes are associated with subsequent development of breast cancer (Lo & Sukumar, 2008). The prognostic significance of aberrant DNA methylation has been investigated by Muller et al. (2003) after screening 39 genes in DNA from serum of normal control patients and patients with primary or metastatic breast cancer, they identified two genes, RASSF1A and APC, whose methylation has a statistically significant association with poor outcome. Other methylated genes, such as GSTP1, SFRP1, have also been identified to be associated with poor prognosis (Arai et al., 2006;Veeck et al., 2006).

In breast cancer, multiple genes are hypermethylated compared to non-cancerous tissue (Agrawal & Murphy, 2007). These include genes involved in evasion of apoptosis (RASSF1A, HOXA5, TWIST1), limitless replication potential (CCND2, p16, BRCA1, RARβ), growth (ERα, PGR), and tissue invasion and metastasis (CDH1) (Han et al., 2007; Yan et al., 2001; Widschwendter & Jones, 2002). These genes are not only hypermethylated in tumor cells, but show increased epigenetic silencing in normal epithelium surrounding the tumor site. The first observations of this phenomenon were in oral cancer. Slaughter et al (1953) was the first group to use the term "field cancerization" which refers to the presence of cancer causing changes in apparently normal tissue surrounding a neoplasm. They theorized the existence of (pre-) neoplastic processes at multiple sites, with the unproven assumption that these have developed independently (Slaughter et al., 1953). In subsequent years, the presence of field cancerization has been described in head and neck squamous cell carcinoma, lung, esophagus, vulva, cervix, colon, bladder, skin, and breast cancers (Yan et al., 2006). Studies have demonstrated that normal adjacent cells to tumors frequently harbor loss of heterozygosity, microsatellite and chromosome instability, and gene mutations (Braakhuis et al., 2003). Recently DNA methylation has been added to list as hypermethylated normal tissue immediately adjacent to tumor sites has been found (Ushijima, 2007).

CpG-island-containing gene promoters are usually unmethylated in normal cells to maintain euchromatic structure, which is the transcriptionally active conformation allowing gene expression. Yet, during cancer development, many of these genes are hypermethylated at their CpG-island-containing promoters to inactivate their expression by changing open euchromatic structure to compact heterochromatic structure (Baylin & Ohm, 2006; Esteller, 2007; Jones & Baylin, 2002; Jones & Baylin, 2007). These genes are selectively hypermethylated in tumorigenesis for inactivation owing to their functional involvement in various cellular pathways that prevent cancer formation. Some of the methylated genes identified in human cancers are classic tumor suppressor genes in which one mutationally inactivated allele is inherited. According to Knudson's two-hit model, complete inactivation of a tumor suppressor gene requires loss-of-function of both gene copies (Knudson, 2000). Epigenetic silencing of the remaining wild-type allele of the tumor suppressor gene, thus, can be considered as the second hit in this model. For example, some well-known tumor suppressor genes, such as p16INK4a, APC and BRCA1, are mutationally inactivated in the germline occasionally lose function of the remaining functional allele in breast epithelial cells through DNA hypermethylation (Birgisdottir et al., 2006; Jin et al., 2001; Knudson, 2000). Since the consequence of aberrant DNA methylation is transcriptional silencing, novel tumor suppressor genes can be identified using methylated CpG islands as a marker.

As a result of that, hypermethylated genes identified from breast neoplasms now form a long list. Their biological functions encompass cell cycle regulation (p16INK4a, p14ARF, 14–3–3σ, cyclin D2, p57KIP2), apoptosis (APC, DAPK1, HIC1, HOXA5, TWIST, TMS1), DNA repair (GSTP1, MGMT, BRCA1), hormone regulation (ERα, PR), cell adhesion and invasion (CDH1, APC, TIMP3), angiogenesis (maspin, THBS1), cellular growth-inhibitory signaling (RARβ, RASSF1A, SYK, TGFβRII, HIN1, NES1, SOCS1, SFRP1 and WIF1). In addition to protein-coding genes, recent studies showed that microRNAs with tumor-suppressor function could be silenced in breast cancer cells through DNA methylation (Lehmann et al., 2008). These breast-genome methylation patterns have been developed as biomarkers for early detection and the classification of subtype of breast tumors, as predictors for risk assessment and for monitoring prognosis, and as indicators of susceptibility or response to therapy (Widschwendter & Jones, 2002;Lo & Sukumar, 2008).

These advances in the knowledge of the breast methylome strongly indicate that DNA hypermethylation plays a crucial role in initiation, promotion and maintenance of breast carcinogenesis, which cooperatively and synergistically interact with other genetic alterations to promote the development of breast cancer. For example, human mammary epithelial cells (HMECs) that gained the ability to emerge from the first transient growth plateau lost p16INK4A expression concurrently with hypermethylation of p16INK4A promoter, indicating that loss of tumor-suppressor function of p16INK4A is required for HMECs to gain growth competency by successfully bypassing the stage of cell senescence (Widschwendter & Jones, 2002; Tlsty et al., 2004). This finding is consistent with other studies where the life span of stem cells could be extended by germline loss of this gene (Janzen et al., 2006). Deregulation of cell cycle control by inhibiting the function of the cyclin-dependent kinase inhibitor, p16INK4A, could create a context for facilitating early abnormal clonal expansion of cells at risk for cancer. It is believed that loss of p16INK4A gene is permissive for enabling such expanding cells to develop genomic instability (Kiyono et al, 1998).

In addition to cell-cycle regulatory genes, DNA methylation-mediated silencing of DNA repair genes, such as BRCA1 and MGMT, could result in further inactivation of tumor suppressor genes or activation of oncogenes, which further drive breast tumorigenesis

(Esteller et al., 2000). More recently, the genes that function as inhibitors of WNT oncogenic pathway, such as SFRP1 and WIF1, have been found to be frequently hypermethylated in primary breast tumors (Ai et al., 2006; Lo et al., 2006).). Thus, in addition to the genetic mutation-mediated mechanism, epigenetic gene silencing is another mechanism that fosters malignant transformation of the mammary gland by aberrantly activating oncogenic signaling pathways (Lo & Sukumar, 2008).

10. Breast cancer epigenetic markers

There are two main reasons RASSF1A methylation is a good biomarker for breast cancer. First, RASSF1A methylation is rare in normal tissue providing a marker with high specificity. Second, the frequency of methylation is observed in 60 to 77% of cells from a tumor which provides a high frequency of diagnostic coverage (Campan et al., 2006; Muller et al., 2003). In addition to breast tumors, hypermethylation of RASSF1A can be detected in non-malignant breast cells and patient sera. In one study, hypermethylation of sera in breast cancer patients was detected in six out of 26 cases (Pfeifer & Dammann, 2005). Promoter methylation of RASSF1A was observed in 70% of samples from women at high-risk of developing breast cancer versus only 29% of samples from women at low-risk. Women with a previous history of benign breast growths are statistically more likely to have RASSF1A methylation (Lewis et al., 2005). Thus, hypermethylation of RASSFIA could be used as a form of breast cancer screening to detect breast cancer at its earliest stages (Dworkin et al., 2009).

However, it is well reported that prolonged exposure of undifferentiated (immature) breast cells to estrogen or estrogen-mimetic compounds during early development increases breast cancer risk in adult life. This phenomenon is called estrogen imprinting (Fenton, 2006). These studies can explain why, in addition to genetic factors, the risk of breast cancer is affected by pregnancy, lifestyle in terms of intake of food and drink, and environment. Although the tumorigenic mechanism underlying this phenomenon and its connection with epigenetic regulation are still largely unknown, recently published findings provide insight into this mechanism. One line of evidence is from the study of DNA methylation patterns in several subtypes of breast cells. Bloushtain-Qimron et al. found that several transcription factor genes involved in stem cell function were hypomethylated and highly expressed in breast progenitor/stem (undifferentiated) cells compared with differentiated breast epithelial cells (Bloushtain-Qimron et al., 2008), suggesting the epigenetic programs define mammary epithelial cell phenotypes. Since breast progenitor/stem cells possess self-renewal and proliferating ability and more sensitively respond to estrogenic action, this subtype of cells has been thought to be potent targets of malignant transformation (Shipitsin et al., 2007). The second line of evidence is from the study of the effects of estrogen exposure on breast progenitor/stem cells, using a primary culture system to decipher the phenomenon of estrogen imprinting. Recent study compared the DNA methylation profiles of epithelial progeny of estrogen-exposed breast progenitor cells with those of epithelial progeny of nonestrogen-exposed progenitor cells. They found that estrogen exposure caused epithelial progeny to exhibit a cancer-like methylome, leading to silencing of some tumor suppressor genes (Cheng et al., 2008). Even though the dose of estradiol (E2) used in their study was higher than normal physiological levels, their findings suggest abnormal exposure to estrogen or estrogenic chemicals induces epigenetic alterations in breast progenitor cells, which have been previously implicated in breast cancer (Lo & Sukumar, 2008).

Even though the aberrant activation of estrogen signaling can lead to tumor-associated alterations in the epigenome of breast progenitor cells, approximately 30% of diagnosed breast cancer cases lack estrogen signaling due to loss or downregulation of estrogen receptor (ER)-α, also subject to epigenetic silencing (Lapidus et al., 1998; Ottaviano et al., 1994). ER-negative breast cancers exhibit more aggressive characteristics than ER-positive breast cancers and are resistant to anti-estrogen therapy. How ER-negative breast cancer cells acquire more aggressive properties after loss of estrogen signaling is a very important issue in the field of breast cancer research. Another study provides evidence to link loss of ER signaling to epigenetic silencing of ERα downstream target genes (Leu et al., 2004). Their study showed that abrogation of ERα signaling by small interfering RNA-mediated knockdown of ERα expression resulted in epigenetic inactivation of ERα targets, which began from recruiting PcG repressors and HDACs to their promoters and was then progressively followed by DNA methylation of their promoters (Leu et al., 2004). Their results suggest that epigenetic regulation on ERα target genes is required for establishing ERα-independent growth and other characteristics of ER-negative breast cancer cells (Lo & Sukumar, 2008).

Other post-translational modifications of ERα such as phosphorylation, ubiquitination, glycosylation, and acetylation are believed to play a role in breast cancer promotion. ERα is modified by p300 on two lysine residues (302 and 303) located in the hinge region (between DNA- and ligand binding domains). When these lysine residues are mutated, ERα had increased hormone sensitivity. Thirty-four percent of atypical breast hyperplasia samples have mutations of the lysine at 303 (K303R) of the ERα (Margueron et al., 2004; Popov et al., 2007; Wang et al., 2001) explaining a functional role of these mutations in breast cancer promotion.

Furthermore, BRCA1 is a tumor suppressor gene for both breast and ovarian cancer (Campan et al., 2006). It encodes a multifunctional protein with roles in DNA repair, cell cycle check point control, protein ubiquitization, and chromatin remodeling (Mirza et al., 2007). In vitro experiments showed that decreased BRCA1 expression in cells led to increased levels of tumor growth, while increased expression of BRCA1 led to growth arrest and apoptosis. Recent studies indicate that BRCA1 methylation is an important marker for prognosis. The magnitude of the decrease of functional BRCA1 protein correlates with disease prognosis (Mirza et al., 2007; Vincent-Salomon et al., 2007). Tumors with BRCA1 mutations are usually more likely to be higher-grade, poorly differentiated, highly proliferative, estrogen receptor (ER) negative, and progesterone receptor (PR) negative, and harbor p53 mutations. BRCA1 mutated breast cancers are also associated with poor survival in some studies (Chappuis et al., 2000; Robson et al., 2004; Stoppa-Lyonnet et al., 2000). Phenotypically, BRCA1-methylated tumors are similar to tumors from carriers of germline BRCA1 mutations.

BRCA1 is thought to be a classical tumor suppressor gene for which Knudson's two-hit hypothesis holds true. About 20% of individuals with a strong personal and family history of breast and ovarian cancer carry germline mutations in the BRCA1 gene (Birgisdottir et al., 2006; Tapia et al., 2008). A second hit is thought to be required in the wild-type BRCA1 allele for the development of BRCA-associated cancer (Chenevix-Trench et al., 2006; Osorio et al., 2002; Osorio et al., 2007). However, about 20% of all tumors from BRCA mutation carriers do not show LOH of the wildtype BRCA1 (Chenevix-Trench et al., 2006; Meric-Bernstam, 2007; Osorio et al., 2002; Osorio et al., 2007).). Other studies have looked at the rate of BRCA1 methylation in germline carriers. BRCA1 promoter hypermethylation was observed in one of two tumors from BRCA1 carriers lacking LOH (Esteller et al., 2001). In other study of population-based ovarian tumors, two of eight tumors with germline BRCA1 mutations showed neither LOH nor promoter methylation (Press et al., 2008). Another study of 47 breast tumors from hereditary breast cancer families identified three BRCA1 carriers of which two showed BRCA1 promoter methylation in their tumors (Birgisdottir et al., 2006). All these investigated studies suggest that methylation of BRCA1 may be serve as a second hit in tumors from a subset of BRCA1 mutation carriers (Dworkin et al., 2009).

Furthermore, BRCA1 promoter methylation was more frequent in invasive than in situ carcinoma and there were no correlation between BRCA1 promoter methylation and ER/PR status in a subset population (Xu et al., 2008). However, they also found a higher prevalence of BRCA1 promoter methylation in cases with at least one node involved and with tumor size greater than 2cm. Based on their findings higher methylation levels may correlate with more advanced tumor stage at diagnosis. They also observed a 45% increase in mortality of individuals with BRCA1 methylation positive tumors compared those who had unmethylated BRCA1 promoters (Xu et al., 2008). Another recent study conducted a familial breast cancer based study and found contradicting results. They found no overall correlation of ER, PR, or grade with hypermethylation of BRCA1 in the tumors from BRCA1 mutation negative families. However, seven individuals had both promoter hypermethylation and LOH; the majority of these tumors had a basal-like phenotype and were triple negative (Honrado et al., 2007).

11. Analysis of DNA methylation in breast cancer

Moreover, much of the research effort to date has concentrated on the identification of silenced genes implicated in breast tumorigenesis. Evron et al. successfully used a three-gene panel (Cyclin D2, RARβ and TWIST) to detect malignant breast cancer cells in ductal fluid from routine operative breast endoscopy (ROBE) and ductal lavage (Evron et al., 2001). Fackler et al. improved this method and tested a four-gene panel (RASSF1A, TWIST, HIN1 and Cyclin D2) using the QM-MSP assay to examine clinical tissue samples (Fackler et al., 2004). The cumulative methylation of these four genes is commonly observed to be higher in primary invasive breast cancers compared with reduction mammoplasty specimens from healthy women (Fackler et al., 2004). Fackler et al. further used the same technique but adopted a nine-gene panel (RASSF1A, TWIST, HIN1, Cyclin D2, RARβ, APC, BRCA1, BRCA2 and p16) to examine ductal lavage samples from women with or without breast cancer. This trial demonstrated that methylation-marker detection was twice as sensitive as cytological diagnosis of ductal lavage cells (Fackler et al., 2006). In addition to biopsied tissue sections and ductal fluid, methylated DNA is also detected in blood since the blood of patients with manifest breast cancer contains detectable amounts of circulating methylated DNA (Widschwendte & Menon, 2006). The blood detection of tumor-specific methylated DNA has been pursued for its potential for prognostic prediction and monitoring relapse of breast cancer after therapy (Widschwendte & Menon, 2006; Muller et al., 2003; Silva et al., 2002).

The analysis of methylation profiles in human cancer indicates that hypermethylation of some of the CpG islands is shared by multiple tumour types, whereas others are methylated in a tumour type-specific manner (Bae et al., 2004; Costello et al., 2000; Esteller et al., 2001; Nass et al., 2000; Parrella et al., 2004; Parrella, 2010). Promoter-aberrant methylation seems to be an early event in tumorigenesis, and an increase in the number of methylated genes during progression has been observed in several tumour types including breast cancer (Lehmann et al., 2002; Subramaniam et al., 2009). Hoque et al (2009) have shown there were differences in the patterns of methylation in pre-invasive breast lesions (atypical ductal hyperplesia and ductal carcinoma in situ) as compared with invasive breast cancers. They suggested that DNA methylation may represent an interesting target for the development of new molecular markers for the detection of breast cancer cells in tumours and bodily fluids. The most widely used analytical approach for the determination of methylation status is methylation-specific-PCR (MSP). This method is based on bisulphite conversion of unmethylated cytosin to thymidine while methylated cytosines are protected from conversion. PCR primers are designed to specifically amplify the modified methylated sequence (Hoque et al., 2009). Semiquantitative approaches which combine the advantages of MSP which is applicable and highly sensitive to any CpGs and RT-PCR were also developed and used for methylation detection in tumours and bodily fluids (Herman et al., 1996; Lo et al., 1999).

12. Conclusion

Both DNA methylation and histone modifications play a crucial role in the maintenance of normal cell function and cellular identity of cancer cells. In breast cancer cells these epigenetic modification become massively perturbed, leading to significant changes in expression profiles which confer advantage to the development of a malignant phenotype. DNMTs are the enzymes responsible for setting up and maintaining DNA methylation patterns in eukaryotic cells. Intriguingly, DNMTs were found to be overexpressed in cancerous cells, which is believed to partly explain the hypermethylation phenomenon commonly observed in tumors. Thus, epigenetic modifications are clearly involved in breast cancer initiation and progression. Early studies focused on single genes important in prognosis and prediction, but newer genome-wide methods are identifying many genes whose regulation is epigenetically altered during breast cancer progression. Detection of hypermethylation in specific genes like RASSF1A could be used as a form of surveillance to detect early stage breast cancer, however future studies may find that the addition of multiple genes and the inclusion of histone alterations to predictive panels may improve sensitivity and specificity. In addition to the use of epigenetic alterations as a means of screening, epigenetic alterations in a tumor or adjacent tissues may also help clinicians in determining prognosis and treatment in breast cancer patients. As we understand specific epigenetic alterations contributing to breast tumorigenesis and prognosis, these discoveries will lead in future to significant advances for breast cancer treatment.

13. References

Aapola, U., Kawasaki, K., Scott, HS., Ollila, J., Vihinen, M., .Heino, M., Shintani, A., Kawasaki, K., Minoshima, S., Krohn, K., Antonarakis, SE., Shimizu, N., Kudoh, J., & Peterson, P. (2000). Isolation and initial characterization of a novel zinc finger gene, DNMT3L, on 21q22.3, related to the cytosine-5-methyltransferase 3 gene family. *Genomics*, 65. 293–298.

Agrawal, A., & Murphy, RF., (2007). Agrawal, DK. DNA methylation in breast and colorectal cancers. *Modern Pathology*, 20. 711–721.

Ai, L., Tao, Q., Zhong, S., Fields, CR., Kim, WJ., Lee, MW., Cui, Y., Brown, KD., & Robertson, KD. (2006). Inactivation of Wnt inhibitory factor-1 (WIF1) expression by epigenetic silencing is a common event in breast cancer. *Carcinogenesis*, 27. 1341-1348.

Allfrey, VG., Faulknerr, R, & Mirsky, AE. (1964). Acetylation and methylation the histones and their possible role in the regulation of RNA synthesis. *Proceedings of the National Academy of Sciences of the United States of America*, 51. 786-794.

Arai, T., Miyoshi, Y., Kim, SJ., Taguchi, T., Tamaki, Y., & Noguchi, S. (2006). Association of GSTP1 CpG islands hypermethylation with poor prognosis in human breast cancers. *Breast Cancer Research and Treatment*, 100, 169–176.

Avner, P., & Heard, E. (2001). X-chromosome inactivation: counting, choice and initiation. *Nature Review of Genetic*, 2. 59-67.

Bae, YK., Brown, A., Garrett, E., Bornman, D., Fackler, MJ., Sukumar, S., Herman, JG., Gabrielson, E. (2004). Hypermethylation in histologically distinct classes of breast cancer. *Clinical Cancer Research*, 10. 5998–6005.

Bakker, J., Lin, X., & Nelson, WG. (2002) Methyl-CpG binding domain protein 2 represses transcription from hypermethylated pi-class glutathione S-transferase gene promoters in hepatocellular carcinoma cells. *Journal Biology Chemistry*, 277. 22573–22580.

Balch, C., Montgomery, JS., Paik, HI., Kim, S., Kim, S., Huang, TH., & Nephew, KP. (2005) New anti-cancer strategies: epigenetic therapies and biomarkers. *Frontier in Biosciences*, 10. 1897–931.

Balch, C., Huang, THM., & Nephew, KP. (2007). High-Throughput Assessments of Epigenetics in Human Disease. In: Kim S, Mardis ER, Tang H, editors. Advances in Genome Sequencing Technology and Algorithms. Artech House Publishers, Inc; 2007.

Barlow, DP., Stoger, R., Herrmann, BG., Saito, K., & Schweifer, N. (1991). The mouse insulin-like growth factor type-2 receptor is imprinted and closely linked to the Tme locus. *Nature*, 349. 84-87.

Bartel, DP. (2004). MicroRNAs: genomics, biogenesis, mechanism, and function. *Cell*, 116, 281-297.

Baylin, SB., & Ohm, JE. (2006). Epigenetic gene silencing in cancer – a mechanism for early oncogenic pathway addiction? *Nature Review of Cancer*, 6. 107–116.

Benetti, R., Gonzalo, S., Jaco, I., Muñoz, P., Gonzalez,S., Murcheftner, S., Murchison, E., Andl, T., Chen, T., Klatt, P., Li, E., Serrano, M., Millar, S., Hannon, G., & Blasco, MA. (2008). A mammalian microRNA cluster controls DNA methylation and telomere recombination via Rbl2-dependent regulation of DNA methyltransferases. *Nature Structural Molecular Biology*, 15. 268–279.

Berdasco, M & Esteller, M. (2010). Aberrant epigenetic landscape in cancer: how cellular identity goes awry. *Developmental cell*, 19. 698-711.

Bestor, TH. (2000). The DNA methyltransferases of mammals. *Human Molecular Genetic*, 9. 2395-2402.

Bird, AP. (1986). CpG-rich islands and the function of DNA methylation. *Nature*, 321. 209-213.

Birgisdottir, V., Stefansson, OA., Bodvarsdottir, SK., Hilmarsdottir, H., Jonasson, JG., & Eyfjord, JE. (2006). Epigenetic silencing and deletion of the BRCA1 gene in sporadic breast cancer. *Breast Cancer Research*, 8. R38.

Bloushtain-Qimron, N., Yao, J., Snyder, EL., Shipitsin, M., Campbell, LL., Mani, SA., Hu, M., Chen, H., Ustyansky, V., Antosiewicz, JE., Argani, P., Halushka, MK., Thomson,

JA., Pharoah, P., Porgador, A., Sukumar, S., Parsons, R., Richardson, AL., Stampfer, MR., Gelman, RS., Nikolskaya, T., Nikolsky, Y., & Polyak K. (2008). Cell type-specific DNA methylation patterns in the human breast. *Proceedings of the National Academy of Sciences of the United States of America*, 105. 14076–14081.

Braakhuis, BJ., Tabor, MP., Kummer, JA., Leemans, CR., & Brakenhoff, RH. (2003). A genetic explanation of Slaughter's concept of field cancerization: evidence and clinical implications. *Cancer Research, 63.* 1727–1730.

Brannan, CI., & Bartolomei, MS. (1999). Mechanisms of genomic imprinting. *Current Opinion in Genetic and Development, 9.* 164-170.

Brehm, A., Miska, EA., McCance, DJ., Reid, JL., Bannister, AJ., & Kouzarides, T. (1998). Retinoblastoma protein recruits histone deacetylase to repress transcription. *Nature,* 391. 597-601.

Brena, RM., Huang, TH., Plass, C. (2006). Quantitative assessment of DNA methylation: Potential applications for disease diagnosis, classification, and prognosis in clinical settings. *Journal of Molecular Medicine, 84.* 365–77.

Campan, M., Weisenberger, DJ., & Laird, PW. (2006). DNA methylation profiles of female steroid hormone-driven human malignancies. *Current topics in microbiology and immunology,* 310. 141–78.

Cao, R., Wang, L., Wang, H., Xia, L., Erdjument-Bromage, H., Tempst, P., Jones, RS., & Zhang, Y. (2002). Role of histone H3 lysine 27 methylation in Polycomb-group silencing. *Science,* 298. 1039–1043.

Cao, R., & Zhang, Y. (2004). The functions of E(Z)/EZH2-mediated methylation of lysine 27 in histone H3. *Current Opinion in Genetic and Development,* 14. 155–164.

Chappuis, PO., Kapusta, L., Begin, LR., Wong, N., Brunet, JS., Narod, SA., Slingerland, J., Foulkes, WD., (2000). Germline BRCA1/2 mutations and p27(Kip1) protein levels independently predict outcome after breast cancer. *Journal of Clinical Oncology,* 18. 4045–4052.

Chedin, F., Lieber, MR., & Hsieh, CL. (2002). The DNA methyltransferase-like protein DNMT3L stimulates de novo methylation by Dnmt3a. *Proceeding National Academy of Science USA,* 99.16916–16921.

Chen, RZ., Pettersson, U., Beard, C., Jackson-Grusby, L., & Jaenisch, R. (1998). DNA hypomethylation leads to elevated mutation rates. *Nature,* 395. 89–93.

Chenevix-Trench, G., Healey, S., Lakhani, S., Waring, P., Cummings, M., Brinkworth, R., Deffenbaugh, AM., Burbidge, LA., Pruss, D., Judkins, T., Scholl, T., Bekessy, A., Marsh, A., Lovelock, P., Wong, M., Tesoriero, A., Renard, H., Southey, M., Hopper, JL., Yannoukakos, K., Brown, M., Easton, D., Tavtigian SV., Goldgar, D., & Spurdle, AB. (2006). Genetic and histopathologic evaluation of BRCA1 and BRCA2 DNA sequence variants of unknown clinical significance. *Cancer Research,* 66. 2019–2027.

Cheng, AS., Culhane, AC., Chan, MW., Venkataramu, CR., Ehrich, M., Nasir, A., Rodriguez, BA., Liu, J., Yan, PS., Quackenbush, J., Nephew, KP., Yeatman. TJ., & Huang. TH. (2008). Epithelial progeny of estrogen-exposed breast progenitor cells display a cancer-like methylome. *Cancer Research,* 68, 1786–1796.

Clouaire, T. & Stancheva, I. (2008) Methyl-CpG binding proteins: specialized transcriptional repressors or structural components of chromatin? *Cellular and Molecular Life Science,* 65. 1509–1522.

Costello, JF., Fruhwald, MC., Smiraglia, DJ., Rush, LJ., Robertson, GP., Gao, X., Wright, FA., Feramisco, JD., Peltomaki, P., Lang, JC. (2000). Aberrant CpG-island methylation has non-random and tumour-type-specific patterns. *Nature* Genetics, 24. 132–138.

Crabb, SJ., Howell, M., Rogers, H., Ishfaq, M., Yurek-George, A., Carey, K., Pickering, BM., East, P., Mitter, R., Maeda, S., Johnson, PW., Townsend, P, Shin-ya, K., Yoshida, M., Ganesan, A., & Packham, G. (2008). C,aracterisation of the in vitro activity of the depsipeptide histone deacetylase inhibitor spiruchostatin A. *Biochemical Pharmacology*, 76. 463-475.

de Ruijter, AJ., van Gennip, AH., Caron, HN., Kemp, S., & van Kuilenburg, AB. (2003). Histone deacetylases (HDACs): characterization of the classical HDAC family. *Biochemistry Journal,* 370. 737-749.

DeChiara, TM., Robertson, EJ., & Efstratiadis, A. (1991). Parental imprinting of the mouse insulin-like growth factor II gene. *Cell,* 64. 849-859.

Delaval, K. & Feil, R. (2004). Epigenetic regulation of mammalian genomic imprinting. *Current Opinion in Genet and Development,* 14. 188-195.

Dennis, C. (2002). The brave new world of RNA. *Nature,* 418. 122-124.

Dimri, GP., Martinez, JL., Jacobs, JJ., Keblusek, P., Itahana, K., Van Lohuizen, M., Campisi, J., Wazer, DE., Band, V., (2002). The Bmi-1 oncogene induces telomerase activity and immortalizes human mammary epithelial cells. *Cancer Research,* 62. 4736–4745.

Dong, A., Yoder, JA., Zhang, X., Zhou, L., Bestor, TH., & Cheng, X. (2001). Structure of human DNMT2, an enigmatic DNA methyltransferase homolog that displays denaturant-resistant binding to DNA. *Nucleic Acids Research,* 29. 439–448.

Dworkin, AM., Huang, TH-M., & Tolandbcd, AE. (2009) Epigenetic alterations in the breast: Implications for breast cancer detection, prognosis and treatment. *Seminar in Cancer Biology,* 3. 165-171.

Eden, A., Gaudet, F., Waghmare, A., & Jaenisch, R. (2003). Chromosomal instability and tumors promoted by DNA hypomethylation. *Science,* 300. 455.

Ehrlich, M. (2002). DNA hypomethylation, cancer, the immunodeficiency, centromeric region instability, facial anomalies syndrome and chromosomal rearrangements. *Journal of Nutrition,* 132. S2424–S2429.

Esteller, M. (2000). Epigenetic lesions causing genetic lesions in human cancer: promoter hypermethylation of DNA repair genes. *European Journal of Cancer*, 36. 2294–2300.

Esteller, M. (2007). Cancer epigenomics: DNA methylomes and histone-modification maps. *Nature Review of Genetics*, 8. 286–298.

Esteller, M. (2007). Epigenetic gene silencing in cancer: the DNA hypermethylome. *Human molecular genetics,* 16. R50–R59.

Esteller, M., & Almouzni, G. (2005). How epigenetics integrates nuclear functions. Workshop on epigenetics and chromatin: transcriptional regulation and beyond. *EMBO Report,* 6. 624–628.

Esteller, M., Corn, PG., Baylin, SB., & Herman, JG. (2001). A gene hypermethylation profile of human cancer. Cancer Research, 61. 3225–3229.

Esteller, M., Fraga, MF., Guo, M., et al. (2001). DNA methylation patterns in hereditary human cancers mimic sporadic tumorigenesis. *Human molecular genetics,* 10. 3001–3007.

Evron, E., Dooley, WC., Umbricht, CB., et al. (2001). Detection of breast cancer cells in ductal lavage fluid by methylation-specific PCR. *Lancet, 357.*1335–1336.

Fackler, MJ., Malone, K., Zhang, Z., et al. (2006). Quantitative multiplex methylation-specific PCR analysis doubles detection of tumor cells in breast ductal fluid. Clin. *Cancer Research,* 12. 3306–3310.

Fackler, MJ., McVeigh, M., Mehrotra, J., et al. (2004). Quantitative multiplex methylation-specific PCR assay for the detection of promoter hypermethylation in multiple genes in breast cancer. *Cancer Research,* 64.4442–4452.

Fan, M., Yan, PS., Hartman-Frey, C., et al. (2006). Diverse gene expression and DNA methylation profiles correlate with differential adaptation of breast cancer cells to the antiestrogens tamoxifen and fulvestrant. *Cancer Research,* 66. 11954–11966.

Feinberg, AP., & Tycko, B. (2004). The history of cancer epigenetics. *Nature Review of Cancer,* 4. 143–153.

Feinberg, AP., Vogelstein, B. (1983). Hypomethylation distinguishes genes of some human cancers from their normal counterparts. *Nature,* 301. 89–92.

Feng, W., Shen, L., Wen, S., et al. (2007). Correlation between CpG methylation profiles and hormone receptor status in breast cancers. *Breast Cancer Research,* 9. R57.

Feng, Q., & Zhang, Y. (2001). The MeCP1 complex represses transcription through preferential binding, remodeling, and deacetylating methylated nucleosomes. *Genes and Development,* 15, 827–832.

Fenton, SE. (2006). Endocrine-disrupting compounds and mammary gland development: early exposure and later life consequences. *Endocrinology,* 147. S18–S24.

Fischle, W., Wang, Y., Jacobs, SA., Kim. Y., Allis, CD., & Khorasanizadeh, S. (2003). Molecular basis for the discrimination of repressive methyllysine marks in histone H3 by Polycomb and HP1 chromodomains. *Genes Development,* 17. 1870–1881.

Fujita, N., Watanabe, S., Ichimura, T., et al. (2003). Methyl-CpG binding domain 1 (MBD1) interacts with the Suv39h1-HP1 heterochromatic complex for DNA methylation-based transcriptional repression. *Journal Biology Chemistry,* 278, 24132–24138.

Fuks, F. (2005). DNA methylation and histone modifications: teaming up to silence genes. *Current Opinion in Genetic and Development,* 15. 490–495.

Fuks, F., Hurd, PJ., Deplus, R., & Kouzarides, T. (2003). The DNA methyltransferases associate with HP1 and the SUV39H1 histone methyltransferase. *Nucleic Acids Research,* 31. 2305–2312.

Fuks, F., Hurd, PJ., Wolf, D., Nan, X., Bird, AP., & Kouzarides, T. (2003). The methyl-CpG-binding protein MeCP2 links DNA methylation to histone methylation. *Journal Biology Chemistry,* 278.4035–4040.

Giacinti, L., Claudio, PP., Lopez, M., & Giordano, A. (2006). Epigenetic information and estrogen receptor alpha expression in breast cancer. *Oncologist,* 11.1–8.

Girault, I., Tozlu, S., Lidereau, R., & Bieche, I. (2003). Expression analysis of DNA methyltransferases 1, 3A, and 3B in sporadic breast carcinomas. *Clinical Cancer Research,* 9. 4415–4422.

Glaser, KB. (2007). HDAC inhibitors: clinical update and mechanism-based potential. *Biochemical Pharmacology,* 74. 659-671.

Goyal, R., Reinhardt, R., & Jeltsch, A. (2006). Accuracy of DNA methylation pattern preservation by the Dnmt1 methyltransferase. *Nucleic Acids Research,*34. 1182-1188.

Grozinger, CM., Hassig, CA., & Schreiber, SL. (1999). Three proteins define a class of human histone deacetylases related to yeast Hda1p. *Proceedin of the National Academy of Science U S A*, 96. 4868-4873.

Guler., G., Iliopoulos, D., Guler, N., Himmetoglu, C., Hayran, M., & Huebner, K. (2007). Wwox and Ap2γ Expression Levels Predict Tamoxifen Response. *Clinical Cancer Research*, 13.

Gupta, A., Godwin, AK., Vanderveer, L., Lu, A., & Liu, J. (2003). Hypomethylation of the synuclein γ gene CpG island promotes its aberrant expression in breast carcinoma and ovarian carcinoma. *Cancer Research*, 63, 664–673.

Han, J., Kim, D., & Morris, KV. (2007). Promoter-associated RNA is required for RNA-directed transcriptional gene silencing in human cells. *Proceedings of the National Academy of Sciences of the United States of America*, 104. 12422–12427.

Hanahan, D., & Weinberg, RA.(2000). The hallmarks of cancer. *Cell*, 100. 57–70.

Harikrishnan, KN, Chow, MZ., Baker, EK., et al. (2005) Brahma links the SWI/SNF chromatin-remodeling complex with MeCP2-dependent transcriptional silencing. *Nature Genetic*, 37,.254–264.

He, L. & Hannon, GJ. (2004). MicroRNAs: small RNAs with a big role in gene regulation. *Nature Review in Genetic*, 5. 522-531.

Heard, E. (2005). Delving into the diversity of facultative heterochromatin: the epigenetics of the inactive X chromosome. *Current Opinion in Genetics and Deveveopment*, 15. 482-489.

Hellebrekers, DM., Griffioen, AW., & van Engeland, M. (2007). Dual targeting of epigenetic therapy in cancer. *Biochimical and Biophysical Acta*, 1775. 76–91.

Herman, JG., Graff, JR., Myohanen, S., Nelkin, BD., Baylin, SB. (1996). Methylation-specific PCR: a novel PCR assay for methylation status of CpG islands. *Proceedings of the National Academy of Sciences of the United States of America*, 93. 9821–9826.

Hoque, MO., Prencipe, M., Poeta, ML., Barbano, R., Valori, VM., Copetti, M., Gallo, AP., Brait, M., Maiello, E., Apicella, A., et al. (2009). Changes in CpG islands promoter methylation patterns during ductal breast carcinoma progression. *Cancer Epidemiology and Biomarkers Prevention*, 18. 2694–2700.

Hong, L., Schroth, GP., Matthews, HR., Yau, P., & Bradbury, EM. (1993). Studies of the DNA binding properties of histone H4 amino terminus. Thermal denaturation studies reveal that acetylation markedly reduces the binding constant of the H4 "tail" to DNA. *Journal of Biological Chemistry*, 268. 305-314.

Honrado, E., Osorio, A., Milne, RL., et al. (2007) Immunohistochemical classification of non-BRCA1/2 tumors identifies different groups that demonstrate the heterogeneity of BRCAX families. *Modern Pathology*, 20. 1298–1306.

Houbaviy, HB., Murray, MF., & Sharp PA. (2003). Embryonic stem cell-specific MicroRNAs. *Developmental Cell*, 5. 351-358.

Howell, CY., Bestor, TH., Ding, F., Latham, KE., Mertineit, C., Trasler, JM., & Chaillet, JR. (2001). Genomic imprinting disrupted by a maternal effect mutation in the Dnmt1 gene. *Cell*, 104. 829-838.

it-Si-Ali, S., Ramirez, S., Barre, FX., Dkhissi, F., Magnaghi-Jaulin, L., Girault, JA., Robin, P., Knibiehler, M., Pritchard, LL., Ducommun, B., Trouche, D., & Harel-Bellan, A.

(1998). Histone acetyltransferase activity of CBP is controlled by cycle-dependent kinases and oncoprotein E1A. *Nature,* 396. 184-186.

Jaenisch, R., & Bird, A. (2003). Epigenetic regulation of gene expression: how the genome integrates intrinsic and environmental signals. *Nature Genetics,* 33 Suppl. 245-254.

Janzen, V., Forkert, R., Fleming, HE., et al. (2006). Stem-cell ageing modified by the cyclin-dependent kinase inhibitor p16INK4a. Nature, 443. 421–426.

Jenuwein, T., & Allis, CD. (2001). Translating the histone code. *Science,* 293. 1074-1080.

Jin, Z., Tamura, G., Tsuchiya, T., et al. (2001). Adenomatous polyposis coli (APC) gene promoter hypermethylation in primary breast cancers. *British Journal of Cancer,* 85. 69–73.

Jones. PA, & Baylin, SB. (2002). The fundamental role of epigenetic events in cancer. *Nature Review in Genetics,* 3. 415-428.

Jones, PA., & Baylin, SB. (2007). The epigenomics of cancer. *Cell,* 2007;128:683–692.

Jones, PA., & Takai, D. (2001). The role of DNA methylation in mammalian epigenetics. *Science,* 293. 1068-1070.

Jones, PL., Veenstra, GJ., Wade, PA., et al. (1998) Methylated DNA and MeCP2 recruit histone deacetylase to repress transcription. *Nature Genetic,* 19.187–191.

Kaneda, A., & Feinberg, AP. (2005). Loss of imprinting of IGF2: a common epigenetic modifier of intestinal tumor risk. *Cancer Research,* 65.11236–11240.

Keshet, I., Schlesinger, Y., Farkash, S., et al. (2006). Evidence for an instructive mechanism of de novo methylation in cancer cells. *Nature Genetic,* 38. 149–153.

Kim, VN. (2005). MicroRNA biogenesis: coordinated cropping and dicing. *Nature Review of Molecular and Cellular* Biology, 6. 376–385.

Kimura, H., & Shiota, K. (2003). Methyl-CpG-binding protein, MeCP2, is a target molecule for maintenance DNA methyltransferase, Dnmt1. *Journal Biology Chemistry,*278, 4806–4812.

Kleer, CG., Cao, Q., Varambally, S., et al. (2003). EZH2 is a marker of aggressive breast cancer and promotes neoplastic transformation of breast epithelial cells. *Proceeding National Academiy of Science USA,* 100. 11606–11611.

Kim, J., Kollhoff, A., Bergmann, A., & Stubbs, L. (2003). Methylation-sensitive binding of transcription factor YY1 to an insulator sequence within the paternally expressed imprinted gene, Peg3. *Human Molecular Genetics,* 12. 233-245.

Kim, JD., Hinz, AK., Choo, JH., Stubbs, L., & Kim, J. (2007). YY1 as a controlling factor for the Peg3 and Gnas imprinted domains. *Genomics,* 89. 262-269.

Kiyono, T., Foster, SA., Koop, JI., McDougall, JK., Galloway, DA., & Klingelhutz, AJ. (1998). Both Rb/p16INK4a inactivation and telomerase activity are required to immortalize human epithelial cells. *Nature,* 396. 84–88.

Klose, RJ., & Bird, AP. (2006). Genomic DNA methylation: the mark and its mediators. *Trends in Biochemical Sci*ence, 31. 89-97.

Knudson, AG. (2000). Chasing the cancer demon. *Annual Review of Genetic,* 34. 1–19.

Kornberg, RD., & Lorch, Y. (1999). Twenty-five years of the nucleosome, fundamental particle of the eukaryote chromosome. *Cell,* 98. 285-294.

Kuo, MH., & Allis, CD. (1998). Roles of histone acetyltransferases and deacetylases in gene regulation. *Bioessays,* 20. 615-626.

Kuzmichev, A., Jenuwein, T., Tempst, P., & Reinberg, D. (2004) Different EZH2-containing complexes target methylation of histone H1 or nucleosomal histone H3. *Mollecular Cell*, 14, 183–193.

Kuzmichev, A., Margueron, R., Vaquero, A., et al. (2005). and histone substrates of polycomb repressive group complexes change during cellular differentiation. *Proceeding National Academiy of Science USA*, 102. 1859–1864.

Kyrylenko, S., Kyrylenko, O., Suuronen, T., & Salminen, A. (2003). Differential regulation of the Sir2 histone deacetylase gene family by inhibitors of class I and II histone deacetylases. *Cellular and molecular life sciences*, 60. 1990-1997.

Lachner, M., O'Carroll, D., Rea, S., Mechtler, K., & Jenuwein, T. (2001). Methylation of histone H3 lysine 9 creates a binding site for HP1 proteins. *Nature*, 410. 116–120.

Lapidus, RG., Nass, SJ., Butash, KA., et al. (1998). Mapping of ER gene CpG island methylation-specific polymerase chain reaction. *Cancer Research*, 58. 2515–2519.

Le Guezennec, X., Vermeulen, M., Brinkman, AB., et al. (2006). MBD2/NuRD and MBD3/NuRD, two distinct complexes with different biochemical and functional properties. *Molecular and Cellular Biology*, 26. 843–851.

Lehmann, U., Hasemeier, B., Christgen, M., et al. (2008). Epigenetic inactivation of microRNA gene hsa-mir-9–1 in human breast cancer. *Journal of Pathology*, 214. 17–24.

Lehmann, U., Langer, F., Feist, H., Glockner, S., Hasemeier, B., & Kreipe, H. (2002) Quantitative assessment of promoter hypermethylation during breast cancer development. American Journal of Pathology, 160, 605–612.

Lehnertz, B., Ueda, Y., Derijck, AA., et al. (2003). Suv39h-mediated histone H3 lysine 9 methylation directs DNA methylation to major satellite repeats at pericentric heterochromatin. *Current Biology*, 13. 1192–1200.

Leu, YW., Yan, PS., Fan, M., et al. (2004). Loss of estrogen receptor signaling triggers epigenetic silencing of downstream targets in breast cancer. *Cancer Research*, 64. 8184–8192.

Leu, YW., Yan, PS., Fan, M., et al. (2004). Loss of estrogen receptor signaling triggers epigenetic silencing of downstream targets in breast cancer. *Cancer Research*, 64. 8184–8192

Lewis, CM., Cler, LR., Bu, DW., et al. (2005) Promoter hypermethylation in benign breast epithelium in relation to predicted breast cancer risk. Clin. *Cancer Research*, 11. 166–172.

Liang, L., Kanduri, C., Pilartz, M., Svensson, K., Song, JH., Wentzel, P., Eriksson, U., & Ohlsson, R. (2000). Dynamic readjustment of parental methylation patterns of the 5'-flank of the mouse H19 gene during in vitro organogenesis. *International Journal of Developmental Biology*, 44. 785-790.

Lo, PK., Mehrotra, J., D'Costa, A., et al. (2006). Epigenetic suppression of secreted frizzled related protein 1 (SFRP1) expression in human breast cancer. *Cancer Biology and Therapeutics*, 5. 281–286.

Lo, PK., & Sukumar, S, (2008). Epigenomics and breast cancer. *Pharmacogenomics*, 12. 1879–1902.

Lo, YM., Wong, IH., Zhang, J., Tein, MS., Ng, MH., (1999). Hjelm, NM. Quantitative analysis of aberrant p16 methylation using real-time quantitative methylation-specific polymerase chain reaction. Cancer Research, 59. 3899–3903.

Lopez-Serra, L., Ballestar, E., Fraga, MF., Alaminos, M., Setien, F., & Esteller, M. (2006). A profile of methyl-CpG binding domain protein occupancy of hypermethylated promoter CpG islands of tumor suppressor genes in human cancer. Cancer Research, 66, 8342–8346.

Luczak, MW., & Jagodzinski, PP. (2006). The role of DNA methylation in cancer development. Folia Histochemical Cytobiology. 44.143–154.

Luedi, PP., Hartemink, AJ., & Jirtle, RL. (2005). Genome-wide prediction of imprinted murine genes. Genome Research, 15. 875–884.

Luger, K., Mader, AW., Richmond, RK., Sargent, DF., & Richmond, TJ. (1997). Crystal structure of the nucleosome core particle at 2.8 A resolution. Nature, 389. 251–260.

Lund, AH., & van Lohuizen, M. (2004) Epigenetics and cancer. Genes and Development, 18. 2315–2335.

Lyon, MF. (1999). X-chromosome inactivation. Current Biology, 9. R235-R237.

Maekita, T., Nakazawa, K., Mihara, M., et al. (2006). High levels of aberrant DNA methylation in Helicobacter pylori-infected gastric mucosae and its possible association with gastric cancer risk. Clinical Cancer Research, 12. 989–995.

Mancini-Dinardo, D., Steele, SJ., Ingram, RS., & Tilghman, SM. (2003). A differentially methylated region within the gene Kcnq1 functions as an imprinted promoter and silencer. Human Molecular Genetics, 12. 283-294.

Margueron, R., Duong, V., Castet, A., & Cavailles, V. (2004). Histone deacetylase inhibition and estrogen signalling in human breast cancer cells. Biochemical pharmacology, 68. 1239–1246.

Martin, C., & Zhang, Y. (2005). The diverse functions of histone lysine methylation. Nature Review of Molecular Cellullar Biology, 6. 838–849.

Mattick, JS, (2001). Non-coding RNAs: the architects of eukaryotic complexity. EMBO Reports, 2. 986-991.

Mattick, JS., & Makunin, IV. (2005). Small regulatory RNAs in mammals. Human Molecular Genetics, 1. R121-R132.

Matarazzo, MR., De Bonis, ML., Strazzullo, M., et al. (2007). Multiple binding of methyl-CpG and polycomb proteins in long-term gene silencing events. Journal of cellular physiology, 210. 711–719.

McGarvey, KM., Fahrner, JA., Greene, E., Martens, J., Jenuwein, T., & Baylin, SB. (2006). Silenced tumor suppressor genes reactivated by DNA demethylation do not return to a fully euchromatic chromatin state. Cancer Research, 66. 3541–3549.

Meehan, RR., Lewis, JD., & Bird, AP, (1992). Characterization of MeCP2, a vertebrate DNA binding protein with affinity for methylated DNA. Nucleic Acids Research, 20. 5085-5092.

Meehan, RR., Lewis, JD., McKay, S., Kleiner, EL., & Bird, AP. (1989). Identification of a mammalian protein that binds specifically to DNA containing methylated CpGs. Cell, 58. 499–507.

Meric-Bernstam, F. (2007). Heterogenic loss of BRCA in breast cancer: the "two-hit" hypothesis takes a hit. *Annals of surgical oncology*, 14. 2428–2429.

Mirza, S., Sharma, G., Prasad, CP., et al. (2007). Promoter hypermethylation of TMS1, BRCA1, ERalpha and PRB in serum and tumor DNA of invasive ductal breast carcinoma patients. *Life Science*, 81. 280–287.

Monk, M. (2002). Mammalian embryonic development--insights from studies on the X chromosome. *Cytogenetic Genome Res*earch, 99. 200-209.

Muller, HM., Widschwendter, A., Fiegl, H., et al. (2003). DNA methylation in serum of breast cancer patients: an independent prognostic marker. *Cancer Research*, 63. 7641–7645.

Nafee, TM., Farrell, WE., Carroll, WD., Fryer, AA., & Ismail, KM. (2008). Epigenetic control of fetal gene expression. *British journal of obstetrics and gynaecology*, 115. 158-168.

Nakayama, T., Watanabe, M., Yamanaka, M., Hirokawa, Y., Suzuki, H., Ito, H., Yatani, R., & Shiraishi, T, (2001b). The role of epigenetic modifications in retinoic acid receptor beta2 gene expression in human prostate cancers. *Lab Investigation*, 81. 1049-1057.

Nan, X., Campoy, FJ., & Bird, A. (1997). MeCP2 is a transcriptional repressor with abundant binding sites in genomic chromatin. *Cell*, 88. 471-481.

Narayan, A., Ji, W., Zhang, XY., et al. (1998). Hypomethylation of pericentromeric DNA in breast adenocarcinomas. *Internation Journal of Cancer*, 77. 833–838.

Nass, SJ., Herman, JG., Gabrielson, E., Iversen, PW., Parl, FF., Davidson, NE., & Graff, JR. (2000). Aberrant methylation of the estrogen receptor and E-cadherin 5' CpG islands increases with malignant progression in human breast cancer. Cancer Research, 60. 4346–4348.

Nguyen, CT., Gonzales, FA., & Jones, PA. (2001). Altered chromatin structure associated with methylation-induced gene silencing in cancer cells: correlation of accessibility, methylation, MeCP2 binding and acetylation. *Nucleic Acids Research*, 29. 4598–4606.

Norton, L. (2005). Conceptual and practical implications of breast tissue geometry: toward a more effective, less toxic therapy. *Oncologist*, 10. 370–381.

Okano, M., Bell, DW., Haber, DA., & Li, E. (1999). DNA methyltransferases Dnmt3a and Dnmt3b are essential for de novo methylation and mammalian development. *Cell*, 99. 247-257.

Okano, M., Xie, S., & Li, E. (1998). Cloning and characterization of a family of novel mammalian DNA (cytosine-5) methyltransferases. *Nature Genetics*, 19. 219-220.

Osorio, A., de la Hoya, M., Rodriguez-Lopez, R., et al. (2002). Loss of heterozygosity analysis at the BRCA loci in tumor samples from patients with familial breast cancer. *International journal of cancer*, 99. 305–309.

Osorio, A., Milne, RL., Honrado, E, et al. (2007). Classification of missense variants of unknown significance in BRCA1 based on clinical and tumor information. *Human mutation*, 28. 477–485.

Ottaviano, YL., Issa, JP., Parl, FF., Smith, HS., & Baylin, SB. Davidson NE. (1994). Methylation of the estrogen receptor gene CpG island marks loss of estrogen receptor expression in human breast cancer cells. *Cancer Research*, 54. 2552–2555.

Pakneshan, P., Szyf, M., Farias-Eisner, R., & Rabbani, SA. (2004). Reversal of the hypomethylation status of urokinase (uPA) promoter blocks breast cancer growth and metastasis. *Journal of Biological Chemistry*, 279. 31735-31744.

Parrella, P. (2010). Epigenetic signature in breast cancer: clinical prespective. *Breast Care*, 5. 66-73.

Parrella, P., Poeta, ML., Gallo, AP., Prencipe, M., Scintu, M., Apicella, A., Rossiello, R., Liguoro, G., Seripa, D., Gravina, C., et al. (2004) Nonrandom distribution of aberrant promoter methylation of cancer-related genes in sporadic breast tumors. Clinical Cancer Research, 10.5349-5354.

Pfeifer, GP., & Dammann, R. (2005). Methylation of the tumor suppressor gene RASSF1A in human tumors. *Biochemistry*, 70. 576-583.

Press, JZ., De Luca, A., Boyd, N., et al. (2008). Ovarian carcinomas with genetic and epigenetic BRCA1 loss have distinct molecular abnormalities. *BMC cancer*, 8. 17.

Polyak, K. (2007). Breast cancer: origins and evolution. *Journal of Clinical Investigation*, 117. 3155-3163.

Popov, VM., Wang, C., Shirley, LA., et al. (2007). The functional significance of nuclear receptor acetylation. *Steroids*, 72. 221-230.

Razin A & Cedar H (1977). Distribution of 5-methylcytosine in chromatin. *Proceeding of the Natlional Academy of Sci ence U S A*, 74. 2725-2728.

Reis-Filho, JS., & Tutt, AN. (2008). Triple negative tumours: a critical review. *Histopathology*, 52. 108-118.

Reynolds, PA., Sigaroudinia, M., Zardo, G., et al. (2006). Tumor suppressor p16INK4A regulates polycomb-mediated DNA hypermethylation in human mammary epithelial cells. *Journal of Biological Chemistry*, 281. 24790-24802.

Richardson, BC. (2002). Role of DNA methylation in the regulation of cell function: autoimmunity, aging and cancer. *Journal of Nutrition*, 132. S2401-S2405.

Riggs, AD. (1975). X inactivation, differentiation, and DNA methylation. *Cytogenetics and Cell Genetics*, 14. 9-25.

Robertson, KD., & Jones, PA. (2000). DNA methylation: past, present and future directions. *Carcinogenesis*, 21. 461-467.

Robson, ME., Chappuis, PO., Satagopan, J., et al. (2004). A combined analysis of outcome following breast cancer: differences in survival based on BRCA1/BRCA2 mutation status and administration of adjuvant treatment. *Breast Cancer Research*, 6. R8-R17.

Roll, JD., Rivenbark, AG., Jones, WD., & Coleman, WB. (2008). DNMT3b overexpression contributes to a hypermethylator phenotype in human breast cancer cell lines. *Molecular Cancer*, 7. 15.

Roth, SY., Denu, JM., & Allis, CD. (2001). Histone acetyltransferases. *Annual Review in Biochemistry*, 70. 81-120.

Saito, Y., & Jones, PA. (2006). Epigenetic activation of tumor suppressor microRNAs in human cancer cells. *Cell Cycle*, 5. 2220-2222.

Saito, Y., Liang, G., Egger, G., Friedman, JM., Chuang, JC., Coetzee, GA., & Jones, PA. (2006). Specific activation of microRNA-127 with downregulation of the proto-oncogene BCL6 by chromatin-modifying drugs in human cancer cells. *Cancer Cell*, 9. 435-443.

Sakuma, M., Akahira, J., Ito, K., Niikura, H., Moriya, T., Okamura, K., Sasano, H., & Yaegashi, N. (2007). Promoter methylation status of the Cyclin D2 gene is associated with poor prognosis in human epithelial ovarian cancer. *Cancer Science*, 98. 380-386.

Sarraf, SA., & Stancheva, I. (2004). Methyl-CpG binding protein MBD1 couples histone H3 methylation at lysine 9 by SETDB1 to DNA replication and chromatin assembly. *Molecular Cell,* 15. 595–605.

Schuettengruber, B., Chourrout, D., Vervoort, M., Leblanc, B., & Cavalli, G. (2007). Genome regulation by polycomb and trithorax proteins. *Cell,* 128. 735-745.

Schlesinger, Y., Straussman, R., Keshet, I., et al. (2007). Polycomb-mediated methylation on Lys27 of histone H3 pre-marks genes for de novo methylation in cancer. *Nature Genetic,* 39. 232–236.

Schultz, DC., Ayyanathan, K., Negorev, D., Maul, GG., & Rauscher, FJ. (2002). 3rd SETDB1: a novel KAP-1-associated histone H3, lysine 9-specific methyltransferase that contributes to HP1-mediated silencing of euchromatic genes by KRAB zinc-finger proteins. *Genes and Development,* 16. 919–932.

Sharma, D., Blum, J., Yang, X., Beaulieu, N., Macleod, AR., & Davidson, NE. (2005). Release of methyl CpG binding proteins and histone deacetylase 1 from the Estrogen receptor alpha (ER) promoter upon reactivation in ER-negative human breast cancer cells. *Molecular Endocrinology,* 19. 1740-51.

Sharma, S., Kelly, TK., & Jones, PA. (2010). Epigenetics in cancer. *Carcinogenesis,* 31. 27-36.

Shipitsin, M., Campbell, LL., Argani, P., et al. (2007). Molecular definition of breast tumor heterogeneity. *Cancer Cell,* 11. 259–273.

Silva, J., Silva, JM., Dominguez, G., et al. (2003). Concomitant expression of p16INK4a and p14ARF in primary breast cancer and analysis of inactivation mechanisms. *Journal Pathology,* 199. 289–297.

Silva, JM., Silva, J., Sanchez, A., et al. (2002).Tumor DNA in plasma at diagnosis of breast cancer patients is a valuable predictor of disease-free survival. *Clinical Cancer Research,* 8. 3761–3766.

Singal, R., & Ginder, GD. (1999). DNA methylation. *Blood,* 93. 4059-4070.

Sinkkonen, L., Hugenschmidt, T., Berninger, P., et al. (2008). MicroRNAs control de novo DNA methylation through regulation of transcriptional repressors in mouse embryonic stem cells. *Nature Structural Molecular* Biology, 15. 259–267.

Soares, J., Pinto, AE., Cunha, CV, et al. (1999). Global DNA hypomethylation in breast carcinoma: correlation with prognostic factors and tumor progression. *Cancer,* 85. 112–118.

Song, F., Smith, JF., Kimura, MT., Morrow, AD., Matsuyama, T., Nagase, H., & Held, WA. (2005). Association of tissue-specific differentially methylated regions (TDMs) with differential gene expression. *Proceeding of the Nationall Academy of Science U S A,* 102. 3336-3341.

Stoppa-Lyonnet, D., Ansquer, Y., Dreyfus, H., et al. (2000). Familial invasive breast cancers: worse outcome related to BRCA1 mutations. *Journal of Clinical Oncology,* 18. 4053–4059.

Strahl, BD., Ohba, R., Cook, RG., & Allis, CD. (1999). Methylation of histone H3 at lysine 4 is highly conserved and correlates with transcriptionally active nuclei in Tetrahymena. *Proceeding of the National Academy of Science U S A,* 96. 14967-14972.

Straussman, R., Nejman, D., Roberts, D., Steinfeld, I., Blum, B., Benvenisty, N., Simon, I., Yakhini, Z., & Cedar, H. (2009). Developmental programming of CpG island methylation profiles in the human genome. *Nature Structural Molecular Bioliology*, 16. 564-571.

Subramaniam, MM., Chan, JY., Soong, R., Ito, K., Ito, Y., Yeoh, KG., Salto-Tellez, M., Putti, TC.. (2009). RUNX3 inactivation by frequent promoter hypermethylation and protein mislocalization constitute an early event in breast cancer progression. *Breast Cancer Research and Treatment*, 113. 113–121.

Sui, M., Huang, Y., Park, BH., Davidson, NE., & Fan, W. (2007). Estrogen receptor alpha mediates breast cancer cell resistance to paclitaxel through inhibition of apoptotic cell death. *Cancer Research*, 67. 5337–44.

Suranim, MA. (1991). Genomic imprinting: developmental significance and molecular mechanism. *Current Opinion in Genetic and Development*, 1. 241-246.

Szyf, M. (2007). The dynamic epigenome and its implications in toxicology. *Toxicology Science*, 100. 7-23.

Szyf, M. (2008). The role of DNA hypermethylation and demethylation in cancer and cancer therapy. *Current Oncology*, 15. 72-75.

Tachibana, M., Ueda, J., Fukuda, M., et al. (2005). Histone methyltransferases G9a and GLP form heteromeric complexes and are both crucial for methylation of euchromatin at H3-K9. *Genes and Development*, 19. 815–826.

Tapia, T., Smalley, SV., Kohen, P., et al. (2008). Promoter hypermethylation of BRCA1 correlates with absence of expression in hereditary breast cancer tumors. *Epigenetics*. 3. 157–163.

Taunton, J., Hassig, CA., & Schreiber, SL. (1996). A mammalian histone deacetylase related to the yeast transcriptional regulator Rpd3p. *Science*, 272. 408-411.

Ting, AH., McGarvey, KM., & Baylin, SB. (2006). The cancer epigenome – components and functional correlates. *Genes and Development*, 20. 3215–3231.

Tlsty, TD., Crawford, YG., Holst, CR., et al. (2004). Genetic and epigenetic changes in mammary epithelial cells may mimic early events in carcinogenesis. *Journal of Mammary Gland Biology, Neoplasia*, 9. 263–274.

Turner, BM. (2000). Histone acetylation and an epigenetic code. *Bioessays*, 22. 836-845.

Ushijima, T. (2007). Epigenetic field for concentration. *Journal of biochemistry and molecular biology*, 40. 142–50.

Vaissiere, T., Sawan, C., & Herceg, Z. (2008). Epigenetic interplay between histone modifications and DNA methylation in gene silencing. *Mutation Research*, 659. 40-48.

Valk-Lingbeek, ME., Bruggeman, SW., & van Lohuizen, M. (2004). Stem cells and cancer; the polycomb connection. *Cell*, 118, 409–418.

Veeck, J., Niederacher, D., An, H., et al. (2006). Aberrant methylation of the Wnt antagonist SFRP1 in breast cancer is associated with unfavourable prognosis. *Oncogene*, 25. 3479–3488.

Vertino, PM., Sekowski, JA., Coll, JM., Applegren, N., Han, S., Hickey, RJ., & Malkas, LH. (2002). DNMT1 is a component of a multiprotein DNA replication complex. *Cell Cycle*, 1. 416-423.

Vigushin, DM., Ali, S., Pace, PE., Mirsaidi, N., Ito, K., Adcock, I., & Coombes, RC. (2001). Trichostatin A is a histone deacetylase inhibitor with potent antitumor activity against breast cancer in vivo. *Clinical Cancer Research*, 7. 971-976.

Vincent-Salomon, A., Ganem-Elbaz, C., Manie, E., et al. (2007). X inactive-specific transcript RNA coating and genetic instability of the X chromosome in BRCA1 breast tumors. *Cancer Research*, 67. 5134–5140.

Visvanathan, K., Sukumar, S., & Davidson, NE. (2006). Epigenetic biomarkers and breast cancer: cause for optimism. *Clinical Cancer Research*, 12. 6591–6593.

Vogelstein, B., & Kinzler, KW. (2004). Cancer genes and the pathways they control. *Nature Medicine*, 10.789–799.

Waddington, CH. (1952). Selection of the genetic basis for an acquired character. *Nature*, 169. 625-626.

Waddington, CH. (1959a). Canalization of development and genetic assimilation of acquired characters. *Nature*, 183. 1654-1655.

Waddington, CH. (1959b). Evolutionary adaptation. *Perspect in Biological Medicine*, 2. 379-401.

Waddington, CH. (1961). Genetic assimilation. *Advance in Genetic*, 10. 257-293.

Waddington, CH., & Robertson, E. (1966). Selection for developmental canalisation. *Genetic Research*, 7. 303-312.

Wade, PA., Gegonne, A., Jones, PL., Ballestar, E., & Aubry, F. (1999). Mi-2 complex couples DNA methylation to chromatin remodelling and histone deacetylation. *Nature Genetic*, 1. 62-66.

Wang, C., Fu, M., Angeletti, RH., Siconolfi-Baez, L., Reutens, AT., Albanese, C., Lisanti, MP., Katzenellenbogen, BS., Kato, S., Hopp, T., Fuqua, SA., Lopez, GN., Kushner, PJ., & Pestell, RG. (2001). Direct acetylation of the estrogen receptor alpha hinge region by p300 regulates transactivation and hormone sensitivity. *The Journal of biological chemistry*, 276. 18375–18383.

Weksberg, R., Smith, AC., Squire, J., & Sadowski, P. (2003). Beckwith-Wiedemann syndrome demonstrates a role for epigenetic control of normal development. *Human Molecular Genetic*, 1. R61-R68.

Widschwendter, M., & Menon U. (2006). Circulating methylated DNA: a new generation of tumor markers. Clin. *Cancer Research*, 12. 7205–7208.

Widschwendter, M., & Jones, PA. (2002). DNA methylation and breast carcinogenesis. *Oncogene*, 21. 5462–5482.

Widschwendter, M., & Jones, PA. (2002). DNA methylation and breast carcinogenesis. *Oncogene*, 21. 5462–82.

Yan, PS., Chen, CM., Shi, H., et al. (2001). Dissecting complex epigenetic alterations in breast cancer using CpG island microarrays. *Cancer Research*, 61. 8375–8380.

Slaughter, DP., Southwick, HW., & Smejkal, W. (1953). Field cancerization in oral stratified squamous epithelium; clinical implications of multicentric origin. *Cancer*, 6. 963-968.

Yan, PS., Venkataramu, C., Ibrahim, A., et al. (2006). Mapping geographic zones of cancer risk with epigenetic biomarkers in normal breast tissue. *Clinical Cancer Research*, 12. 6626–6636.

Yang, Y., Hu, JF., Ulaner, GA., Li, T., Yao, X., Vu, TH., & Hoffman, AR. (2003). Epigenetic regulation of Igf2/H19 imprinting at CTCF insulator binding sites. *Journal of Cellullar Biochemistry*, 90. 1038-1055.

Yoder, JA., Soman, NS., Verdine, GL., & Bestor, TH. (1997). DNA (cytosine-5)-methyltransferases in mouse cells and tissues. Studies with a mechanism-based probe. *Journal of Molecular Biology*, 270. 385-395.

Yoon, HG., Chan, DW., Reynolds, AB., Qin, J., & Wong, J. (2003). N-CoR mediates DNA methylation-dependent repression through a methyl CpG binding protein Kaiso. *Molecular Cell*, 12. 723-734.

Zeschnigk, M., Schmitz, B., Dittrich, B., Buiting, K., Horsthemke, B., & Doerfler, W. (1997). Imprinted segments in the human genome: different DNA methylation patterns in the Prader-Willi/Angelman syndrome region as determined by the genomic sequencing method. *Human Molecular Genetics*, 6. 387-395.

Zhang, Y., Ng, HH., Erdjument-Bromage, H., Tempst, P., Bird, A., & Reinberg, D. (1999). Analysis of the NuRD subunits reveals a histone deacetylase core complex and a connection with DNA methylation. *Genes Development*, 13. 1924-1935.

Zhang, Y. & Reinberg, D. (2001a). Transcription regulation by histone methylation: interplay between different covalent modifications of the core histone tails. *Genes and Development*, 15. 2343-2360.

Zhang, Y. & Reinberg, D. (2001b). Transcription regulation by histone methylation: interplay between different covalent modifications of the core histone tails. *Genes and Development*, 15. 2343-2360.

Zhavoronkova, EN. & Vaniushin, BF. (1987). [DNA methylation and interaction with glucocorticoid receptor complexes in the rat liver]. *Biokhimiia*, 52. 870-877.

Zhou, Q., & Davidson, NE. (2006). Silencing estrogen receptor alpha in breast cancer cells. *Cancer Biology and Therapeutic*, 5. 848-489.

Zhu, B., Zheng, Y., Angliker, H., Schwarz, S., Thiry, S., Siegmann, M., & Jost, JP. (2000). 5-Methylcytosine DNA glycosylase activity is also present in the human MBD4 (G/T mismatch glycosylase) and in a related avian sequence. *Nucleic Acids Research*, 28. 4157-4165.

Xu. X., Gammon, MD., Zhang, Y., Bestor, TH., Zeisel, SH., Wetmur, JG., Wallenstein, S., Bradshaw, PT., Garbowski, G., Teitelbaum, SL., Neugut, AI., Santella, RM., & Chen, J. (2009). BRCA1 promoter methylation is associated with increased mortality among women with breast cancer. *Breast cancer research and treatment*, 115. 397-404.

3

MCF-7 Breast Cancer Cell Line, a Model for the Study of the Association Between Inflammation and ABCG2-Mediated Multi Drug Resistance

Fatemeh Kalalinia, Fatemeh Mosaffa and Javad Behravan
Biotechnology Research Center and Department of Pharmaceutical Biotechnology
Mashhad University of Medical Sciences
Mashhad
Iran

1. Introduction

Breast cancer is one of the most common and serious malignancies worldwide. Despite intensive cancer control efforts, it remains the second-leading cause of cancer death among women (Harris et al., 2000). While the overall response rate can be high, the duration of response is relatively short, and most patients with initially responsive tumors will experience a drug-resistance phenotype. Therefore, a lot of studies have centered on the field of drug resistance to improve cancer chemotherapy and management of cancers Gottesman, 2002).

The development of intrinsic or acquired resistance to a wide variety of anticancer drugs is a major obstacle to successful cancer chemotherapy. Some cancers show primary resistance or natural resistance in which they do not respond to standard chemotherapy drugs from the beginning. On the other hand, many types of sensitive tumors respond well to chemotherapy drugs in the beginning but show acquired resistance later (Choi, 2005). Multidrug resistance (MDR) can be defined as the intrinsic or acquired resistance of cancer cells to multiple classes of structurally and mechanistically unrelated antitumor drugs (Teodori et al., 2002). To date, the most widely studied cellular mechanisms of MDR are those associated with drug efflux involving members of the adenosine triphosohate-binding cassette (ABC) membrane transporter family (Mao et al., 2005).

Recently, several human ABC transporters with a potential role in drug resistance have been discovered. Among them, a novel known protein is ATP-binding cassette sub-family G member 2 (ABCG2). Human ABCG2 (also known as MXR, BCRP, and ABCP) was first cloned by Doyle et al. (Doyle et al., 1998) in the drug-resistant breast cancer cell line (MCF-7). ABCG2 is an efflux pump, which transports a variety of xenobiotics and endogenous compounds across cellular membranes. Tissue localization of ABCG2 in the mammary glands, intestine, kidney, liver, ovary, testis, placenta, endothelium and in hematopoietic stem cells indicates that ABCG2 plays an important role in absorption, distribution, and elimination of its substrates (Krishnamurthy et al., 2004; Mao & Unadkat, 2005). The expression of ABCG2 protein and/or mRNA has been detected in numerous types of human cancers (Diestra et al., 2002; Ross et al., 2000), and a large spectrum of anticancer drugs are effluxed by ABCG2

(Doyle et al., 2003). It has also been shown that ABCG2 expression may be associated with poor response to chemotherapy (van den Heuvel-Eibrink et al., 2002, Steinbach, 2002 #216) . Alteration in ABCG2 expression and function can significantly affect the disposition of the transporter drug substrates, it is possible that its overexpression in cancer cells is responsible for decreasing in drug concentration within the cell and a reduced cancer-chemotherapy efficacy (Glavinas et al., 2004; Mao & Unadkat, 2005).

Inflammation is a state consisting of complex cytological and chemical reactions that occur in affected blood vessels and adjacent tissues in response to an injury or abnormal stimulation caused by physical, chemical or biological agents (Ho et al., 2006; Philip et al., 2004). Although inflammation is essential, it can be harmful to the host and therefore it is subject to multiple levels of biochemical, pharmacological, and molecular controls involving a diverse and potentially huge array of cell types and soluble mediators including cytokines (Haddad, 2002). In fact tumors are similar to healing or desmoplastic tissue in many ways and the micro-environment of the tumor highly resembles an inflammation site (Caruso et al., 2004). Breast cancer is a prototype of these kinds of cancer. Indeed, proinflammatory cytokines have been found to be present within the microenvironment of breast carcinomas and secreted by infiltrating host leukocytes, malignant and/or stromal cells of the breast cancer (Basolo et al., 1996; Jin et al., 1997; Lithgow et al., 2005; Miles et al., 1994).

In recent years, it has been demonstrated that the expression and function of the MDR transporters is altered in numerous tissues during an inflammatory response. The current review focuses on the elucidation of the effects of inflammation on the ABCG2 expression and function, using MCF-7 human breast carcinoma cell line.

2. The role of inflammation on the ABCG2 expression and function

In an overview, the results of several studies on the effect of inflammation on the levels of ABCG2 protein expression and function in MCF-7 cells will be reviewed in this paper. In the first part, the observed effects of the proinflammatory cytokines on the ABCG2 protein expression and function will be expressed. In the next section, the effects of cyclooxygenase 2 on drug resistance due to ABCG2 will be reviewed and eventually the influence of treatment with anti-inflammatory drugs indomethacin and dexamethasone on the incidence of drug resistance phenotype will be expressed.

2.1 Proinflammatory cytokines and ABCG2 expression and function

Proinflammatory cytokines including interleukin-1β (IL-1β), interleukin-6 (IL-6) and tumor necrosis factor-α (TNF-α) are well-known regulators of inflammatory response. Inflammatory components including host leukocytes, chemokines and cytokines are also present in the microenvironment of most probably all tumors including those not casually related to an obvious inflammatory process (Germano et al., 2008).

Numerous in vitro and in vivo investigations reported that inflammation and proinflammatory cytokines are able to modulate the expression or function of different drug transporters including Multi-Drug Resistance transporter 1 (MDR1/ABCB1), Multidrug Resistance-associated Proteins (MRPs/ABCCs) and Lung-resistance Related Protein / Major Vault Protein (LRP/MVP). These modulations appeared to happen at various levels of expression including transcriptional, posttranscriptional, translational, and/or post-translational levels (Bertilsson et al., 2001; Hartmann et al., 2002; Hirsch-Ernst et al., 1998;

MCF-7 Breast Cancer Cell Line, a Model for the Study of the Association Between Inflammation and ABCG2-
Mediated Multi Drug Resistance

57

Piquette-Miller et al., 1998; Stein et al., 1997; Sukhai et al., 2001; Theron et al., 2003; Vos et al., 1998; Walther et al., 1994; Walther et al., 1995).

The influence of proinflammatory cytokines (IL-1β, IL-6 and TNF-α) on ABCG2 expression and function in human MCF-7 breast cancer cell line were studied using real-time PCR and flow cytometry, respectively. The results showed that, the levels of ABCG2 mRNA, protein expression and function in MCF-7 cells increased significantly after treatment with either IL-1β or TNF-α (Fig. 1).

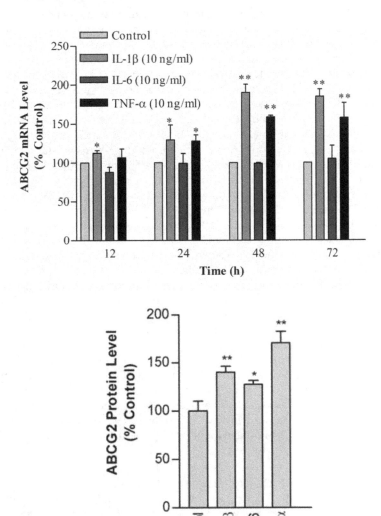

Fig. 1. The effects of proinflammatory cytokines on ABCG2 mRNA expression (A) and protein levels (B) in MCF-7 cells.

A;Cells were treated with 10 ng/ml of each cytokine for 12–72 h and real-time RT-PCR analysis was performed on total RNA extracted from control and treated cells. Values were normalized to the β-actin content of samples and expressed as mean (% control) ±SD (n = 3); *P<0.05; **P<0.01 versus control (0 ng/ml). B; After 72-h incubations with IL-1β (50 ng/ml), IL-6 (50 ng/ml) or TNF-α (50 ng/ml), expression of ABCG2 protein was measured by flow cytometry. Each value represents MFI mean (% control) of at least three independent experiments ± SD; *P<0.05, **P<0.01 versus controls.

Pradhan and colleagues also found that under proinflammatory conditions two transcription factors, estrogen receptor (ER) and NF-κB are cooperatively recruited to the promoter region of the ABCG2 gene at adjacent sites. ER allows the NF-κB family member p65 to access a latent NF-κB response element located near the estrogen response element (ERE) in the gene promoter; in turn, this p65 recruitment is required to stabilize ER occupancy at the functional ERE. Once present together on the ABCG2 promoter, ER and p65 act synergistically to potentiate mRNA and subsequent protein expression. This study has important implications for patients with ER-positive breast tumors, as it reveals a mechanism whereby inflammation enhances the expression of an ER target gene, which in turn can exacerbate breast tumor progression by promoting drug resistance mechanism whereby inflammation enhances the expression of an ER target gene, which in turn can exacerbate breast tumor progression by promoting drug resistance (Pradhan et al., 2010).

On the other hand, while IL-6 had no significant effects on ABCG2 mRNA expression and function in MCF-7 cells, it could slightly increase ABCG2 protein expression in these cells. This shows that IL-6 probably modulates ABCG2 expression by affecting ABCG2 protein translation and/or stability, but not ABCG2 transcription. For unknown reasons, this modulation did not result in the increased activity of the protein (Mosaffa et al., 2009).

In contrast to the results obtained for MCF-7 cells, in its mitoxantrone-resistance derivative, MCF-7/MX cells, none of the cytokines (even at high concentrations and long incubation times) exerted significant effects on ABCG2 mRNA levels. Because MCF-7/MX cells overexpress ABCG2 mRNA, it is likely that although modulation of the signaling pathway(s) responsible for increased transcription of ABCG2 in IL-1β and TNF-α-treated MCF-7 cells, has already happened in MCF-7/MX cells, but treatment with these cytokines could not cause further induction in ABCG2 mRNA levels (Mosaffa et al., 2009).

The results showed that IL-1β increased ABCG2 function and TNF-α enhanced both ABCG2 protein expression and function in MCF-7/MX cells. This lack of correspondence between mRNA and expression/function data suggests that perhaps in addition to the transcriptional regulatory effects of IL-1β and TNF-α, these two cytokines can also mediate ABCG2 expression and function via translational and/or post-translational effects (Mosaffa et al., 2009).

2.2 Cyclooxygenase-2 and ABCG2 expression and function

Cyclooxygenases (COX), also known as prostaglandin endoperoxide synthases or prostaglandin H synthases, comprise a group of enzymes that participate in the conversion of arachidonic acid to prostaglandins (PGs) that affect a number of physiological and pathological states in neoplastic and inflamed tissues (Smith et al., 1996). There are two isoforms of the enzyme that have been identified, COX-1 and COX-2. Constitutively expressed COX-1 supplies normal tissues with prostaglandins required to maintain physiological organ functions (O'Neill et al., 1993), such as cytoprotection of the gastric mucosa (Chan et al., 1995) and regulation of renal blood flow (Tanioka et al., 2003). On the other hand, COX-2 is highly induced by growth factors (epidermal growth factor (EGF)), cytokines (IL-1β, IL6, TNF-α (Davies et al., 2002; Zhang et al., 2006)), and carcinogens (phorbol esters (Liu et al., 1996; Rigas et al., 2005)) via protein kinase C (PKC) and RAS-mediated signaling at sites of inflammation. Therefore, it is assumed that COX-2 plays an important role in the prostaglandin E2 (PGE2) production involved in pathophysiological processes (Trebino et al., 2003). COX-2 may be implicated in tumor promotion through modulating cell proliferation, inhibiting apoptosis, control of cell migration, cell adhesion, tumor invasion and suppression of immune response (Cao et al., 2002). In recent years, it has been reported that COX-2 modulates ABC transporter expression and is involved in the development of the MDR phenotype (Ratnasinghe et al., 2001, Fantappiè O, 2002 #78, Puhlmann, 2005 #103).

Kalalinia et al. studies had aimed to explore the potential link between COX-2 expression and development of multidrug resistance phenotype due to ABCG2 expression in MCF-7 cell line. In one study they used of 12-O-tetradecanoylphorbol-13-acetate (TPA) for induction of COX-2 expression in MCF-7 cells. TPA often employed in biomedical research to activate the signal transduction enzyme protein kinase C (PKC). The effects of TPA on PKC result from its similarity to one of the natural activators of classic PKC isoforms, diacylglycerol (DAG).

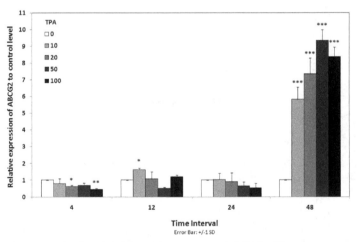

Fig. 2. Effects of TPA on the levels of ABCG2 mRNA in MCF-7 cells.
Cells were treated with TPA (0-100 nM for 4-48 h) and ABCG2 mRNA expression was measured by real-time RT-PCR using total RNA extracted from control and treated cells. Relative expression levels for each gene were normalized to that of the β-actin. The results were expressed as: (target/reference ratio) treated samples / (target/reference ratio) untreated control sample. Values were expressed as mean ± SD (n = 3); *, p < 0.05; **, p < 0.01; ***, p < 0.001.

The real-time PCR analysis showed that COX-2 inducer TPA caused a considerable increase up to 9-fold in ABCG2 mRNA expression in parental MCF-7 cells (Fig. 2). While a slight increase in ABCG2 expression was observed in the resistant cell line MCF-7/MX. The results of flow cytometry showed a slight increase of ABCG2 expression at protein level in MCF-7, while no significant changes in the level of ABCG2 protein expression was observed in MCF-7/MX (Fig. 3). As we mentioned earlier, in the drug resistant MCF-7/MX cells, ABCG2 is already overexpressed, and its expression may be at a threshold maximum level, so an induction with TPA treatment may not be causing any detectable increase in ABCG2 mRNA level. Likewise, a close association between MDR and COX-2 has been reported in non-Hodgkin's lymphomas (Szczuraszek et al., 2009), non-small cell lung cancer (Surowiak et al., 2008) and breast cancer cases (Surowiak et al., 2005). Adenovirus-mediated transfer of rat COX-2 cDNA into renal rat mesangial cells increased P-glycoprotein (P-gp/MDR1) expression, and this was blocked by COX-2 inhibitor NS398, suggesting that COX-2 products may be implicated in this response (Miller et al., 2006; Patel et al., 2002). All of these studies strongly suggest that COX-2 could be involved in the development of the MDR phenotype (Sorokin, 2004).

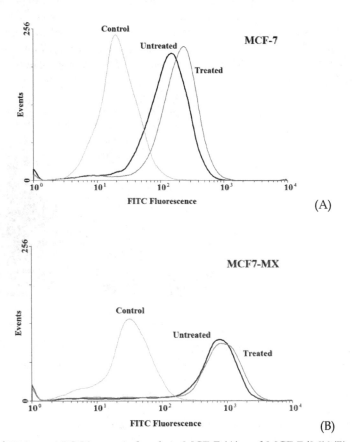

(A)

(B)

Fig. 3. Effect of TPA on ABCG2 protein levels in MCF-7 (A) and MCF-7/MX (B) cells. After 48 h incubation with TPA (10 nM), expression of ABCG2 protein was measured by flow cytometry. Each histogram shows the overlay of the treated sample (dark gray), untreated sample (black) and secondary antibody as negative control (light gray).

Different studies showed that incubation of MDR cells with PKC activator TPA stimulate P-gp phosphorylation, reduce drug accumulation, and enhance drug resistance (Ramachandran et al., 1998). Fine et al. demonstrated that phorbol 12,13-dibutyrate [P(BtO)2] led to an increase in protein kinase C activity and induced a drug-resistance phenotype as a result of increased phosphorylation of an unknown 20-kDa particulate protein (Fine et al., 1988). Similar to TPA treatment, diacylglycerol (DAG), a physiological stimulant of PKC, also increased the expression of MDR1 mRNA and protein. Whereas, protein kinase inhibitor staurosporine suppressed the induction of MDR1 expression by TPA and DAG (Chaudhary et al., 1992). These reports suggest that MDR gene expression in different cell types is regulated by a PKC-mediated pathway.

ABCG2 function was measured by flow cytometric mitoxantrone efflux assay. In long term exposure TPA enhanced the ABCG2 function, which was more considerable in MCF-7/MX than parental MCF-7 cells (Kalalinia et al., 2010). There is considerable precedent that PKC activation is associated with increased transport processes. Fine et al showed that, protein kinase C activity was 7-fold higher in the drug-resistant mutant MCF-7 cells compared with the control MCF-7 cells, sensitive parent cells (Fine et al., 1988). Fine et al reported that exposure of drug-sensitive cells to the phorbol 12, 13-dibutyrate [P (BtO)2] caused an enhanced PKC activity and induced drug-resistance phenotype, whereas drug-resistant cells in the same exposure to P(BtO)2 showed further increased in drug resistance. So phorbol ester might be the reason of decreased drug accumulation by inducing phosphorylation of a drug efflux pump or carrier protein (Fine et al., 1988).

2.3 Celecoxib (a selective inhibitor of COX-2) and ABCG2 expression and function

Numerous studies showed that COX-2 inhibitors (coxibs) enhance the efficacy of different anticancer therapy methods. Different mechanisms have been suggested to contribute to the antitumor activity of coxibs such as the inhibition of cell cycle progression, induction of apoptosis, inhibition of angiogenesis and decreased invasive potential of tumor cells (Fife et al., 2004; Gasparini et al., 2003; Hashitani et al., 2003; Masferrer et al., 2000). Another mechanism by which COX-inhibitors could sensitize cells to chemotherapeutic drugs is functional blockade of membrane transporter proteins of the ABC-transporter family (Patel et al., 2002; Zatelli et al., 2005).

Kalalinia et. al. investigated the relationship between the inhibition of COX-2 and expression of ABCG2 in parental and resistance breast cancer cell lines. They reported that treatment of MCF-7 and MCF-7/MX cells with celecoxib up-regulates ABCG2 expression at mRNA levels. The results also indicated that, celecoxib reversed the inhibitory effects of TPA on ABCG2 protein expression and increased its expression to the basal level in MCF-7/MX, while co-treatment of MCF-7 cells with TPA and celecoxib caused increased ABCG2 protein expression to a small amount more than TPA lonely (Fig. 4). In the same way , Zrieki et al. showed that treatment of human colorectal Caco-2 cell line with COX-1/ COX-2 inhibitor naproxen led to an stimulation of ABCG2 expression which corresponded to the significant decrease of Rho123 retention achieved in activity study. In contrast, treatment with selective COX-2 inhibitors nimesulide did not influence the expression of ABCG2 at protein level (Zrieki et al., 2008). Several studies have shown that specific COX-2 inhibitors could prevent or reduce the development of chemoresistance phenotype by downregulation of the expression and function of P-glycoprotein (MDR1) (Huang et al., 2007; Kim et al., 2004; Roy et al., 2010; Zatelli et al., 2005; Zatelli et al., 2007). Xia et al. found that celecoxib significantly inhibited MDR1 expression without any effects on pump function of P-gp.

They demonstrated that the inhibitory effect of celecoxib on MDR1 was COX-2-independent but directly correlated to hypermethylation of MDR1 gene promoter (Xia et al., 2009). In addition, it is shown that COX-2 inhibitors induced PGH2 generation and NF-κB activation, which result in inhibition of P-gp expression and function in breast cancer cells (Zatelli et al., 2009).

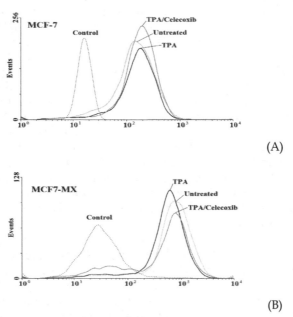

(A)

(B)

Fig. 4. Effects of celecoxib on the expression of ABCG2 at protein levels in MCF-7 (A) and MCF-7/MX (B) cell lines were studied by flow cytometry.
Cells were fixed and permeabilized by formaldehyde and methanol, blocked with BSA and then incubated with primary monoclonal antibody BXP-21. After washing, cells were incubated with a FITC-conjugated goat anti-mouse antibody. Each histogram shows the overlay of the TPA treated sample (black), TPA and celecoxib treated sample (dark gray), untreated sample (ligh gray) and secondary antibody as negative control (broken light gray).

In MCF-7 cell line, celecoxib in presence of TPA 10 nM caused reduction of ABCG2 function in a dose- and time-dependent manner (Kalalinia et al., 2010). Another study provides evidence that NS-398, selective COX-2 inhibitor, sensitizes chemoresistant breast cancer cells to the cytotoxic effects of doxorubicin and notably enhances intracellular DOX accumulation and retention in vitro. It was shown that these effects depended on the inhibition of P-gp expression and function in both native and chemoresistant MCF-7 cells (Zatelli et al., 2007).

2.4 The influence of indomethacin on ABCG2 expression and function
Several preclinical and clinical trials have shown that nonsteroidal anti-inflammatory drugs (NSAIDs), used as classical COX inhibitors, could reduce the incidence of cancers (Cha et al., 2007; Kang et al., 2005; Lin et al., 2005). Although the exact anticancer mechanisms of NSAIDs are not fully understood, it seems to be related closely to their suppression of COX

MCF-7 Breast Cancer Cell Line, a Model for the Study of the Association Between Inflammation and ABCG2-
Mediated Multi Drug Resistance

63

enzyme and subsequent reduction in prostaglandin production (Kismet et al., 2004; Zatelli et al., 2005). Modulation of the efficacy of cancer chemotherapy by NSAIDs has not been examined in detail.

Elahian et. al. investigated the pharmacological silencing of ABCG2 in MCF-7 cells through the use of indomethacin, in the hopes of opening a novel way in management of breast cancer. MTT assay showed that indomethacin did not significantly change the survival of MCF-7 and MCF-7/MX cells, but cotreatment of mitoxantrone with indomethacin increased the mitoxantrone cytotoxicity and reduced the IC50 of mitoxantrone in these cells. Altough indomethacin sensitized MCF-7 cells to mitoxantrone, but it did not alter mitoxantrone accumulation in MCF-7 cells, compared to the control (Elahian et al., 2010). It might suggest that indomethacin exerts the sensitising effects through a mechanism not involving the inhibition of ABCG2, but possibly reducing the synthesis of COX and its end-products (Spugnini et al., 2006; Verdina et al., 2008). Indeed, further studies would be necessary to clarify the molecular mechanisms involved in the potentiation of mitoxantrone cytotoxicity by indomethacin in MCF-7 and MCF-7/MX cells. Real-time PCR results showed that indomethacin-treated MCF-7 cells indicated no significant change in the amount of ABCG2 mRNA expression. This observation has been also confirmed on the level of ABCG2 protein expression (Elahian et al., 2009). As a result, expression of a MDR phenotype in human malignant cells may not always be sensitive to potentiation of drug cytotoxicity by NSAIDs (Roller et al., 1999). The present results also confirmed other studies that show NSAIDs' effects are cell and efflux transporter specific (Nozaki et al., 2007).

2.5 The influence of dexamethasone on ABCG2 expression and function

Glucocorticoides are efficacious in the reducing of chemotherapy adverse side effects and show their intrinsic anticancer activity (Vee et al., 2009) (Pavek et al., 2005). Some glucocorticoids, such as beclomethasone, 6α-methylprednisolone, dexamethasone, and triamcinolone, at micromolar concentrations, are shown to efficiently decrease the transport of ABCG2 substrates (Pavek et al., 2005).

Glucocorticoide receptor agonists regulate gene expression in various ways, at the transcriptional (Adcock, 2001), posttranscriptional (Korhonen et al., 2002), and posttranslational levels (Kritsch et al., 2002). Direct interaction of ligand-activated GR with control elements of target genes could regulate gene transcription in a positive or negative way. However, there are different mechanisms for the negative regulation of gene transcription by glucocorticoides. They could interfere with general transcription factors such as activator protein-1 (AP-1) (Herrlich, 2001) and nuclear factor-κB (NF-κB) (Almawi et al., 2002), resulting in decreased transcription of AP-1- and NF-κB -responsive genes. Genomic organization of the ABCG2 gene revealed the presence of several AP-1 sites in the ABCG2 promoter (Bailey-Dell et al., 2001). So it could be a direct target of transcriptional repression in a similar way. On the other hand, it has been reported that dexamethasone mediates negative regulation of gene expression by destabilizing the mRNA of some target genes (Garcia-Gras et al., 2000; Lasa et al., 2002).

Investigating the effects of dexamethasone on ABCG2 expression in MCF-7 cells showed that dexamethasone decreased the mRNA level of ABCG2 gene in comparison with control in MCF-7 and MCF-7/MX cell lines. Flow cytometry analysis indicated that a decrease in the level of ABCG2 protein was observed in dexamethasone treated MCF-7/MX cells. While the level of ABCG2 protein expressed as a ratio of the corresponding control was unchanged in

MCF-7 treated cells (Elahian et al., 2009). Cotreatment with different concentrations of mitoxantrone and dexamethasone increased the sensitivity of MCF-7 and MCF-7/MX cells to the toxic effects of mitoxantrone. In addition, the flow cytometry results showed that dexamethasone could inhibit the efflux and consequently caused increase in the accumulation of mitoxantrone in MCF-7/MX cells. However, ABCG2 inhibition by dexamethasone was not significant in MCF-7 cells (Elahian et al., 2010).

These studies also confirmed that suppression role of dexamethasone on ABCG2 expression in MCF-7/MX cells was more significant than MCF-7 cells. It could be a confirmation for higher level of ABCG2 in MCF-7/MX cells compared with their parental cells and also confirmed other studies that show hormonal regulation of MDR gene expression is cell type specific (Demeule et al., 1999; Imai et al., 2005).

3. Conclusion

In this review we aimed to focuse on the explanation the role of inflammation on the ABCG2 expression and function, using MCF-7 human breast carcinoma cell line. Pro-inflammatory cytokines have been found to be present within the micro-environment of tumors and inflammation. They are able to modulate the expression and function of different drug transporters. Mosaffa et al. showed that that proinflammatory cytokines IL-1β and TNF-α induce ABCG2 mRNA and protein expression and increase its function in MCF-7 cells. In MCF-7/MX, these cytokines increased ABCG2 protein expression and function, but they have no influence on the transporter mRNA levels.

Cyclooxygenase-2 (COX-2) is induced by mitogenic and inflammatory stimuli such as growth factors and cytokines, which results in enhanced synthesis of PGs in neoplastic and inflamed tissues. Kalalinia et al. studies had aimed to explore the potential link between COX-2 expression and development of multidrug resistance phenotype in MCF-7 cell line. They reported that COX-2 inducer TPA (12-O-tetradecanoylphorbol-13-acetate) caused a considerable increase up to 9-fold in ABCG2 mRNA expression in parental MCF-7 cells, while a slight increase in ABCG2 expression was observed in the resistant cell line MCF-7/MX. They also showed a positive corrolation between ABCG2 protein expression and COX-2 protein level in each cell line. On the other hand, celecoxib (a selective inhibitor of COX-2) up-regulated the expression of ABCG2 mRNA in MCF-7 and MCF-7/MX cells, which was accompanied by increased ABCG2 protein expression. Furthermore, TPA could increase ABCG2 function in all cell lines with the greatest stimulatory effects in MCF-7/MX (more than 6 times the control level). In addition, celecoxib inverted the effects of TPA on ABCG2 function. This effect was more obvious in MCF-7/MX.

Several studies have demonstrated that anti-inflammatory drugs like NSAIDs and some glucocorticoids could be effective in chemosensitizing of the many carcinoma cell lines to cytotoxic agents. The pharmacological modulation of ABCG2 in MCF-7 cells by dexamethasone and indomethacin was investigated by elahian et al. . They showed that dexamethasone induced downregulation of ABCG2 mRNA compared to controls in both MCF-7 and MCF-7/MX cell lines, whereas no changes were noted in the presence of indomethacin. The level of ABCG2 protein was decreased in dexamethasone treated MCF-7/MX cells. Cotreatment of mitoxantrone with different concentrations of dexamethasone and indomethacin sensitized parental and resistant MCF-7 cells to mitoxantrone cytotoxicity. Dexamethasone also increased the accumulation of mitoxantrone in the MCF-7/MX cell line, indicating an inhibitiory effect on the ABCG2 protein.

MCF-7 Breast Cancer Cell Line, a Model for the Study of the Association Between Inflammation and ABCG2-
Mediated Multi Drug Resistance

65

In this review, we describe the effects of proinflammatory cytokines (IL-1β and TNF-α), inflammatory mediator (COX-2) and anti-inflammatory drugs (celecoxib and dexametashone) on the expression of ABCG2 which addressed concerning to finding a new adjutant therapy for patients with cancer experiencing resistance to cancer treatment.

4. References

Adcock, I. M. (2001). Glucocorticoid-regulated transcription factors. Pulm Pharmacol Ther, Vol.14, No.3, pp. 211-219.

Almawi, W. Y., & Melemedjian, O. K. (2002). Negative regulation of nuclear factor-kappaB activation and function by glucocorticoids. J Mol Endocrinol, Vol.28, No.2, pp. 69-78.

Bailey-Dell, K. J., Hassel, B., Doyle, L. A., & Ross, D. D. (2001). Promoter characterization and genomic organization of the human breast cancer resistance protein (ATP-binding cassette transporter G2) gene. Biochim Biophys Acta, Vol.1520, No.3, pp. 234-241.

Basolo, F., Fiore, L., Fontanini, G., Conaldi, P. G., Calvo, S., Falcone, V., & Toniolo, A. (1996). Expression of and response to interleukin 6 (IL6) in human mammary tumors. Cancer Res, Vol.56, No.13, pp. 3118-3122.

Bertilsson, P. M., Olsson, P., & Magnusson, K. E. (2001). Cytokines influence mRNA expression of cytochrome P450 3A4 and MDRI in intestinal cells. J Pharm Sci, Vol.90, No.5, pp. 638-646.

Cao, Y., & Prescott, S. M. (2002). Many actions of cyclooxygenase-2 in cellular dynamics and in cancer. J Cell Physiol, Vol.190, No.3, pp. 279-286.

Caruso, C., Lio, D., Cavallone, L., & Franceschi, C. (2004). Aging, longevity, inflammation, and cancer. Ann N Y Acad Sci, Vol.1028, pp. 1-13.

Cha, Y. I., & DuBois, R. N. (2007). NSAIDs and cancer prevention: targets downstream of COX-2. Annu Rev Med, Vol.58, pp. 239-252.

Chan, C. C., Boyce, S., Brideau, C., Ford-Hutchinson, A. W., Gordon, R., Guay, D., Hill, R. G., Li, C. S., Mancini, J., Penneton, M., & et al. (1995). Pharmacology of a selective cyclooxygenase-2 inhibitor, L-745,337: a novel nonsteroidal anti-inflammatory agent with an ulcerogenic sparing effect in rat and nonhuman primate stomach. J Pharmacol Exp Ther, Vol.274, No.3, pp. 1531-1537.

Chaudhary, P. M., & Roninson, I. B. (1992). Activation of MDR1 (P-glycoprotein) gene expression in human cells by protein kinase C agonists. Oncol Res, Vol.4, No.7, pp. 281-290.

Choi, C. H. (2005). ABC transporters as multidrug resistance mechanisms and the development of chemosensitizers for their reversal. Cancer Cell Int, Vol.5, pp. 30.

Davies, G., Martin, L. A., Sacks, N., & Dowsett, M. (2002). Cyclooxygenase-2 (COX-2), aromatase and breast cancer: a possible role for COX-2 inhibitors in breast cancer chemoprevention. Ann Oncol, Vol.13, No.5, pp. 669-678.

Demeule, M., Jodoin, J., Beaulieu, E., Brossard, M., & Beliveau, R. (1999). Dexamethasone modulation of multidrug transporters in normal tissues. FEBS Lett, Vol.442, No.2-3, pp. 208-214.

Diestra, J. E., Scheffer, G. L., Catala, I., Maliepaard, M., Schellens, J. H., Scheper, R. J., Germa-Lluch, J. R., & Izquierdo, M. A. (2002). Frequent expression of the multi-drug resistance-associated protein BCRP/MXR/ABCP/ABCG2 in human tumours detected by the BXP-21 monoclonal antibody in paraffin-embedded material. J Pathol, Vol.198, No.2, pp. 213-219.

Doyle, L. A., & Ross, D. D. (2003). Multidrug resistance mediated by the breast cancer resistance protein BCRP (ABCG2). Oncogene, Vol.22, No.47, pp. 7340-7358.

Doyle, L. A., Yang, W., Abruzzo, L. V., Krogmann, T., Gao, Y., Rishi, A. K., & Ross, D. D. (1998). A multidrug resistance transporter from human MCF-7 breast cancer cells. Proc Natl Acad Sci U S A, Vol.95, No.26, pp. 15665-15670.

Elahian, F., Kalalinia, F., & Behravan, J. (2009). Dexamethasone downregulates BCRP mRNA and protein expression in breast cancer cell lines. Oncol Res, Vol.18, No.1, pp. 9-15.

Elahian, F., Kalalinia, F., & Behravan, J. (2010). Evaluation of indomethacin and dexamethasone effects on BCRP-mediated drug resistance in MCF-7 parental and resistant cell lines. Drug Chem Toxicol, Vol.33, No.2, pp. 113-119.

Fife, R. S., Stott, B., & Carr, R. E. (2004). Effects of a selective cyclooxygenase-2 inhibitor on cancer cells in vitro. Cancer Biol Ther, Vol.3, No.2, pp. 228-232.

Fine, R. L., Patel, J., & Chabner, B. A. (1988). Phorbol esters induce multidrug resistance in human breast cancer cells. Proc Natl Acad Sci U S A, Vol.85, No.2, pp. 582-586.

Garcia-Gras, E. A., Chi, P., & Thompson, E. A. (2000). Glucocorticoid-mediated destabilization of cyclin D3 mRNA involves RNA-protein interactions in the 3'-untranslated region of the mRNA. J Biol Chem, Vol.275, No.29, pp. 22001-22008.

Gasparini, G., Longo, R., Sarmiento, R., & Morabito, A. (2003). Inhibitors of cyclo-oxygenase 2: a new class of anticancer agents? Lancet Oncol, Vol.4, No.10, pp. 605-615.

Germano, G., Allavena, P., & Mantovani, A. (2008). Cytokines as a key component of cancer-related inflammation. Cytokine.

Glavinas, H., Krajcsi, P., Cserepes, J., & Sarkadi, B. (2004). The role of ABC transporters in drug resistance, metabolism and toxicity. Curr Drug Deliv, Vol.1, No.1, pp. 27-42.

Gottesman, M. M. (2002). Mechanisms of cancer drug resistance. Annu Rev Med, Vol.53, pp. 615-627.

Haddad, J. J. (2002). Cytokines and related receptor-mediated signaling pathways. Biochem Biophys Res Commun, Vol.297, No.4, pp. 700-713.

Harris, R. E., Alshafie, G. A., Abou-Issa, H., & Seibert, K. (2000). Chemoprevention of breast cancer in rats by celecoxib, a cyclooxygenase 2 inhibitor. Cancer Res, Vol.60, No.8, pp. 2101-2103.

Hartmann, G., Cheung, A. K., & Piquette-Miller, M. (2002). Inflammatory cytokines, but not bile acids, regulate expression of murine hepatic anion transporters in endotoxemia. J Pharmacol Exp Ther, Vol.303, No.1, pp. 273-281.

Hashitani, S., Urade, M., Nishimura, N., Maeda, T., Takaoka, K., Noguchi, K., & Sakurai, K. (2003). Apoptosis induction and enhancement of cytotoxicity of anticancer drugs by celecoxib, a selective cyclooxygenase-2 inhibitor, in human head and neck carcinoma cell lines. Int J Oncol, Vol.23, No.3, pp. 665-672.

Herrlich, P. (2001). Cross-talk between glucocorticoid receptor and AP-1. Oncogene, Vol.20, No.19, pp. 2465-2475.

Hirsch-Ernst, K. I., Ziemann, C., Foth, H., Kozian, D., Schmitz-Salue, C., & Kahl, G. F. (1998). Induction of mdr1b mRNA and P-glycoprotein expression by tumor necrosis factor alpha in primary rat hepatocyte cultures. J Cell Physiol, Vol.176, No.3, pp. 506-515.

Ho, E. A., & Piquette-Miller, M. (2006). Regulation of multidrug resistance by pro-inflammatory cytokines. Curr Cancer Drug Targets, Vol.6, No.4, pp. 295-311.

Huang, L., Wang, C., Zheng, W., Liu, R., Yang, J., & Tang, C. (2007). Effects of celecoxib on the reversal of multidrug resistance in human gastric carcinoma by downregulation of the expression and activity of P-glycoprotein. Anticancer Drugs, Vol.18, No.9, pp. 1075-1080.

MCF-7 Breast Cancer Cell Line, a Model for the Study of the Association Between Inflammation and ABCG2-Mediated Multi Drug Resistance

67

Imai, Y., Ishikawa, E., Asada, S., & Sugimoto, Y. (2005). Estrogen-mediated post transcriptional down-regulation of breast cancer resistance protein/ABCG2. Cancer Res, Vol.65, No.2, pp. 596-604.

Jin, L., Yuan, R. Q., Fuchs, A., Yao, Y., Joseph, A., Schwall, R., Schnitt, S. J., Guida, A., Hastings, H. M., Andres, J., Turkel, G., Polverini, P. J., Goldberg, I. D., & Rosen, E. M. (1997). Expression of interleukin-1beta in human breast carcinoma. Cancer, Vol.80, No.3, pp. 421-434.

Kalalinia, F., Elahian, F., & Behravan, J. (2010). Potential role of cyclooxygenase-2 on the regulation of the drug efflux transporter ABCG2 in breast cancer cell lines. J Cancer Res Clin Oncol.

Kang, H. K., Lee, E., Pyo, H., & Lim, S. J. (2005). Cyclooxygenase-independent down-regulation of multidrug resistance-associated protein-1 expression by celecoxib in human lung cancer cells. Mol Cancer Ther, Vol.4, No.9, pp. 1358-1363.

Kim, S. K., Lim, S. Y., Wang, K. C., Kim, Y. Y., Chi, J. G., Choi, Y. L., Shin, H. J., & Cho, B. K. (2004). Overexpression of cyclooxygenase-2 in childhood ependymomas: role of COX-2 inhibitor in growth and multi-drug resistance in vitro. Oncol Rep, Vol.12, No.2, pp. 403-409.

Kismet, K., Akay, M. T., Abbasoglu, O., & Ercan, A. (2004). Celecoxib: a potent cyclooxygenase-2 inhibitor in cancer prevention. Cancer Detect Prev, Vol.28, No.2, pp. 127-142.

Korhonen, R., Lahti, A., Hamalainen, M., Kankaanranta, H., & Moilanen, E. (2002). Dexamethasone inhibits inducible nitric-oxide synthase expression and nitric oxide production by destabilizing mRNA in lipopolysaccharide-treated macrophages. Mol Pharmacol, Vol.62, No.3, pp. 698-704.

Krishnamurthy, P., Ross, D. D., Nakanishi, T., Bailey-Dell, K., Zhou, S., Mercer, K. E., Sarkadi, B., Sorrentino, B. P., & Schuetz, J. D. (2004). The stem cell marker Bcrp/ABCG2 enhances hypoxic cell survival through interactions with heme. J Biol Chem, Vol.279, No.23, pp. 24218-24225.

Kritsch, K. R., Murali, S., Adamo, M. L., & Ney, D. M. (2002). Dexamethasone decreases serum and liver IGF-I and maintains liver IGF-I mRNA in parenterally fed rats. Am J Physiol Regul Integr Comp Physiol, Vol.282, No.2, pp. R528-536.

Lasa, M., Abraham, S. M., Boucheron, C., Saklatvala, J., & Clark, A. R. (2002). Dexamethasone causes sustained expression of mitogen-activated protein kinase (MAPK) phosphatase 1 and phosphatase-mediated inhibition of MAPK p38. Mol Cell Biol, Vol.22, No.22, pp. 7802-7811.

Lin, J., Hsiao, P. W., Chiu, T. H., & Chao, J. I. (2005). Combination of cyclooxygenase-2 inhibitors and oxaliplatin increases the growth inhibition and death in human colon cancer cells. Biochem Pharmacol, Vol.70, No.5, pp. 658-667.

Lithgow, D., & Covington, C. (2005). Chronic inflammation and breast pathology: a theoretical model. Biol Res Nurs, Vol.7, No.2, pp. 118-129.

Liu, X. H., & Rose, D. P. (1996). Differential expression and regulation of cyclooxygenase-1 and -2 in two human breast cancer cell lines. Cancer Res, Vol.56, No.22, pp. 5125-5127.

Mao, Q., & Unadkat, J. D. (2005). Role of the breast cancer resistance protein (ABCG2) in drug transport. Aaps J, Vol.7, No.1, pp. E118-133.

Masferrer, J. L., Leahy, K. M., Koki, A. T., Zweifel, B. S., Settle, S. L., Woerner, B. M., Edwards, D. A., Flickinger, A. G., Moore, R. J., & Seibert, K. (2000). Antiangiogenic and antitumor activities of cyclooxygenase-2 inhibitors. Cancer Res, Vol.60, No.5, pp. 1306-1311.

Miles, D. W., Happerfield, L. C., Naylor, M. S., Bobrow, L. G., Rubens, R. D., & Balkwill, F. R. (1994). Expression of tumour necrosis factor (TNF alpha) and its receptors in benign and malignant breast tissue. Int J Cancer, Vol.56, No.6, pp. 777-782.

Miller, B., Patel, V. A., & Sorokin, A. (2006). Cyclooxygenase-2 rescues rat mesangial cells from apoptosis induced by adriamycin via upregulation of multidrug resistance protein 1 (P-glycoprotein). J Am Soc Nephrol, Vol.17, No.4, pp. 977-985.

Mosaffa, F., Lage, H., Afshari, J. T., & Behravan, J. (2009). Interleukin-1 beta and tumor necrosis factor-alpha increase ABCG2 expression in MCF-7 breast carcinoma cell line and its mitoxantrone-resistant derivative, MCF-7/MX. Inflamm Res, Vol.58, No.10, pp. 669-676.

Nozaki, Y., Kusuhara, H., Kondo, T., Iwaki, M., Shiroyanagi, Y., Nakayama, H., Horita, S., Nakazawa, H., Okano, T., & Sugiyama, Y. (2007). Species difference in the inhibitory effect of nonsteroidal anti-inflammatory drugs on the uptake of methotrexate by human kidney slices. J Pharmacol Exp Ther, Vol.322, No.3, pp. 1162-1170.

O'Neill, G. P., & Ford-Hutchinson, A. W. (1993). Expression of mRNA for cyclooxygenase-1 and cyclooxygenase-2 in human tissues. FEBS Lett, Vol.330, No.2, pp. 156-160.

Patel, V. A., Dunn, M. J., & Sorokin, A. (2002). Regulation of MDR-1 (P-glycoprotein) by cyclooxygenase-2. J Biol Chem, Vol.277, No.41, pp. 38915-38920.

Pavek, P., Merino, G., Wagenaar, E., Bolscher, E., Novotna, M., Jonker, J. W., & Schinkel, A. H. (2005). Human breast cancer resistance protein: interactions with steroid drugs, hormones, the dietary carcinogen 2-amino-1-methyl-6-phenylimidazo(4,5-b)pyridine, and transport of cimetidine. J Pharmacol Exp Ther, Vol.312, No.1, pp. 144-152.

Philip, M., Rowley, D. A., & Schreiber, H. (2004). Inflammation as a tumor promoter in cancer induction. Semin Cancer Biol, Vol.14, No.6, pp. 433-439.

Piquette-Miller, M., Pak, A., Kim, H., Anari, R., & Shahzamani, A. (1998). Decreased expression and activity of P-glycoprotein in rat liver during acute inflammation. Pharm Res, Vol.15, No.5, pp. 706-711.

Pradhan, M., Bembinster, L. A., Baumgarten, S. C., & Frasor, J. (2010). Proinflammatory cytokines enhance estrogen-dependent expression of the multidrug transporter gene ABCG2 through estrogen receptor and NF{kappa}B cooperativity at adjacent response elements. J Biol Chem, Vol.285, No.41, pp. 31100-31106.

Ramachandran, C., Kunikane, H., You, W., & Krishan, A. (1998). Phorbol ester-induced P-glycoprotein phosphorylation and functionality in the HTB-123 human breast cancer cell line. Biochem Pharmacol, Vol.56, No.6, pp. 709-718.

Ratnasinghe, D., Daschner, P. J., Anver, M. R., Kasprzak, B. H., Taylor, P. R., Yeh, G. C., & Tangrea, J. A. (2001). Cyclooxygenase-2, P-glycoprotein-170 and drug resistance; is chemoprevention against multidrug resistance possible? Anticancer Res, Vol.21, No.3C, pp. 2141-2147.

Rigas, B., & Kashfi, K. (2005). Cancer prevention: a new era beyond cyclooxygenase-2. J Pharmacol Exp Ther, Vol.314, No.1, pp. 1-8.

Roller, A., Bahr, O. R., Streffer, J., Winter, S., Heneka, M., Deininger, M., Meyermann, R., Naumann, U., Gulbins, E., & Weller, M. (1999). Selective potentiation of drug cytotoxicity by NSAID in human glioma cells: the role of COX-1 and MRP. Biochem Biophys Res Commun, Vol.259, No.3, pp. 600-605.

Ross, D. D., Karp, J. E., Chen, T. T., & Doyle, L. A. (2000). Expression of breast cancer resistance protein in blast cells from patients with acute leukemia. Blood, Vol.96, No.1, pp. 365-368.

MCF-7 Breast Cancer Cell Line, a Model for the Study of the Association Between Inflammation and ABCG2-Mediated Multi Drug Resistance

69

Roy, K. R., Reddy, G. V., Maitreyi, L., Agarwal, S., Achari, C., Vali, S., & Reddanna, P. (2010). Celecoxib inhibits MDR1 expression through COX-2-dependent mechanism in human hepatocellular carcinoma (HepG2) cell line. Cancer Chemother Pharmacol, Vol.65, No.5, pp. 903-911.

Smith, W. L., & Dewitt, D. L. (1996). Prostaglandin endoperoxide H synthases-1 and -2. Adv Immunol, Vol.62, pp. 167-215.

Sorokin, A. (2004). Cyclooxygenase-2: potential role in regulation of drug efflux and multidrug resistance phenotype. Curr Pharm Des, Vol.10, No.6, pp. 647-657.

Spugnini, E. P., Cardillo, I., Verdina, A., Crispi, S., Saviozzi, S., Calogero, R., Nebbioso, A., Altucci, L., Cortese, G., Galati, R., Chien, J., Shridhar, V., Vincenzi, B., Citro, G., Cognetti, F., Sacchi, A., & Baldi, A. (2006). Piroxicam and cisplatin in a mouse model of peritoneal mesothelioma. Clin Cancer Res, Vol.12, No.20 Pt 1, pp. 6133-6143.

Stein, U., Walther, W., Laurencot, C. M., Scheffer, G. L., Scheper, R. J., & Shoemaker, R. H. (1997). Tumor necrosis factor-alpha and expression of the multidrug resistance-associated genes LRP and MRP. J Natl Cancer Inst, Vol.89, No.11, pp. 807-813.

Sukhai, M., Yong, A., Pak, A., & Piquette-Miller, M. (2001). Decreased expression of P-glycoprotein in interleukin-1beta and interleukin-6 treated rat hepatocytes. Inflamm Res, Vol.50, No.7, pp. 362-370.

Surowiak, P., Materna, V., Matkowski, R., Szczuraszek, K., Kornafel, J., Wojnar, A., Pudelko, M., Dietel, M., Denkert, C., Zabel, M., & Lage, H. (2005). Relationship between the expression of cyclooxygenase 2 and MDR1/P-glycoprotein in invasive breast cancers and their prognostic significance. Breast Cancer Res, Vol.7, No.5, pp. R862-870.

Surowiak, P., Pawelczyk, K., Maciejczyk, A., Pudelko, M., Kolodziej, J., Zabel, M., Murawa, D., Drag, M., Gansukh, T., Dietel, M., & Lage, H. (2008). Positive correlation between cyclooxygenase 2 and the expression of ABC transporters in non-small cell lung cancer. Anticancer Res, Vol.28, No.5B, pp. 2967-2974.

Szczuraszek, K., Materna, V., Halon, A., Mazur, G., Wrobel, T., Kuliczkowski, K., Maciejczyk, A., Zabel, M., Drag, M., Dietel, M., Lage, H., & Surowiak, P. (2009). Positive correlation between cyclooxygenase-2 and ABC-transporter expression in non-Hodgkin's lymphomas. Oncol Rep, Vol.22, No.6, pp. 1315-1323.

Tanioka, T., Nakatani, Y., Kobayashi, T., Tsujimoto, M., Oh-ishi, S., Murakami, M., & Kudo, I. (2003). Regulation of cytosolic prostaglandin E2 synthase by 90-kDa heat shock protein. Biochem Biophys Res Commun, Vol.303, No.4, pp. 1018-1023.

Teodori, E., Dei, S., Scapecchi, S., & Gualtieri, F. (2002). The medicinal chemistry of multidrug resistance (MDR) reversing drugs. Farmaco, Vol.57, No.5, pp. 385-415.

Theron, D., Barraud de Lagerie, S., Tardivel, S., Pelerin, H., Demeuse, P., Mercier, C., Mabondzo, A., Farinotti, R., Lacour, B., Roux, F., & Gimenez, F. (2003). Influence of tumor necrosis factor-alpha on the expression and function of P-glycoprotein in an immortalised rat brain capillary endothelial cell line, GPNT. Biochem Pharmacol, Vol.66, No.4, pp. 579-587.

Trebino, C. E., Stock, J. L., Gibbons, C. P., Naiman, B. M., Wachtmann, T. S., Umland, J. P., Pandher, K., Lapointe, J. M., Saha, S., Roach, M. L., Carter, D., Thomas, N. A., Durtschi, B. A., McNeish, J. D., Hambor, J. E., Jakobsson, P. J., Carty, T. J., Perez, J. R., & Audoly, L. P. (2003). Impaired inflammatory and pain responses in mice lacking an inducible prostaglandin E synthase. Proc Natl Acad Sci U S A, Vol.100, No.15, pp. 9044-9049.

van den Heuvel-Eibrink, M. M., Wiemer, E. A., Prins, A., Meijerink, J. P., Vossebeld, P. J., van der Holt, B., Pieters, R., & Sonneveld, P. (2002). Increased expression of the breast cancer resistance protein (BCRP) in relapsed or refractory acute myeloid leukemia (AML). Leukemia, Vol.16, No.5, pp. 833-839.

Vee, M. L., Lecureur, V., Stieger, B., & Fardel, O. (2009). Regulation of drug transporter expression in human hepatocytes exposed to the proinflammatory cytokines tumor necrosis factor-alpha or interleukin-6. Drug Metab Dispos, Vol.37, No.3, pp. 685-693.

Verdina, A., Cardillo, I., Nebbioso, A., Galati, R., Menegozzo, S., Altucci, L., Sacchi, A., & Baldi, A. (2008). Molecular analysis of the effects of Piroxicam and Cisplatin on mesothelioma cells growth and viability. J Transl Med, Vol.6, pp. 27.

Vos, T. A., Hooiveld, G. J., Koning, H., Childs, S., Meijer, D. K., Moshage, H., Jansen, P. L., & Muller, M. (1998). Up-regulation of the multidrug resistance genes, Mrp1 and Mdr1b, and down-regulation of the organic anion transporter, Mrp2, and the bile salt transporter, Spgp, in endotoxemic rat liver. Hepatology, Vol.28, No.6, pp. 1637-1644.

Walther, W., & Stein, U. (1994). Influence of cytokines on mdr1 expression in human colon carcinoma cell lines: increased cytotoxicity of MDR relevant drugs. J Cancer Res Clin Oncol, Vol.120, No.8, pp. 471-478.

Walther, W., Stein, U., & Pfeil, D. (1995). Gene transfer of human TNF alpha into glioblastoma cells permits modulation of mdr1 expression and potentiation of chemosensitivity. Int J Cancer, Vol.61, No.6, pp. 832-839.

Xia, W., Zhao, T., Lv, J., Xu, S., Shi, J., Wang, S., Han, X., & Sun, Y. (2009). Celecoxib enhanced the sensitivity of cancer cells to anticancer drugs by inhibition of the expression of P-glycoprotein through a COX-2-independent manner. J Cell Biochem, Vol.108, No.1, pp. 181-194.

Zatelli, M. C., Luchin, A., Piccin, D., Tagliati, F., Bottoni, A., Vignali, C., Bondanelli, M., & degli Uberti, E. C. (2005). Cyclooxygenase-2 inhibitors reverse chemoresistance phenotype in medullary thyroid carcinoma by a permeability glycoprotein-mediated mechanism. J Clin Endocrinol Metab, Vol.90, No.10, pp. 5754-5760.

Zatelli, M. C., Luchin, A., Tagliati, F., Leoni, S., Piccin, D., Bondanelli, M., Rossi, R., & degli Uberti, E. C. (2007). Cyclooxygenase-2 inhibitors prevent the development of chemoresistance phenotype in a breast cancer cell line by inhibiting glycoprotein p-170 expression. Endocr Relat Cancer, Vol.14, No.4, pp. 1029-1038.

Zatelli, M. C., Mole, D., Tagliati, F., Minoia, M., Ambrosio, M. R., & degli Uberti, E. (2009). Cyclo-oxygenase 2 modulates chemoresistance in breast cancer cells involving NF-kappaB. Cell Oncol, Vol.31, No.6, pp. 457-465.

Zhang, G. S., Liu, D. S., Dai, C. W., & Li, R. J. (2006). Antitumor effects of celecoxib on K562 leukemia cells are mediated by cell-cycle arrest, caspase-3 activation, and downregulation of Cox-2 expression and are synergistic with hydroxyurea or imatinib. Am J Hematol, Vol.81, No.4, pp. 242-255.

Zrieki, A., Farinotti, R., & Buyse, M. (2008). Cyclooxygenase inhibitors down regulate P-glycoprotein in human colorectal Caco-2 cell line. Pharm Res, Vol.25, No.9, pp. 1991-2001.

Part 2

Breast Cancer Cell Interaction, Invasion and Metastasis

4

Interaction of Alkylphospholipid Formulations with Breast Cancer Cells in the Context of Anticancer Drug Development

Tilen Koklic[1,2], Rok Podlipec[1,2], Janez Mravljak[3],
Maja Garvas[1], Marjeta Šentjurc[1] and Reiner Zeisig[4]
[1]Jozef Stefan Institute, Ljubljana
[2]Center of Excellence NAMASTE, Ljubljana
[3]Faculty of Pharmacy, University of Ljubljana, Ljubljana
[4]Max-Delbrück-Centre for Molecular Medicine, Berlin-Buch,
[1,2,3]Slovenia
[4]Germany

1. Introduction

Alkylphospholipids have shown promising results in several clinical studies (Mollinedo 2007) and among them Perifosine (octadecyl(1,1-di-methyl-4-piperidinium-4-yl)phosphate, OPP), and miltefosine (hexadecylphosphatidylcholine (HPC)) seems to be most promising for breast cancer therapy (Fichtner, Zeisig et al. 1994). For this type of tumor, an antitumor effect was found only for hormone receptor negative tumors *in vivo*, while no effect was found for receptor positive tumors. The reason for this difference is not yet understood and requires further studies. The exact mechanism of action of alkylphospholipids on the molecular level is still not well known in detail. It is clear that they do not target DNA, but they insert into the plasma membrane and subsequently induce a broad range of biological effects, ultimately leading to cell death.

Unfortunately, administration of free (micellar) alkylphospholipids results in unwanted side effects, reflected in gastrointestinal toxicity and hemolytic activity, which limits the application of higher doses of alkylphospholipids. To achieve better therapeutic effects of alkylphospholipids *in vivo* with less side effects, different liposomal formulations of alkylphospholipids have been tested and showed diminished hemolytic activity. On the other hand, in most cases, cytotoxic activity of liposomes was also lower as compared to free alkylphospholipids (Zeisig et al., 1998).

For efficient application of liposomes as nanocarriers in breast cancer therapy it is not only necessary to investigate the properties of the nanocarrier, which has to transport the drug to the (target) cell, but also the properties of the target cell. The main difference between Perifosine (OPP) resistent MCF7 cells and OPP sensitive MT-3 cells is in the uptake of OPP liposomes by cells and the transport of OPP across plasma membrane. At physiological temperatures the rate of transfer of OPP across plasma membrane increases to greater extent in OPP resistant MCF7 cells, while the uptake of liposomal OPP formulations is lower for

OPP resistant MCF7 cells as compared to OPP sensitive MT3 breast cancer cells. On the other hand the properties of an efficient OPP formulation are mainly determined by cholesterol concentration, which should be below 50 mol%.

2. Alkylphospholipids in clinical trials

In the late 1970's and early 1980's systemic investigations of structure – activity relationship were performed to screen lysophospholipids, alkylphospholipids and etherlipids to identify new candidates for cancer treatment. Among them, especially Miltefosine (Fig. 1), basically a simple phosphorus acid diester, displayed high inhibitory activity against chemically induced mammary carcinomas in rats (Eibl & Unger, 1990). It became the first drug based on a phospholipid structure demonstrating the high potential of this simple structured molecule class. The main advantage of this class of drugs is the target. In contrast to most anti-cancer drugs, which interfere at the DNA level with cell proliferation, alkylphospholipids act at the cell membrane, where they disturb the PI3K/Akt/mTOR signal transduction pathway (Fig. 2). Initial preclinical tests were promising, indicating a good anti-cancer activity against several human tumour xenograft models in the mouse (Arndt et al., 1997; Fichtner et al., 1994), including different breast cancer cell lines like: MT-3 (Zeisig et al., 1998), MDA-MB 435 and MDA-MB 231 (Sobottka & Berger, 1992), MaTu (Arndt et al., 1999), MT-1 (Naundorf et al., 1992), C3H, Ca 755 (Zeisig et al., 1991) and also syngeneic models like murine P388 leukemia, and B 16 melanoma (Zeisig et al., 1991). Preclinical experiments further demonstrated that alkylphospholipids, if used in liposomal form, are able to abolish multi drug resistance in human breast cancer xenografts (Zeisig et al., 2004) and inhibit metastasis if combined with an aggregation inhibitor inside liposomes in murine syngene (Wenzel et al., 2010) and human xenograft breast cancer models (Wenzel et al., 2009). Perifosine in combination with dioleylphosphoethanolamine, as a component of the liposome bilayer, also enhances transport of drugs across the blood brain barrier and in this way improves the treatment of intracerebral tumours and metastases (Orthmann et al., 2010). Miltefosine was also tested as an alternative approach for the treatment of patients with progressive cutaneous lesions from breast cancer in Phase I and II studies, which indicated that Miltefosine (either used alone or in conjunction with other therapies for distant metastases) is an effective and tolerable local treatment for cutaneous breast cancer (Clive et al., 1999; Unger & Eibl, 1991).

Only small changes in the molecular structure (slightly longer alkyl chain, a modified head group) while maintaining molecular size and shape resulted in Perifosine (OPP). Gills et al. (Gills & Dennis, 2009) summarised the clinical trials with Perifosine as single agent until 2009. Seven Phase 1 single agent studies of Perifosine have been completed. The trials demonstrated that Perifosine can be safely given to humans with a manageable toxicity profile. The dose limiting toxicity in the Phase I studies was, similar to Miltefosine, gastrointestinal: nausea, vomiting and diarrhea. Perifosine as single agent has been further evaluated in Phase II studies for the treatment of most common cancers, including breast, prostate, head and neck, pancreatic cancers, melanoma, renal cell carcinoma, advanced brain tumours, soft-tissue sarcomas, hepatocellular carcinoma, as well as in haematological malignancies including multiple myeloma and Waldenstrom's macroglobulinemia (WM). Potent activity with Perifosine, given as single-agent, has been observed so far in sarcoma and WM patients.

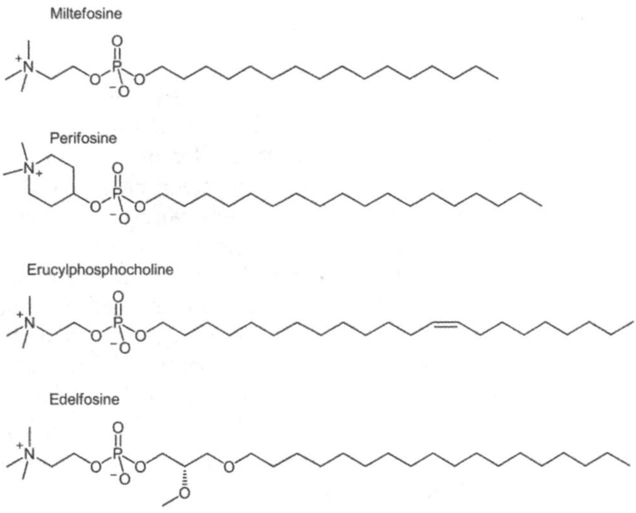

Miltefosine

Perifosine

Erucylphosphocholine

Edelfosine

Fig. 1. Structural formula of pharmaceutically tested alkylphospholipids.

Name	Abbreviation(s) CAS-number	IUPAC-name	Formula, molecular weight (g/mol), reference
Miltefosine	HPC, HePC, 58066-85-6	Hexadecyl-2-(trimethylazaniumyl) ethylphosphat	$C_{21}H_{46}NO_4P$, 407.57, (Eibl & Unger, 1990; Unger et al., 1988)
Perifosine	OPP, D21266 57716-52-4	(1,1-dimethylpiperidin-1-ium-4-yl) octadecyl phosphate	$C_{25}H_{52}NO_4P$, 461.66, (Hilgard et al., 1997)
Erucyl phosphocholine	EuPC; C22:1-PC 143317-74-2	[(Z)-docos-13-enyl] 2-(trimethylazaniumyl) ethyl phosphate	$C_{27}H_{56}NO_4P$, 489.71, (Erdlenbruch et al., 1998)
Edelfosine	ET-18-OCH3 77286-66-9	(2-methoxy-3-octadecyloxypropyl) 2-(trimethylazaniumyl) ethyl phosphate	$C_{27}H_{58}NO_6P$, 523.73, (Heesbeen et al., 1991)

Table 1. Names, abbreviation, IUPAC names, formula, molecular weights and references of most common alkylphospholipids

Erucylphosphocholine is an alkylphospholipids derivative with a 22 carbon atom chain and a cis-13,14 double bond. Although it differs from miltefosine only in alkyl chain length and the presence of a double bond (Fig. 1), significant differences were found in pharmacological properties. This structural modification increases hydrophobicity resulting in the formation of lamellar supramolecular structures, which abolished hemolytic side effects and allows Erucylphosphocholine to be administrated intravenously (Erdlenbruch et al., 1999; Kaufmann-Kolle et al., 1996; van Blitterswijk & Verheij, 2008). It is a potent inducer of apoptosis (Jendrossek et al., 2003) that exerts more potent antineoplastic effects *in vitro* and *in vivo* than Miltefosine.

3. Mode of action of APL

Anti-cancer mechanisms of alkylphospholipids have been described and extensively discussed in some recent reviews (Danker et al., 2010; Gajate & Mollinedo, 2002; Gills & Dennis, 2009; van Blitterswijk & Verheij, 2008). Early interest focussed on immune stimulating activity of alkylphospholipids. It could be demonstrated that Miltefosine and other lipids of this class are able to activate T-cells and macrophages to express and release chemokines like GM-CSF (Vehmeyer et al., 1992), IFgamma (Hochhuth et al., 1992) and/or nitric oxide (NO) (Zeisig et al., 1995). This effect could be improved if the alkylphospholipids were used in liposomal form. Because of their amphiphilic structure, alkylphospholipids are able to form lamellar bilayers, if combined with lipids of opposite molecular shape. Liposomes were taken up by macrophages much better than the free, micellar lipids and induced, after cellular uptake, the release of IF gamma and NO (Eue et al., 1995). But their potency as immune stimulator was limited and not sufficient enough amount of chemokines was released for a complete inhibition of tumor cell proliferation.

3.1 Uptake and absorption of alkylphospholipids

Due to their amphiphilic nature alkylphospholipids are easily incorporated into cell membranes in substantial amounts and then spread among intracellular membrane compartments, where they accumulate and interfere with a wide variety of key enzymes (Unger et al., 1992; van Blitterswijk et al., 1987). At lower, clinically relevant concentrations alkylphospholipids interfere with phospholipid turnover and lipid-based signal transduction pathways. In mouse S49 lymphoma cells alkylphospholipids accumulate in detergent-resistant, sphingolipid- and cholesterol-enriched lipid raft domains and are rapidly internalized by clathrin-independent, raft-mediated endocytosis (van der Luit et al., 2007). Alkylphospholipid uptake in KB carcinoma cells, however, appears to be raft-independent and mediated by a yet unidentified ATP-dependent lipid transporter (Vink et al., 2007). In leukemic cells treatment with alkylphospholipids induces the formation of membrane raft aggregates containing Fas/CD95 death receptor and the adaptor molecule Fas-associated death domain-containing protein (FADD), which are critical in the triggering of apoptosis (Gajate et al., 2009). Miltefosine and other alkylphospholipids also alter intracellular cholesterol traffic and metabolism leading to an increased uptake, synthesis and accumulation of cholesterol in the cell (Carrasco et al., 2008; Jimenez-Lopez et al., 2006; Marco et al., 2009). As cholesterol and sphingomyelin content are critical for the integrity and functionality of membrane lipid rafts, the disturbance of the cholesterol/sphingomyelin ratio could alter signaling pathways associated with these membrane domains.

3.2 Inhibition of phosphatidylcholine biosinthesis

Inhibition of phosphatidylcholine (PC) biosynthesis is a major alkylphospholipid target (Fig. 2). Inhibition of the biosynthesis of PC causes stress on cells sufficient to trigger apoptosis. In the endoplasmic reticulum, alkylphospholipids inhibit CTP (phosphocholine cytidyltransferase, CT), which chatalyses the rate-limiting step of the *de novo* PC synthesis. Alkylphospholipids inhibit CT in all exponentially growing tumor and normal cells, including leukemic and endothelial cells (Zerp et al., 2008). Synthesis of PC is essential for cell proliferation and is upregulated in tumor cells. PC is not only the most abundant membrane lipid and crucial for new membrane formation, but also the precursor for the second messengers diacylglycerol (DAG) and phosphatidic acid (PA) and for sphingomyelin (SM) in membrane lipid rafts. Inhibition of PC biosynthesis blocks the downstream sphingomyeline synthase (SMS) that catalyzes synthesis of sphingomyelin and diacylglycerol in the trans-Golgi (van Blitterswijk et al., 2003). Possible consequence is the accumulation of the ceramide, which is a second SMS substrate and can trigger apoptosis (Wieder et al., 1998). Another consequence of the PC shortage is the oxidative stress with reactive oxygen species (ROS) formation (Smets et al., 1999; Vrablic et al., 2001; Wagner et al., 1993).

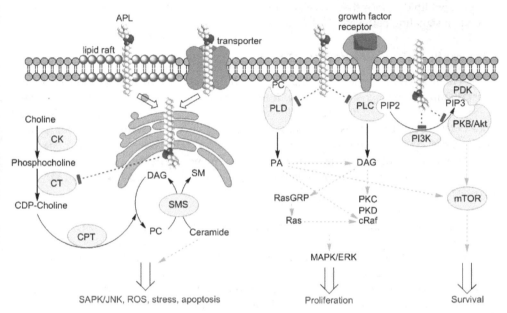

Fig. 2. Alkylphospholipid targets in lipid metabolism and signalling pathways summarized after van Blitterswijk et al. (van Blitterswijk & Verheij, 2008).

3.3 Influence of alkylphospholipids on major signaling pathways

Alkylphospholipids interfere with phosphatidylinositol-3-kinase (PI3K)/protein kinase B (PKB)/Akt survival pathway, which is important for proliferation, differentiation, survival and intracellular trafficking (Fig. 2). They inhibit phosphorylation and recruitment of PKB/Akt to the membrane, which is essential for its activation (Elrod et al., 2007; Kondapaka et al., 2003; Rahmani et al., 2005; Tazzari et al., 2008) probably by decreased production of PIP_3 (Gills & Dennis, 2009; van Blitterswijk & Verheij, 2008).

Alkylphospholipids inhibit PC hydrolysis to phosphatidic acid (PA) by phospholipase D and further to diacylgycerol (DAG) (Kiss & Crilly, 1997; Lucas et al., 2001). PA and DAG are second messengers, essential for the mitogen-activated protein kinase (MAPK) pathways, which regulate mitosis, metabolism, survival, apoptosis and differentiation (Chen et al., 2001; Kyriakis & Avruch, 2001; Pearson et al., 2001). PA is also involved in the activation of protein kinase C-ζ (Limatola et al., 1994), mTOR (Fang et al., 2001) and c-Raf (Rizzo et al., 2000). DAG activates proteins with the C1 domain, such as protein kinases C and D, Ras guanine-releasing protein (RasGRP) and indirectly MAPK/ERK pathway (Carrasco &

Merida, 2007; van Dijk et al., 1997; Yang & Kazanietz, 2003). Alkylphospholipids also inhibit DAG formation by phospholipase C (Maly et al., 1995; Ruiter et al., 2001; Strassheim et al., 2000). Alkylphospholipids also activate the stress-activated protein kinase/Jun N-terminal kinase (SAPK/JNK) pathway responsible for apoptosis in tumor cells (Gajate et al., 1998; Nieto-Miguel et al., 2007; Nieto-Miguel et al., 2008; Nieto-Miguel et al., 2006; Ruiter et al., 2001; Ruiter et al., 1999). Apoptosis can be triggered by imbalance between apoptotic and survival signals (Ruiter et al., 2001; Ruiter et al., 1999), which can be influenced by alkylphospholipids, since they have an influence on cross-talk between several membrane dependent signaling pathways.

4. Interaction of free Perifosine (OPP) with breast cancer cells

In this chapter the investigation of the interaction of Perifosine (octadecyl(1,1-di-methyl-4-piperidinium-4-yl)phosphate – OPP), with ER positive (ER+) and ER negative (ER-) breast cancer cell lines is emphasized. Perifosine was chosen since it is one of the most cancerostatically active lipids, with strong antitumor effect on xenotransplanted human breast cancer. We summarize results obtained mostly by the electron paramagnetic resonance (EPR) method in order to measure the influence of Perifosine on cell membrane fluidity and to measure transport of free and liposome incorporated Perifosine into breast cancer cells.

4.1 Influence of Perifosine (OPP) on cell membrane fluidity as studied by EPR

To get the information about the influence of a biologically active substance on cell membrane by EPR it is necessary to introduce a lipophilic paramagnetic probe into the membrane bilayer. This so called spin probe serves as a marker, which reflects the motion of the alkyl chains in the vicinity of the nitroxide group of the spin probe and in this way gives information about its surrounding. Motional characteristics that determine membrane fluidity are reflected in the EPR spectra line-shape. Main parameters obtained directly from the line-shape of the EPR spectra are order parameter (S) and correlation time (τ_c). Order parameter describes the orientational order of the phospholipids alkyl chains with S = 1 for perfectly ordered chains and S = 0 for isotropic alignment, and rotational correlation time (τ_c) describes the dynamics of the spin probe motion; more fluid membranes are characterized by a small τ_c. The changes in the EPR spectra line-shape give direct information about the external influences (temperature, interactions, damages) on cell membrane fluidity. More exact information about the membrane alterations can be obtained by computer simulation of the EPR spectra taking into account that the membrane is heterogeneous, composed of several coexisting domains with different fluidity characteristics. Therefore the EPR spectrum is composed of several spectral components reflecting different modes of restricted rotational motion of the spin probe molecules in different membrane environments (Pabst et al., 2007; Stopar et al., 2006; Strancar et al., 2003; Strancar et al., 2005).

In order to see how Perifosine (OPP) influences the plasma membrane fluidity of ER+ MCF7 and ER- MT-3 breast cancer cells, the cells were labeled with the spin probe 5P. This is a spin labeled OPP (5P), containing the nitroxide group at the 5th C atom (counting from the polar head group), (Mravljak et al., 2005). Structural formula of 5P is shown in Fig. 3.

It enters the plasma membrane easily but due to its charge, it only slowly crosses from outer to inner side of cell membrane, therefore it is suitable spin probe for detecting changes in the properties of the outer layer of plasma membrane. For spin labeling of cell membranes, MCF7 and MT-3 cells were mixed with 5P (2 µM) as a spin probe and with different amounts of Perifosine (OPP) to achieve final concentrations of OPP in extracellular medium: 0 µM, 25 µM, 50 µM or 150 µM.

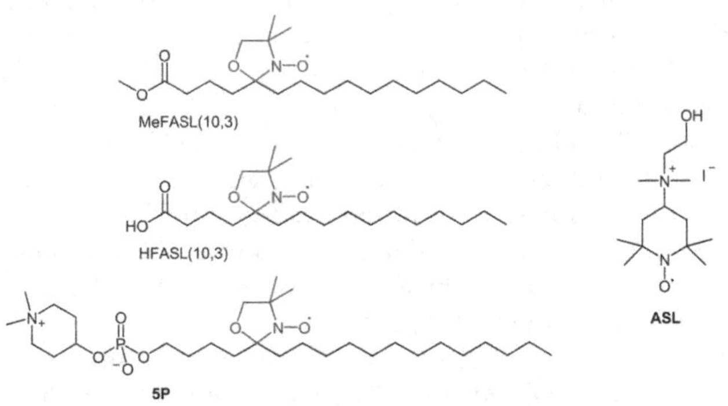

Fig. 3. Structural formulas of spin probes. MeFASL(10,3) – 5-doxylpalmitoyl methylester; HFASL(10,3) – 5-doxyl-palmitic acid, ASL - spin labeled tempocholine; 5P – spin labeled OPP, containing the doxyl group at the 5th C atom (counting from the polar head group).

From the spectra the order parameter was calculated. In the absence of OPP, S = 0.66 for MT-3 and S = 0.68 for MCF7 cells were obtained. After addition of 150 µM OPP, the order parameter decreased to S = 0.57 for MT-3 and to 0.60 for MCF7 cells. At lower concentrations of Perifosine no significant differences in order parameter were observed. This result indicates that OPP increases membrane fluidity of both cell lines at concentrations higher than 50 µM. The influence of OPP is less pronounced for MCF7 as for MT-3 cells. This indicates that OPP either doesn't incorporate into the alkylphospholipid resistant, ER+ MCF7 cell membranes as well as into alkylphospholipid sensitive, ER- MT-3 cells, or it doesn't concentrate in plasma membrane of MCF7 cells at such high concentrations as it does in MT-3 cells.

4.2 Transport of Perifosine (OPP) into the cell

To get information about the transport of Perifosine (OPP) into breast cancer cells by EPR, several spin labeled OPPs were synthesized in our group (Mravljak et al., 2005), which have an EPR detectable nitroxide group at various positions along the alkyl chain. We have chosen spin labeled OPP (5P) (structural formula in Fig. 3) with the lowest critical micellar concentration (CMC) of all synthesized spin labeled OPPs (Mravljak et al., 2005). Its CMC is around 10 µM, while 14P (spin labeled OPP, containing the nitroxide group at the 14th C atom) exhibited the CMC of around 200 µM (Mravljak et al., 2005). Edelfosine and OPP disperse in water in the form of micelles, due to their inverted-cone shape (Busto et al., 2007), displaying a CMC at 2.5 - 3 µM (Rakotomanga et al., 2004). It appears that addition of the doxyl group to OPP distorts the inverted-cone shape of molecule to greater extent when it is placed further away from the polar head group, which results in increased CMC. Since the CMC of 5P is similar to CMC of other similar alkylphospholipids one can assume that the disturbance caused by attaching doxyl group to OPP is small. Therefore we asumed that from all of synthesized spin labeled OPPs, 5P is the best candidate as a model molecule for studying behavior of Perifosine (OPP).

When 5P is transported into the cell, the EPR spectra intensity decreases due to the reduction of the nitroxide group to the corresponding EPR non-visible hydroxylamine by oxy-redoxy systems inside the cells (Chen et al., 1988; Swartz et al., 1986; Ueda et al., 2003) and can be detected by measuring the amplitude of the middle line of EPR spectra with time. From the kinetics of EPR spectra intensity decrease, information about the transport and/or interaction of spin probe with cells can be obtained. Reduction kinetics of 5P was found to be much slower as for spin probes usually used in EPR investigations of cell membranes MeFASL(10,3) and HFASL(10,3) (Chen et al., 1988; Yonar et al., 2010) indicating that its transport into the cell cytoplasm and organelles is slower as for the other probes. This is not surprising due to the charge at the head group of 5P (Fig. 3), which prevents passive transport of OPP across the membrane. For human KB carcinoma cells it has been demonstrated that OPP is internalized by an ATP-dependent translocase activity across the plasma membrane (Munoz-Martinez et al., 2008).

In order to investigate whether there is a difference in the uptake of OPP by alkylphospholipid (APL) resistant MCF7 cells (estrogen receptor positive, ER+) and APL sensitive MT-3 cells (estrogen receptor negative, ER-), both cell lines were incubated with 5P and EPR spectra intensity decrease was measured with time after incubation (Fig. 4).

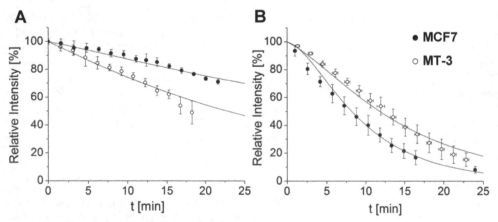

Fig. 4. EPR spectra intensity decrease with time after incubation of MCF7 cells ($\bullet$), and MT-3 ($\circ$) cells with 5P at A) room temperature and B) 37 °C MCF7 (estrogen receptor positive) and MT-3 (estrogen receptor negative) breast cancer cells (5-7 x 10^6 MCF7 cells and 12-20 x 10^6 MT-3 cells) were incubated with 5P (2-3 µM concentration, depending on the estimated number of total cell membrane bilayer lipids), which was adsorbed to the wall of a glass tube in order to achieve gradual accumulation of OPP in cells during 10 min incubation at room temperature and EPR spectra intensity decrease was measured with time after incubation.

From the kinetics of EPR spectra intensity decrease (Fig. 4) the rate of transfer of spin labeled OPP (5P) across the cell membrane was calculated using a similar model as described previously (Koklic et al., 2008). The rate of nitroxide reduction inside the cells does not differ significantly between the two cell lines and is faster at physiological temperature as at room temperature, while by increasing the temperature from room to physiological temperature the rate of transfer remains in the range of error for MT-3 cells (estrogen receptor negative), but increases significantly for estrogen receptor positive MCF7 cells (Podlipec et al., manuscript in preparation).

5. Interaction of liposomal Perifosine (OPP) with breast cancer cells

5.1 Effect of supramolecular organization of liposomal OPP formulations on their interaction with breast cancer cells

Alkylphospholipids are amphiphilic molecules and usually form micelles under physiological conditions. Unfortunately, administration of free (micellar) alkylphospholipids results in unwanted side effects, reflected in gastrointestinal toxicity and hemolytic activity, which limits the application of higher doses of alkylphospholipids. To achieve better therapeutic effects of alkylphospholipids *in vivo* with less side effects, different liposomal formulations of alkylphospholipids were prepared. This is possible only in the presence of lipids or other amphiphiles with a complimentary molecular shape. Usually cholesterol fulfills this role and enables the preparation of stable liposomal formulations from alkylphospholipids and lipids of different chain length and head groups. Among different alkylphospholipids, most investigations with liposomal formulations were performed with Perifosine (OPP). *In vivo* data show that the hemolytic effect of OPP is significantly diminished in liposomal formulations, but unfortunately in most cases, cytotoxic activity of OPP liposomes was also lower than of free OPP (Zeisig et al., 1998).

In an early study (Zeisig et al., 2001) we investigated the influence of cholesterol in liposomes consisting of Perifosine (OPP), dicetylphosphate and cholesterol (CH) on liposome stability and in vitro cytotoxicity. It was found that the ratio between the alkylphospholipid and cholesterol affects the cytotoxicity of the liposomes (Table 2). An increase in the OPP/CH ratio correlated directly with an increase in cytotoxicity against breast cancer cells. In the same time it was shown that a portion of 10 – 30% of OPP was present as micelles in liposomal formulations with OPP/CH ratio between 10:10 and 10:5, while the remaining OPP was stabilised by CH and forms liposomes. This was concluded, using ^{1}H-NMR spectroscopy, by the analysis of lipid composition after centrifugation of liposomal formulations, where micelles remain in supernatant in comparison to the initial sample. This micellar part of OPP molecules can easily be exchanged with the external environment and is able to become incorporated into other (bi)layers, as monolayer incorporation experiments demonstrated. It was assumed that this part of OPP is also mainly responsible for the cytotoxicity against tumor cells, which are not able to internalize the vesicles very well (Zeisig et al., 2001). A similar composition dependent effect was found *in vivo*, when the hemolytic effect of differently composed liposomes was followed. Again, liposomes with higher OPP/CH ratio, and thus containing a higher proportion of micellar OPP, were more hemolytically active than liposomal OPP formulations with a lower CH content (Zeisig et al., 1998).

Recently we developed a new method achieving more accurate estimates of the relative proportion of micelles, in comparison to the previously used methods (Koklic et al., 2010). The method is based on the spectral decomposition of EPR spectra. We confirmed findings of previous studies, which showed that the amount of micelles in liposomal OPP formulations increases with decreasing amount of cholesterol (Table 2).

According to the results presented in Table 2 we concluded that the amount of micelles in OPP liposome formulations is too small to be the main reason for better efficiency of liposomes with low amount of cholesterol in experimental breast cancer therapy (Koklic et al., 2010). Therefore we proposed that better efficiency of liposomes with lower amount of cholesterol depends also on the physical and chemical characteristics of liposome membranes and their interaction with cells.

Code	Molar ratio OPP:CH:X:PEG	OPP*	CH*	X*	Micelles** (%)	Hemolysis increase# (%)	Cytotoxicity $IC_{50\ MT-3}$#
N5 PEG	10:5:2:1	55.6	27.8	11.1	18 ± 7	179 ±23	23 ± 1
N5	10:5:2:0	58.8	29.4	11.8	20 ± 9	126 ± 30	18 ± 3
N7.5	10:7.5:2:0	51.3	38.5	10.2	11 ± 4	147 ± 32	18 ± 3
N10	10:10:2:0	45.5	45.5	9	5 ± 2	127 ± 29	28 ± 5
P10	10:10:2:0	45.5	45.5	9	0.5 ± 0.6	nd	19 ±2
N15	10:15:2:0	37.0	55.6	7.4	0 ± 1	nd	n.d.
Micelles	100:0:0:0	100	0	0	100	248 ± 11	17 ±9

N and P denote charge of the formulation (- or +, respectively)
X is a charged compound (DCP (dicetylphosphate) for N formulations and DDAB (dimethylioctadecylammonium bromide) for P formulation)
PEG are stearically stabilized liposomes with $PEG_{2000}DSPE$ (1,2-distearoyl-sn-glycero-3-phosphoethanolamine-N-[cyanur(polyethylene glycol)-2000])
*   mol% of total lipids
**   reference (Koklic et al., 2010)
# IC_{50} concentration (μM) required for 50% inhibition of cell growth for MT-3 breast cancer cells, (Zeisig et al., 1998)

Table 2. Composition of OPP liposomes, relative portion of micelles obtained by EPR and their hemolytic and cytotoxic activity.

5.2 Membrane domain structure of liposomal OPP formulations

For a better understanding of the interaction between liposomal OPP formulations and tumor cells, a deeper understanding of liposomal bilayer organization is necessary. Therefore, EPR with spin labels was used to study the influence of cholesterol, charge and sterical stabilization by PEG_{2000} DSPE on physical and chemical characteristics of liposomal OPP formulations. For this purpose liposomes with the composition presented in Table 2 were spin labeled with 5-doxylpalmitoyl methyl ester (MeFASL(10,3), Fig. 3) and EPR spectra were measured. By computer simulation of the EPR spectra line-shape, information about membrane fluidity and membrane domain structure was obtained, taking into account that the membrane is heterogeneous, composed of regions with different fluidity characteristics (Koklic et al., 2002; Koklic et al., 2008). Typical spectra are presented in Fig. 5A.

It was found that in general the experimental spectra are composed of at least three spectral components. Each spectral component corresponds to a mode of motion of a portion of spin probes partitioned in different parts of the membrane with the same physical properties and characterizes a certain type of lateral membrane domains with different fluidity characteristics. EPR parameters (order parameter S, rotational correlation time τ_c , polarity correction factor p_A), which describe the motional modes of nitroxide in a certain domain

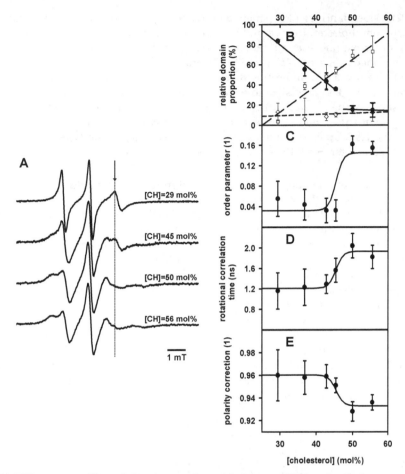

Fig. 5. A) EPR spectra of lipophilic spin-probe methyl ester of 5-doxylpalmitate (MeFASL(10,3)) in the membrane of OPP liposomes with different concentrations of cholesterol (the amount of cholesterol is indicated in mol%) in PBS buffer at 39 °C. The arrow points to a peak, which vanishes at around 50 mol% of cholesterol in the liposome membrane. B) - E) Dependence of EPR spectral parameters of spectral components on cholesterol concentration ([cholesterol]). Spectral parameters of EPR spectra of spin-probe MeFASL(10,3) in membranes of liposomal OPP formulations were derived by fitting of the calculated to the experimental spectra. B) Relative proportions of spectral components with: the lowest order parameter – domain type 1 (●); middle order parameter – domain type 2 (◊); and the highest order parameter – domain type 3 (□). Solid black line is a linear fit to the relative proportion of domain type 1, C) Order parameter, D) rotational correlation time, and E) polarity correction factor of the less ordered domain type (domain type 1). (republished with permission from (Koklic et al., 2008)).

type and reflect the fluidity characteristics of the domains as well as the proportion of spin probes in each domain type were determined. They were found to depend mainly on the amount of cholesterol, and only to a minor part on charge and sterical stabilization (Koklic et al., 2002). Dependance of EPR parameters, reflecting the properties of the least ordered domain type on cholesterol concentration is presented in Fig. 5 B, C, and D. A sudden increase in order parameter and rotational correlation time was observed when cholesterol concentration increases from 45 mol% to 50 mol%, while at the same time the polarity correction factor decreased, indicating that the spin probes in the domain type with lowest order parameter are less accessible to water. Relative proportion of this domain type (Fig. 5B) decreases at higher cholesterol concentrations, whereas the relative proportion of the domain type with the highest order parameter increases. It seems that above 50 mol% cholesterol the least ordered domains are transformed into a new type of domains with higher order parameter (S = 0.15) and with proportion of 15 %.

5.3 Release of liposome encapsulated material during the interaction of Perifosine (OPP) liposomal formulations with breast cancer cells

In order to better understand the factors that determine the therapeutic activity of liposomal OPP formulations, the interaction of liposomal OPP formulations at different cholesterol/Perifosine (CH/OPP) ratios with MT-3 and MCF7 breast cancer cells was measured and correlated with the membrane domain structure of liposomal OPP formulations (Koklic et al., 2008). For this purpose, spin labeled tempocholine (ASL) (Fig. 3), which cannot penetrate an intact liposome membrane easily, was entrapped into the liposomes. Labeled liposomal formulations were mixed with the cells and the kinetics of ASL reduction in the presence of human breast cancer cells was measured by EPR. ASL gets reduced to EPR non-visible hydroxylamine when it is released from liposomes and exposed to the oxy-redoxy systems inside the cells (Chen et al., 1988; Swartz et al., 1986; Ueda et al., 2003), which is reflected in an EPR spectra intensity decrease. Therefore, from the kinetics of EPR spectra intensity decrease information about the interaction of liposomes with cells can be obtained. Results are presented in Fig. 6.

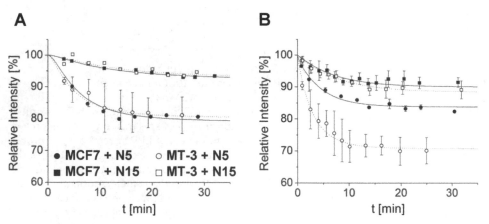

Fig. 6. EPR spectra intensity decrease after mixing of MCF7 cells (closed signs) or MT-3 cells (open signs) with Perifosine (OPP) liposomal formulations with two concentrations of cholesterol: 29 mol% (N5) (circles) and 56 mol% (N15) (squares) at A) room temperature and B) 37 °C. Symbols represent mean values of two to three measurements with error bars representing standard deviations.

For liposomal OPP formulation with low cholesterol content N5 (circles) a fast decrease of the EPR signal was observed in first 10 minutes after mixing liposomes with cells (Fig. 6), indicating that about 30% of spin-probes were released fast from the liposome interior into the cell cytoplasm. On the other hand, for liposomal OPP formulation with high cholesterol content N15 (Fig. 6 sguares), only a very small amount of liposome entrapped ASL was released into the cells, since the intensity decrease was less than 10% at room and physiological temperature. This indicates that the liposomes remained intact either in the extracellular space or entered the cells by endocythosis, but remained intact at least for the time of measurement. It is important to note that at room temperature both cell lines behave similarly, while at physiological temperature significantly higher amount of liposomes with low CH (N5) interact with alkylphospholipid sensitive, estrogen receptor negative, MT-3 cells (open circles in Fig. 6B) than with alkylphospholipid resistant, estrogen receptor positive, MCF7 cells (Podlipec et al., manuscript in preparation). These results, obtained on trypsinated cells, which are presented here, agree well with the results published by Koklic et al. (Koklic et al., 2008), which were obtained on scraped MT-3 cells, although small differences could originate from different procedures of removal of cells from the culture flasks (Batista et al., 2010).

In order to investigate interaction of OPP liposomes with breast cancer cells in more detail, we have added 0.5 mol% of a phospholipid fluorescent probe C6-NBD-PC, where 7-nitrobenz-2-oxa-1,3-diazol-4-yl (NBD) is attached to the phosphatidylcholine phospholipid (16:0-06:0 NBD PC, Avanti polar lipids, Alabaster, AL, USA) to OPP liposomes as described previously (Arsov et al., 2011). Results with the lipophilic fluorescence probe C6-NBD-PC (Fig. 7) confirm the EPR measurements, indicating that liposomes with high amount of

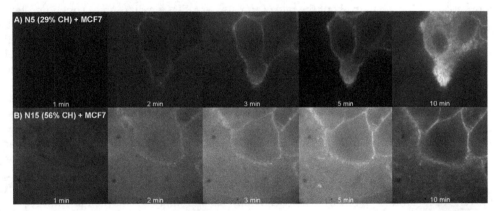

Fig. 7. Interaction of fluorescently labeled Perifosine (OPP) liposomal formulations with MCF7 breast cancer cells. Fluorescence microscopy was performed to localize C6-NBD-PC labeled liposomal formulation immediately after addition to cells, at room temperature.
A) Negatively charged liposomal OPP formulation (N5) with 29 mol % of cholesterol (1 mM final total lipid concentration) were added to MCF7 cells attached to the bottom of a well and the distribution of the lipophilic fluorescent probe C6-NBD-PC was followed with time as indicated at the bottom of each image.
B) Negatively charged liposomal OPP formulation (N15) with 56 mol % cholesterol were added to MCF7 cells and measured under same conditions as in experiment A.

cholesterol do not interact with cells. Fluorescence microscopy clearly shows that OPP liposomes with high amount of CH (N15) remain outside the cells, while low cholesterol – containing, N5 liposomes interact with cell membranes because the fluorescent probe distributes in the cell interior. In addition for liposomes with low amount of cholesterol (N5), for which C6-NBD-PC distributes inside the cells, maximum of fluorescence emission spectrum shifts for a few nanometers, indicating that either micelles or liposomes interacted with cells and delivered C6-NBD-PC into lipophilic compartments of MCF7 cells, where the environment of the fluorescent probe changed (Arsov et al., 2011).

Comparing liposome membrane characteristics, derived from EPR spectra (Fig. 5) and summarized in Table 2, with liposome cell interaction experiments (Fig. 6 and Fig. 7) we can see that the propensity of Perifosine (OPP) liposomal formulations for interaction with tumor cells and for delivery of OPP into cells coincides with the existence of disordered domains as well as with the existence of micelles. We have shown that by increasing the concentration of cholesterol above 50 mol% the domains with the lowest order parameter (between 0.06 and 0.03, Fig. 5) are transformed into a new type of domains with higher order parameter (S = 0.15). This suggests that disordered motion of lipid alkyl chains within the liquid-disordered domains, which coexist with liquid-ordered domains, is necessary for fast delivery of liposome encapsulated probe into the cells. On the other hand, the presence of micelles in liposome formulations with concentration of cholesterol below approximately 50 mol% suggests that micelles are necessary for efficient delivery of liposome encapsulated probe into cells.

5.4 Transport of spin labeled Perifosine (OPP) from liposomes to cell membrane does not depend on the liposome cell interaction

In order to get information about the rate of transfer of OPP from liposomes containing two different concentrations of cholesterol to cells, a portion of OPP molecules in liposomal OPP formulations was replaced with spin labeled OPP (5P), so that the final concentration of 5P in OPP liposomes was 17 mol%. Because of such high amount of P5 in the liposomal formulations, the EPR lines are highly broadened (Fig. 8A) due to the spin exchange interaction between paramagnetic probes.

EPR spectra in Fig. 8B are similar as obtained for MCF7 cells labeled with 5P, indicating that high amount of 5P from liposomal OPP formulation was transferred to cell membranes in a time shorter than 2 minutes. It was not possible to resolve any difference in the rate of transfer from N5 or N15 liposomes after 2 minutes of mixing liposomes with cells. Very fast transfer was also observed when giant liposomes (composition: POPC:POPE:POPS:CH molar ratios 40:20:10:40), which represent a model for cell membrane, were incubated with N5 or N15 liposomes (Mravljak et al., 2010), proving that spin labeled OPP molecules are transferred from one type of membrane to other membranes within several minutes, and the rate of transport does not depend significantly on the membrane composition. We can conclude from the above experiment that analkylphospholipid-like molecule can easily exchange between membranes and can accumulate in cells when they are in contact with liposomal OPP formulations. This is in agreement with lipid monolayer experiments, which showed that alkylphospholipids, below the critical micellar concentration (CMC), insert progressively into lipid monolayers as monomers from the aqueous medium, while above CMC, not only monomers but also groups of monomers (micelles) are transferred into the monolayers (Rakotomanga et al., 2004). It was also shown that, while the alkylphospholipid HePC is miscible with POPC, there is high affinity between HePC and sterols (ergosterol, and cholesterol) and that maximum condensation is reached at a ratio of HePC/sterol around 50:50 (mol/mol) (Rakotomanga et al., 2004). This kind of behavior is generally known as the condensing effect of cholesterol towards phospholipids (Chapman et al., 1969; Ghosh & Tinoco, 1972). Micelles constituted a reservoir of monomers both for monomer insertion between condensed phospholipids and for insertion of groups of monomers between fluid phospholipids. Since biological membranes are composed of dynamically condensed domains surrounded by fluid domains, it has been suggested that, above the CMC, alkylphospholipids can insert into both kinds of phases: as monomers into the condensed phase and as a group of monomers into the fluid phase. (Rakotomanga et al., 2005). The presence of albumin in the medium has the effect of increasing the CMC value by binding molecules of lipids and, hence, reducing the concentration of free monomers in the medium (Kim et al., 2007). Like albumin acts as an alkylphospholipid reservoir - it binds reversibly to the cell surface and may release the drug gradually - the role of liposomes seems to be similar.

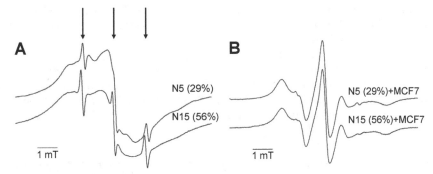

Fig. 8. EPR spectra of lipophilic spin-probe – spin labeled OPP (5P)
A) in the membrane of liposomal OPP formulation with different concentrations of cholesterol (the amount of cholesterol is indicated in mol%) in PBS buffer at room temperature. The arrows point to peaks corresponding to free 5P, which is neither incorporated in liposomes, neither in micelles. A broad spectrum corresponds to supramolecular structures of OPP (liposomes and micelles);
B) in the membrane of MCF7 cells. Spectra were recorded 2 minutes after mixing of spin labeled OPP liposomes (1.5 μL) with pellet of MCF7 cells (1.5 μL with 5 -10 x 10^6 cells).

At first glance these results are in stark contrast with the experiments with fluorescently labeled liposomal OPP formulations (Fig. 7) and with OPP liposomes with the entrapped hydrophilic probe (Fig. 6), since those experiments suggest that OPP liposomes with high amount of cholesterol almost do not interact with breast cancer cells. Fast transfer of OPP from liposomes to other membranes would lead to destabilization of liposomes, which was not the case for N15 liposomes with high amount of CH. It seems that OPP differs from spin labeled OPP (5P), which is not surprising with respect to the doxyl group attached to the alkyl chain, which probably prevents the condensing effect of cholesterol.

6. Summary of differences between MT-3 and MCF7 breast cancer cell lines

Main differences between OPP sensitive MT-3 and OPP resistant MCF7 cells are:
1. Plasma membrane fluidity is slightly larger for estrogen receptor negative (ER-) MT-3 as for estrogen receptor positive (ER+) MCF7.

2. OPP increases plasma membrane fluidity of both cell lines at concentrations higher than 50 μM. The influence of Perifosine (OPP) is less pronounced for MCF7 as for MT-3 cells. This indicates that OPP either doesn't incorporate into alkylphospholipid resistant, ER+ MCF7 cells as well as it incorporates into alkylphospholipid sensitive, ER- MT-3 cells, or it doesn't concentrate in plasma membrane of MCF7 cells at such high concentrations as it does in MT-3 cells.
3. Transport of alkylphospholipids across plasma membrane and subsequent reduction in breast cancer cells (Fig. 4) showed that the transport and the reduction of spin labeled OPP is faster for MT-3 than for MCF7 cells at room temperature, whereas it is just the opposite at physiological temperature. The main difference between MCF7 and MT-3 cells is the transport of OPP across the plasma membrane, which increases significantly for MCF7 cells at physiologic temperature, but remains almost unchanged for MT-3 cells. Because of this we suspect that OPP uptake by OPP resistant MCF7 cells might be mediated, similarly as in the case of KB carcinoma cells (Vink et al., 2007), by a lipid transporter. This observation could explain lower influence of OPP on cell membrane fluidity of MCF7 cells and support the hypothesis that OPP doesn't concentrate in the plasma membrane of MCF7 cells.
4. Liposomal OPP formulations with low CH concentration (N5) quickly release a portion of their content when mixed with breast cancer cells. At room temperature the release is comparable for MT-3 and MCF7 cells (Fig. 6). However, at physiological temperature the amount of released content increases for OPP sensitive MT-3 cells, but remain in the same range for MCF7 cells.

7. Conclusions with respect to experimental breast cancer therapy with alkylphospholipids

For efficient application of liposomes as nanocarriers in breast cancer therapy it is not only necessary to investigate in detail the physical properties of the nanocarrier, which has to transport the drug to the (target) cell, but also the properties of the target cell. In the case of application of alkylphospholipids, where plasma membrane is the specific target, one has to know the properties of the plasma membrane and differences among membranes of different breast cancer cell lines. We have shown that plasma membrane of MT-3 cells is more fluid (lower order parameter) as the membrane of MCF7 cells and was influenced more by OPP. Besides, it should be taken into account also that the properties of plasma membrane depend on external factors. For example, it has been shown that confluent MT-3 breast cancer cells have significantly higher membrane fluidity and higher relative proportion of disordered membrane domains as compared to cells harvested during exponential growth (Koklic et al., 2005). The fluidity of plasma membrane of MT-3 breast cancer cells also has an important role in metastasis development. The increase in membrane fluidity of MT-3 breast cancer cells was correlated with 2-fold increase in sialyl Lewis X and/or A ligand-mediated adhesion of these cells and a higher motility of ligands in the membrane of confluent cells, together with an accumulation of these ligands in distinct areas on a cell membrane (Zeisig et al., 2007).

In order to better understand the interaction of OPP micelles or liposomes with breast cancer cells, one has to take into account the following main characteristics of alkylphospholipids and of liposomal formulations:

1. In mouse S49 lymphoma cells, alkylphospholipids accumulate in detergent-resistant, sphingolipid- and cholesterol-enriched lipid raft domains and are rapidly internalized by clathrin-independent, raft-mediated endocytosis (van der Luit et al., 2007).

2. Alkylphospholipid uptake in KB carcinoma cells appears to be raft-independent and mediated by a yet unidentified ATP-dependent lipid transporter (Vink et al., 2007).

3. Lipid monolayer experiments showed that alkylphospholipids, below the critical micellar concentration (CMC), insert progressively into lipid monolayers as monomers from the aqueous medium, while above CMC, not only monomers but also groups of monomers (micelles) are transferred into the monolayers (Rakotomanga et al., 2004).

4. While alkylphospholipid HePC is miscible with POPC, there is high affinity between HePC and sterols (ergosterol, and cholesterol) and that maximum condensation is reached at a ratio of HePC/sterol around 50:50 (mol/mol) (Rakotomanga et al., 2004). This kind of behavior is generally known as the condensing effect of cholesterol towards phospholipids (Chapman et al., 1969; Ghosh & Tinoco, 1972).

5. Alkylphospholipid OPP increases membrane fluidity of both MCF7 and MT-3 cell line at concentrations higher than 50 μM, indicating that OPP incorporates into the membrane of breast cancer cells and is slowly transferred into the cell interior as it was detected by reduction kinetics of spin labeled OPP (Fig. 4). OPP transfer increases at physiologic temperature for OPP resistant MCF7 cells, but remains almost the same for OPP sensitive MT-3 cells. We believe that OPP uptake by OPP resistant MCF7 cells might be mediated, similarly as in the case of KB carcinoma cells (Vink et al., 2007), by a lipid transporter.

6. Liposomal OPP formulations efficient in experimental breast cancer therapy should have cholesterol concentration below 50 mol%.

7. *In vivo* data show that hemolytic effects of liposomal OPP formulations is diminished as compared to free OPP, but cytotoxic activity of liposomal formulations is also lower (Zeisig et al., 1998).

8. Liposomal formulations with lower cholesterol/OPP ratio containing higher proportion of micellar OPP, are hemolytically more active than liposomal formulations with lower cholesterol concentration (Zeisig et al., 1998). At approximately 55 mol% cholesterol liposomal formulations do not contain any OPP micelles (Koklic et al., 2010). While there is almost no release of content from liposomal OPP formulations with 56 mol% cholesterol for both cell lines, liposomal formulations with low cholesterol concentration quickly release a portion of their content when mixed with breast cancer cells (Fig. 6). Similarly lipid phase of liposomal OPP formulations with low cholesterol concentration quickly enters and crosses plasma membrane of OPP resistant MCF7 cells, but remains outside of cells in the case of liposomal formulations with 56 mol% cholesterol, as measured by C6-NBD-PC labeled liposomal formulations.

9. Fluidity characteristics of liposomal OPP formulations depend mainly on the amount of cholesterol, and only to a minor part on charge and sterical stabilization (Koklic et al., 2002). A sudden increase in order parameter of most disordered domain type occurs at cholesterol concentration around 50 mol%, while at the same time the polarity correction factor decreases, indicating that the spin probes are located in an environment less accessible to water.

10. Surface activity of an alkylphospholipid Edelfosine is decreased by other lipids, especially sterols, which indicates that Edelfosine is slowly released from the lipid mixture to the aqueous environment (Busto et al., 2008).

Based on all of the above mentioned properties, there are two competing hypothesis of OPP liposome formulation – breast cancer cell interaction, which still need further experimental validation. Either OPP liposome formulations with low cholesterol concentration are able to deliver OPP into breast cancer cells by fusing with plasma membrane of breast cancer cells, due to liposome membrane properties, or alkylphospholipids whether in free or micellar form insert with high affinity into cholesterol containing target membranes (cells) as long as liposomal carriers contain low amounts of cholesterol. Once the remaining liposomal carriers have cholesterol concentration above around 50 mol% the remaining alkylphospholipids are stabilized in liposomes and do not interact with cells anymore. In this way liposomes serve as a reservoir capable of releasing alkylphospholipids and preventing side effect associated with high alkylphospholipid concentrations.

8. References

Arndt, D., Zeisig, R., Eue, I., Sternberg, B., & Fichtner, I. (1997). Antineoplastic activity of sterically stabilized alkylphosphocholine liposomes in human breast carcinomas. *Breast Cancer Res Treat*, Vol. 43, No. 3, (May), pp. 237-46, 0167-6806

Arndt, D., Zeisig, R., Fichtner, I., Teppke, A.D., & Fahr, A. (1999). Pharmacokinetics of sterically stabilized hexadecylphosphocholine liposomes versus conventional liposomes and free hexadecylphosphocholine in tumor-free and human breast carcinoma bearing mice. *Breast Cancer Res Treat*, Vol. 58, No. 1, (Nov), pp. 71-80, 0167-6806

Arsov, Z., Urbančič, I., Garvas, M., Biglino, D., Ljubetič, A., Koklič, T., & Štrancar, J. (2011). Fluorescence microspectroscopy as a tool to study mechanism of nanoparticles delivery into living cancer cells. *Biomed Opt Express*, Vol. submited for review, No. pp. 2083-2095, 2156-7085

Batista, U., Garvas, M., Nemec, M., Schara, M., Veranic, P., & Koklic, T. (2010). Effects of different detachment procedures on viability, nitroxide reduction kinetics and plasma membrane heterogeneity of V-79 cells. *Cell Biol Int*, Vol. 2, No. 8, (Jun), pp. 663-8, 1095-8355

Busto, J.V., Del Canto-Janez, E., Goni, F.M., Mollinedo, F., & Alonso, A. (2008). Combination of the anti-tumour cell ether lipid edelfosine with sterols abolishes haemolytic side effects of the drug. *J Chem Biol*, Vol. 1, No. 1-4, (Nov), pp. 89-94, 1864-6158

Busto, J.V., Sot, J., Goñi, F.M., Mollinedo, F., & Alonso, A. (2007). Surface-active properties of the antitumour ether lipid 1-O-octadecyl-2-O-methyl-rac-glycero-3-phosphocholine (edelfosine). *Biochimica et Biophysica Acta (BBA) - Biomembranes*, Vol. 1768, No. 7, pp. 1855-60, 0005-2736

Carrasco, M.P., Jimenez-Lopez, J.M., Segovia, J.L., & Marco, C. (2008). Hexadecylphosphocholine interferes with the intracellular transport of cholesterol in HepG2 cells. *FEBS J*, Vol. 275, No. 8, (Apr), pp. 1675-86, 1742-464X

Carrasco, S., & Merida, I. (2007). Diacylglycerol, when simplicity becomes complex. *Trends Biochem Sci*, Vol. 32, No. 1, (Jan), pp. 27-36, 0968-0004

Chapman, D., Owens, N.F., Phillips, M.C., & Walker, D.A. (1969). Mixed monolayers of phospholipids and cholesterol. *Biochim Biophys Acta*, Vol. 183, No. 3, pp. 458-65, 0006-3002

Chen, K., Morse, P.D., 2nd, & Swartz, H.M. (1988). Kinetics of enzyme-mediated reduction of lipid soluble nitroxide spin labels by living cells. *Biochim Biophys Acta*, Vol. 943, No. 3, (Sep 1), pp. 477-84, 0006-3002

Chen, Z., Gibson, T.B., Robinson, F., Silvestro, L., Pearson, G., Xu, B., Wright, A., Vanderbilt, C., & Cobb, M.H. (2001). MAP kinases. *Chem Rev*, Vol. 101, No. 8, (Aug), pp. 2449-76, 0009-2665

Clive, S., Gardiner, J., & Leonard, R.C.F. (1999). Miltefosine as a topical treatment for cutaneous metastases in breast carcinoma. *Cancer Chemotherapy and Pharmacology*, Vol. 44, No. 7, pp. S29-S30, 0344-5704

Danker, K., Reutter, W., & Semini, G. (2010). Glycosidated phospholipids: uncoupling of signalling pathways at the plasma membrane. *British Journal of Pharmacology*, Vol. 160, No. 1, pp. 36-47, 0007-1188

Eibl, H., & Unger, C. (1990). Hexadecylphosphocholine: a new and selective antitumor drug. *Cancer Treat Rev*, Vol. 17, No. 2-3, (Sep), pp. 233-42, 0305-7372

Elrod, H.A., Lin, Y.D., Yue, P., Wang, X., Lonial, S., Khuri, F.R., & Sun, S.Y. (2007). The alkylphospholipid perifosine induces apoptosis of human lung cancer cells requiring inhibition of Akt and activation of the extrinsic apoptotic pathway. *Mol Cancer Ther*, Vol. 6, No. 7, (Jul), pp. 2029-38, 1535-7163

Erdlenbruch, B., Jendrossek, V., Gerriets, A., Vetterlein, F., Eibl, H., & Lakomek, M. (1999). Erucylphosphocholine: pharmacokinetics, biodistribution and CNS-accumulation in the rat after intravenous administration. *Cancer Chemother Pharmacol*, Vol. 44, No. 6, pp. 484-90, 0344-5704

Erdlenbruch, B., Jendrossek, V., Marx, M., Hunold, A., Eibl, H., & Lakomek, M. (1998). Antitumor effects of erucylphosphocholine on brain tumor cells in vitro and in vivo. *Anticancer Res*, Vol. 18, No. 4A, (Jul-Aug), pp. 2551-7, 0250-7005

Eue, I., Zeisig, R., & Arndt, D. (1995). Alkylphosphocholine-induced production of nitric oxide and tumor necrosis factor alpha by U 937 cells. *J Cancer Res Clin Oncol*, Vol. 121, No. 6, pp. 350-6, 0171-5216

Fang, Y., Vilella-Bach, M., Bachmann, R., Flanigan, A., & Chen, J. (2001). Phosphatidic acid-mediated mitogenic activation of mTOR signaling. *Science*, Vol. 294, No. 5548, (Nov 30), pp. 1942-5, 0036-8075

Fichtner, I., Zeisig, R., Naundorf, H., Jungmann, S., Arndt, D., Asongwe, G., Double, J.A., & Bibby, M.C. (1994). Antineoplastic activity of alkylphosphocholines (APC) in human breast carcinomas in vivo and in vitro; use of liposomes. *Breast Cancer Res Treat*, Vol. 32, No. 3, pp. 269-79, 0167-6806

Gajate, C., Gonzalez-Camacho, F., & Mollinedo, F. (2009). Lipid raft connection between extrinsic and intrinsic apoptotic pathways. *Biochem Biophys Res Commun*, Vol. 380, No. 4, (Mar 20), pp. 780-4, 1090-2104

Gajate, C., & Mollinedo, F. (2002). Biological activities, mechanisms of action and biomedical prospect of the antitumor ether phospholipid ET-18-OCH(3) (edelfosine), a proapoptotic agent in tumor cells. *Curr Drug Metab*, Vol. 3, No. 5, (Oct), pp. 491-525, 1389-2002

Gajate, C., Santos-Beneit, A., Modolell, M., & Mollinedo, F. (1998). Involvement of c-Jun NH2-terminal kinase activation and c-Jun in the induction of apoptosis by the ether phospholipid 1-O-octadecyl-2-O-methyl-rac-glycero-3-phosphocholine. *Mol Pharmacol*, Vol. 53, No. 4, (Apr), pp. 602-12, 0026-895X

Ghosh, D., & Tinoco, J. (1972). Monolayer interactions of individual lecithins with natural sterols. *Biochim Biophys Acta*, Vol. 266, No. 1, (Apr 14), pp. 41-9, 0006-3002

Gills, J.J., & Dennis, P.A. (2009). Perifosine: Update on a Novel Akt Inhibitor. *Current Oncology Reports*, Vol. 11, No. 2, (Mar), pp. 102-10, 1523-3790

Heesbeen, E.C., Verdonck, L.F., Hermans, S.W., van Heugten, H.G., Staal, G.E., & Rijksen, G. (1991). Alkyllysophospholipid ET-18-OCH3 acts as an activator of protein kinase C in HL-60 cells. *FEBS Lett,* Vol. 290, No. 1-2, (Sep 23), pp. 231-4, 0014-5793

Hilgard, P., Klenner, T., Stekar, J., Nossner, G., Kutscher, B., & Engel, J. (1997). D-21266, a new heterocyclic alkylphospholipid with antitumour activity. *Eur J Cancer,* Vol. 33, No. 3, (Mar), pp. 442-6, 0959-8049

Hochhuth, C.H., Vehmeyer, K., Eibl, H., & Unger, C. (1992). Hexadecylphosphocholine induces interferon-gamma secretion and expression of GM-CSF mRNA in human mononuclear cells. *Cell Immunol,* Vol. 141, No. 1, (Apr 15), pp. 161-8, 0008-8749

Jendrossek, V., Muller, I., Eibl, H., & Belka, C. (2003). Intracellular mediators of erucylphosphocholine-induced apoptosis. *Oncogene,* Vol. 22, No. 17, (May 1), pp. 2621-31, 0950-9232

Jimenez-Lopez, J.M., Carrasco, M.P., Marco, C., & Segovia, J.L. (2006). Hexadecylphosphocholine disrupts cholesterol homeostasis and induces the accumulation of free cholesterol in HepG2 tumour cells. *Biochem Pharmacol,* Vol. 71, No. 8, (Apr 14), pp. 1114-21, 0006-2952

Kaufmann-Kolle, P., Berger, M.R., Unger, C., & Eibl, H. (1996). Systemic administration of alkylphosphocholines. Erucylphosphocholine and liposomal hexadecylphosphocholine. *Adv Exp Med Biol,* Vol. 416, No. pp. 165-8, 0065-2598

Kim, Y.L., Im, Y.J., Ha, N.C., & Im, D.S. (2007). Albumin inhibits cytotoxic activity of lysophosphatidylcholine by direct binding. *Prostaglandins Other Lipid Mediat,* Vol. 83, No. 1-2, (Feb), pp. 130-8, 1098-8823

Kiss, Z., & Crilly, K.S. (1997). Alkyl lysophospholipids inhibit phorbol ester-stimulated phospholipase D activity and DNA synthesis in fibroblasts. *FEBS Lett,* Vol. 412, No. 2, (Jul 28), pp. 313-7, 0014-5793

Koklic, T., Pirs, M., Zeisig, R., Abramovic, Z., & Sentjurc, M. (2005). Membrane switch hypothesis. 1. Cell density influences lateral domain structure of tumor cell membranes. *J Chem Inf Model,* Vol. 45, No. 6, (Nov-Dec), pp. 1701-7, 1549-9596

Koklic, T., Sentjurc, M., & Zeisig, R. (2002). The influence of cholesterol and charge on the membrane domains of alkylphospholipid liposomes as studied by EPR. *J Liposome Res,* Vol. 12, No. 4, (Nov), pp. 335-52, 0898-2104

Koklic, T., Sentjurc, M., & Zeisig, R. (2010). Determination of the amount of micelles in alkylphospholipid liposome formulations with electron paramagnetic resonance method. *J Liposome Res,* Vol. 21, No. 1, (Mar), pp. 1-8, 1532-2394

Koklic, T., Zeisig, R., & Sentjurc, M. (2008). Interaction of alkylphospholipid liposomes with MT-3 breast-cancer cells depends critically on cholesterol concentration. *Biochimica et Biophysica Acta (BBA) - Biomembranes,* Vol. 1778, No. 12, pp. 2682-9, 0005-2736

Kondapaka, S.B., Singh, S.S., Dasmahapatra, G.P., Sausville, E.A., & Roy, K.K. (2003). Perifosine, a novel alkylphospholipid, inhibits protein kinase B activation. *Mol Cancer Ther,* Vol. 2, No. 11, (Nov), pp. 1093-103, 1535-7163

Kyriakis, J.M., & Avruch, J. (2001). Mammalian mitogen-activated protein kinase signal transduction pathways activated by stress and inflammation. *Physiol Rev,* Vol. 81, No. 2, (Apr), pp. 807-69, 0031-9333

Limatola, C., Schaap, D., Moolenaar, W.H., & van Blitterswijk, W.J. (1994). Phosphatidic acid activation of protein kinase C-zeta overexpressed in COS cells: comparison with other protein kinase C isotypes and other acidic lipids. *Biochem J,* Vol. 304 (Pt 3), No. (Dec 15), pp. 1001-8, 0264-6021

Lucas, L., Hernandez-Alcoceba, R., Penalva, V., & Lacal, J.C. (2001). Modulation of phospholipase D by hexadecylphosphorylcholine: a putative novel mechanism for its antitumoral activity. *Oncogene*, Vol. 20, No. 9, (Mar 1), pp. 1110-7, 0950-9232

Maly, K., Uberall, F., Schubert, C., Kindler, E., Stekar, J., Brachwitz, H., & Grunicke, H.H. (1995). Interference of new alkylphospholipid analogues with mitogenic signal transduction. *Anticancer Drug Des*, Vol. 10, No. 5, (Jul), pp. 411-25, 0266-9536

Marco, C., Jimenez-Lopez, J.M., Rios-Marco, P., Segovia, J.L., & Carrasco, M.P. (2009). Hexadecylphosphocholine alters nonvesicular cholesterol traffic from the plasma membrane to the endoplasmic reticulum and inhibits the synthesis of sphingomyelin in HepG2 cells. *Int J Biochem Cell Biol*, Vol. 41, No. 6, (Jun), pp. 1296-303, 1878-5875

Mravljak, J., Podlipec, R., Koklič, T., Pečar, S., & Šentjurc, M. (2010). Interaction of spin-labeled derivatives of a cancerostatic alkylphospholipid, perifosine, with model and cell membranes. *VIIIth International Workshop on EPR(ESR) in Biology and Medicine*, Vol. Krakow, Poland, 4.-7. October 2010

Mravljak, J., Zeisig, R., & Pecar, S. (2005). Synthesis and biological evaluation of spin-labeled alkylphospholipid analogs. *Journal of Medicinal Chemistry*, Vol. 48, No. 20, (Oct), pp. 6393-9, 0022-2623

Munoz-Martinez, F., Torres, C., Castanys, S., & Gamarro, F. (2008). The anti-tumor alkylphospholipid perifosine is internalized by an ATP-dependent translocase activity across the plasma membrane of human KB carcinoma cells. *Biochimica Et Biophysica Acta-Biomembranes*, Vol. 1778, No. 2, (Feb), pp. 530-40, 0005-2736

Naundorf, H., Rewasowa, E.C., Fichtner, I., Buttner, B., Becker, M., & Gorlich, M. (1992). Characterization of two human mammary carcinomas, MT-1 and MT-3, suitable for in vivo testing of ether lipids and their derivatives. *Breast Cancer Res Treat*, Vol. 23, No. 1-2, pp. 87-95, 0167-6806

Nieto-Miguel, T., Fonteriz, R.I., Vay, L., Gajate, C., Lopez-Hernandez, S., & Mollinedo, F. (2007). Endoplasmic reticulum stress in the proapoptotic action of edelfosine in solid tumor cells. *Cancer Res*, Vol. 67, No. 21, (Nov 1), pp. 10368-78, 1538-7445

Nieto-Miguel, T., Gajate, C., Gonzalez-Camacho, F., & Mollinedo, F. (2008). Proapoptotic role of Hsp90 by its interaction with c-Jun N-terminal kinase in lipid rafts in edelfosine-mediated antileukemic therapy. *Oncogene*, Vol. 27, No. 12, (Mar 13), pp. 1779-87, 1476-5594

Nieto-Miguel, T., Gajate, C., & Mollinedo, F. (2006). Differential targets and subcellular localization of antitumor alkyl-lysophospholipid in leukemic versus solid tumor cells. *J Biol Chem*, Vol. 281, No. 21, (May 26), pp. 14833-40, 0021-9258

Orthmann, A., Zeisig, R., Koklic, T., Sentjurc, M., Wiesner, B., Lemm, M., & Fichtner, I. (2010). Impact of membrane properties on uptake and transcytosis of colloidal nanocarriers across an epithelial cell barrier model. *J Pharm Sci*, Vol. 99, No. 5, (May), pp. 2423-33, 1520-6017

Pabst, G., Hodzic, A., Strancar, J., Danner, S., Rappolt, M., & Laggner, P. (2007). Rigidification of neutral lipid bilayers in the presence of salts. *Biophysical Journal*, Vol. 93, No. 8, (Oct), pp. 2688-96, 0006-3495

Pearson, G., Robinson, F., Beers Gibson, T., Xu, B.E., Karandikar, M., Berman, K., & Cobb, M.H. (2001). Mitogen-activated protein (MAP) kinase pathways: regulation and physiological functions. *Endocr Rev*, Vol. 22, No. 2, (Apr), pp. 153-83, 0163-769X

Rahmani, M., Reese, E., Dai, Y., Bauer, C., Payne, S.G., Dent, P., Spiegel, S., & Grant, S. (2005). Coadministration of histone deacetylase inhibitors and perifosine

synergistically induces apoptosis in human leukemia cells through Akt and
    ERK1/2 inactivation and the generation of ceramide and reactive oxygen species.
    Cancer Res, Vol. 65, No. 6, (Mar 15), pp. 2422-32, 0008-5472
Rakotomanga,   M.,   Loiseau,   P.M.,   &   Saint-Pierre-Chazalet,   M.   (2004).
    Hexadecylphosphocholine interaction with lipid monolayers. *Biochimica Et
    Biophysica Acta-Biomembranes*, Vol. 1661, No. 2, (Mar), pp. 212-8, 0005-2736
Rakotomanga, M., Saint-Pierre-Chazalet, M., & Loiseau, P.M. (2005). Alteration of fatty acid
    and sterol metabolism in miltefosine-resistant Leishmania donovani promastigotes
    and consequences for drug-membrane interactions. *Antimicrobial Agents and
    Chemotherapy*, Vol. 49, No. 7, (Jul), pp. 2677-86, 0066-4804
Rizzo, M.A., Shome, K., Watkins, S.C., & Romero, G. (2000). The recruitment of Raf-1 to
    membranes is mediated by direct interaction with phosphatidic acid and is
    independent of association with Ras. *J Biol Chem*, Vol. 275, No. 31, (Aug 4), pp.
    23911-8, 0021-9258
Ruiter, G.A., Verheij, M., Zerp, S.F., & van Blitterswijk, W.J. (2001). Alkyl-lysophospholipids
    as anticancer agents and enhancers of radiation-induced apoptosis. *Int J Radiat
    Oncol Biol Phys*, Vol. 49, No. 2, (Feb 1), pp. 415-9, 0360-3016
Ruiter, G.A., Zerp, S.F., Bartelink, H., van Blitterswijk, W.J., & Verheij, M. (1999). Alkyl-
    lysophospholipids activate the SAPK/JNK pathway and enhance radiation-
    induced apoptosis. *Cancer Res*, Vol. 59, No. 10, (May 15), pp. 2457-63, 0008-5472
Smets, L.A., Van Rooij, H., & Salomons, G.S. (1999). Signalling steps in apoptosis by ether
    lipids. *Apoptosis*, Vol. 4, No. 6, (Dec), pp. 419-27, 1360-8185
Sobottka, S.B., & Berger, M.R. (1992). Assessment of antineoplastic agents by MTT assay:
    partial underestimation of antiproliferative properties. *Cancer Chemother Pharmacol*,
    Vol. 30, No. 5, pp. 385-93, 0344-5704
Stopar, D., Strancar, J., Spruijt, R.B., & Hemminga, M.A. (2006). Motional restrictions of
    membrane proteins: A site-directed spin labeling study. *Biophysical Journal*, Vol. 91,
    No. 9, (Nov), pp. 3341-8, 0006-3495
Strancar, J., Koklic, T., & Arsov, Z. (2003). Soft picture of lateral heterogeneity in
    biomembranes. *Journal of Membrane Biology*, Vol. 196, No. 2, (Nov 15), pp. 135-46,
    0022-2631
Strancar, J., Koklic, T., Arsov, Z., Filipic, B., Stopar, D., & Hemminga, M.A. (2005). Spin label
    EPR-based characterization of biosystem complexity. *Journal of Chemical Information
    and Modeling*, Vol. 45, No. 2, (Mar-Apr), pp. 394-406, 1549-9596
Strassheim, D., Shafer, S.H., Phelps, S.H., & Williams, C.L. (2000). Small cell lung carcinoma
    exhibits greater phospholipase C-beta1 expression and edelfosine resistance
    compared with non-small cell lung carcinoma. *Cancer Res*, Vol. 60, No. 10, (May 15),
    pp. 2730-6, 0008-5472
Swartz, H.M., Sentjurc, M., & Morse, P.D., 2nd (1986). Cellular metabolism of water-soluble
    nitroxides: effect on rate of reduction of cell/nitroxide ratio, oxygen concentrations and
    permeability of nitroxides. *Biochim Biophys Acta*, Vol. 888, No. 1, (Aug 29), pp. 82-90,
Tazzari, P.L., Tabellini, G., Ricci, F., Papa, V., Bortul, R., Chiarini, F., Evangelisti, C.,
    Martinelli, G., Bontadini, A., Cocco, L., *et al.* (2008). Synergistic proapoptotic
    activity of recombinant TRAIL plus the Akt inhibitor Perifosine in acute
    myelogenous leukemia cells. *Cancer Res*, Vol. 68, No. 22, (Nov 15), pp. 9394-403,
    1538-7445 (Electronic) 0008-5472 (Linking)

Ueda, A., Nagase, S., Yokoyama, H., Tada, M., Noda, H., Ohya, H., Kamada, H., Hirayama, A., & Koyama, A. (2003). Importance of renal mitochondria in the reduction of TEMPOL, a nitroxide radical. *Mol Cell Biochem,* Vol. 244, No. 1-2, (Feb), pp. 119-24,

Unger, C., & Eibl, H. (1991). Hexadecylphosphocholine: Preclinical and the first clinical results of a new antitumor drug. *Lipids,* Vol. 26, No. 12, pp. 1412-7, 0024-4201

Unger, C., Eibl, H., Breiser, A., von Heyden, H.W., Engel, J., Hilgard, P., Sindermann, H., Peukert, M., & Nagel, G.A. (1988). Hexadecylphosphocholine (D 18506) in the topical treatment of skin metastases: a phase-I trial. *Onkologie,* Vol. 11, No. 6, (Dec), pp. 295-6, 0378-584X

Unger, C., Sindermann, H., Peukert, M., Hilgard, P., Engel, J., & Eibl, H. (1992). Hexadecylphosphocholine in the topical treatment of skin metastases in breast cancer patients. *Prog Exp Tumor Res,* Vol. 34, No. pp. 153-9, 0079-6263

van Blitterswijk, W.J., van der Luit, A.H., Veldman, R.J., Verheij, M., & Borst, J. (2003). Ceramide: second messenger or modulator of membrane structure and dynamics? *Biochem J,* Vol. 369, No. Pt 2, (Jan 15), pp. 199-211, 0264-6021

van Blitterswijk, W.J., van der Meer, B.W., & Hilkmann, H. (1987). Quantitative contributions of cholesterol and the individual classes of phospholipids and their degree of fatty acyl (un)saturation to membrane fluidity measured by fluorescence polarization. *Biochemistry,* Vol. 26, No. 6, (Mar 24), pp. 1746-56, 0006-2960

van Blitterswijk, W.J., & Verheij, M. (2008). Anticancer alkylphospholipids: Mechanisms of action, cellular sensitivity and resistance, and clinical prospects. *Current Pharmaceutical Design,* Vol. 14, No. 21, (Jul), pp. 2061-74, 1381-6128

van der Luit, A.H., Vink, S.R., Klarenbeek, J.B., Perrissoud, D., Solary, E., Verheij, M., & van Blitterswijk, W.J. (2007). A new class of anticancer alkylphospholipids uses lipid rafts as membrane gateways to induce apoptosis in lymphoma cells. *Molecular Cancer Therapeutics,* Vol. 6, No. 8, pp. 2337-45, 1535-7163

van Dijk, M.C., Muriana, F.J., de Widt, J., Hilkmann, H., & van Blitterswijk, W.J. (1997). Involvement of phosphatidylcholine-specific phospholipase C in platelet-derived growth factor-induced activation of the mitogen-activated protein kinase pathway in Rat-1 fibroblasts. *J Biol Chem,* Vol. 272, No. 17, (Apr 25), pp. 11011-6, 0021-9258

Vehmeyer, K., Eibl, H., & Unger, C. (1992). Hexadecylphosphocholine stimulates the colony-stimulating factor-dependent growth of hemopoietic progenitor cells. *Exp Hematol,* Vol. 20, No. 1, (Jan), pp. 1-5, 0301-472X

Vink, S.R., van der Luit, A.H., Klarenbeek, J.B., Verheij, M., & van Blitterswijk, W.J. (2007). Lipid rafts and metabolic energy differentially determine uptake of anti-cancer alkylphospholipids in lymphoma versus carcinoma cells. *Biochem Pharmacol,* Vol. 74, No. 10, (Nov 15), pp. 1456-65, 0006-2952

Vrablic, A.S., Albright, C.D., Craciunescu, C.N., Salganik, R.I., & Zeisel, S.H. (2001). Altered mitochondrial function and overgeneration of reactive oxygen species precede the induction of apoptosis by 1-O-octadecyl-2-methyl-rac-glycero-3-phosphocholine in p53-defective hepatocytes. *FASEB J,* Vol. 15, No. 10, (Aug), pp. 1739-44, 0892-6638

Wagner, B.A., Buettner, G.R., & Burns, C.P. (1993). Increased generation of lipid-derived and ascorbate free radicals by L1210 cells exposed to the ether lipid edelfosine. *Cancer Res,* Vol. 53, No. 4, (Feb 15), pp. 711-3, 0008-5472

Wenzel, J., Zeisig, R., & Fichtner, I. (2009). Inhibition of metastasis in a murine 4T1 breast cancer model by liposomes preventing tumor cell-platelet interactions. *Clin Exp Metastasis,* Vol. 27, No. 1, pp. 25-34, 1573-7276

Wenzel, J., Zeisig, R., & Fichtner, I. (2010). Inhibition of metastasis in a murine 4T1 breast cancer model by liposomes preventing tumor cell-platelet interactions. *Clin Exp Metastasis*, Vol. 27, No. 1, pp. 25-34, 1573-7276

Wieder, T., Orfanos, C.E., & Geilen, C.C. (1998). Induction of ceramide-mediated apoptosis by the anticancer phospholipid analog, hexadecylphosphocholine. *J Biol Chem*, Vol. 273, No. 18, (May 1), pp. 11025-31, 0021-9258

Yang, C., & Kazanietz, M.G. (2003). Divergence and complexities in DAG signaling: looking beyond PKC. *Trends Pharmacol Sci*, Vol. 24, No. 11, (Nov), pp. 602-8, 0165-6147

Yonar, D., Paktas, D.D., Horasan, N., Strancar, J., Sentjurc, M., & Sunnetcioglu, M.M. (2010). EPR investigation of clomipramine interaction with phosphatidylcholine membranes in presence and absence of cholesterol. *J Liposome Res*, Vol. No. (Jul 12), pp. 1532-2394

Zeisig, R., Arndt, D., Stahn, R., & Fichtner, I. (1998). Physical properties and pharmacological activity in vitro and in vivo of optimised liposomes prepared from a new cancerostatic alkylphospholipid. *Biochim Biophys Acta*, Vol. 1414, No. 1-2, (Nov 11), pp. 238-48, 0006-3002

Zeisig, R., Fichtner, I., Arndt, D., & Jungmann, S. (1991). Antitumor effects of alkylphosphocholines in different murine tumor models: use of liposomal preparations. *Anticancer Drugs*, Vol. 2, No. 4, (Aug), pp. 411-7, 0959-4973

Zeisig, R., Koklic, T., Wiesner, B., Fichtner, I., & Sentjurc, M. (2007). Increase in fluidity in the membrane of MT3 breast cancer cells correlates with enhanced cell adhesion in vitro and increased lung metastasis in NOD/SCID mice. *Archives of Biochemistry and Biophysics*, Vol. 459, No. 1, pp. 98-106, 0003-9861

Zeisig, R., Muller, K., Maurer, N., Arndt, D., & Fahr, A. (2001). The composition-dependent presence of free (micellar) alkylphospholipid in liposomal formulations of octadecyl-1,1-dimethyl-piperidino-4-yl-phosphate affects its cytotoxic activity in vitro. *J Membr Biol*, Vol. 182, No. 1, (Jul 1), pp. 61-9, 0022-2631

Zeisig, R., Rückerl, D., & Fichtner, I. (2004). Reduction of tamoxifen resistance in human breast carcinomas by tamoxifen-containing liposomes in vivo. *Anti-Cancer Drugs*, Vol. 15, No. 7, pp. 707-14, 0959-4973

Zeisig, R., Rudolf, M., Eue, I., & Arndt, D. (1995). Influence of hexadecylphosphocholine on the release of tumor necrosis factor and nitroxide from peritoneal macrophages in vitro. *J Cancer Res Clin Oncol*, Vol. 121, No. 2, pp. 69-75, 0171-5216

Zerp, S.F., Vink, S.R., Ruiter, G.A., Koolwijk, P., Peters, E., van der Luit, A.H., de Jong, D., Budde, M., Bartelink, H., van Blitterswijk, W.J., et al. (2008). Alkylphospholipids inhibit capillary-like endothelial tube formation in vitro: antiangiogenic properties of a new class of antitumor agents. *Anticancer Drugs*, Vol. 19, No. 1, (Jan), pp. 65-75, 0959-4973

5

Fibrillar Human Serum Albumin Suppresses Breast Cancer Cell Growth and Metastasis

Shao-Wen Hung, Chiao-Li Chu,
Yu-Ching Chang and Shu-Mei Liang
Agricultural Biotechnology Research Center, Academia Sinica, Taipei
Taiwan

1. Introduction

1.1 Breast cancer classification

Breast cancer is one of the most common cancers among women worldwide and approximately one-third of women diagnosed will eventually develop metastases and die (Jemal et al, 2010). Breast cancer is heterogeneous at the molecular, histopathologic and clinical levels and is commonly classified into several categories according to multiple schemes, each based on different criteria. A typical description of breast cancer can be comprised of tumor grade, histologic type, tumor stage, and the expression of proteins and genes etc. (McSherry et al, 2007). Normal non-cancerous cells are differentiated and have specific cell shapes and functions; whereas, cancer cells lose differentiation (de-differentiate), have less uniform nuclei, and exhibit uncontrolled cell division. Pathologists, therefore, determine breast cancer by grade according to the degree of differentiation of cells compared to normal breast cells: highly differentiated (low grade), moderately differentiated (intermediate grade), and poorly differentiated (high grade). Cancers classified as high grade generally have a worse prognosis (McSherry et al, 2007). The majority of breast cancers are derived from the epithelium lining the ducts or lobules of the breast. They can be classified histologically according to characteristics seen upon light microscopy of biopsy specimens. Histologic classification is divided into: ductal carcinoma in situ (DCIS), invasive ductal carcinoma, and invasive lobular carcinoma (McSherry et al, 2007). Breast cancer can further be classified using the TMN Classification of Malignant Tumors, TMN stage is based on tumor size, lymph node micrometastasis, and macrometastasis, where 'T' describes tumor size; 'N' indicates whether or not the tumor has spread to the lymph nodes; and 'M' indicates whether or not distant metastasis has occurred. Larger tumor size with lymph nodal spread and distal metastasis has a worse prognosis (Gonzalez-Angulo et al, 2007). Expression of certain proteins and genes can also be used to classify breast cancer (McGrogan et al, 2008; Stickeler et al, 2009). Whole-genome analysis using expression microarray and immunohistochemical analysis has revolutionized the understanding of breast carcinomas in recent years, and led to the discovery of five distinct subtypes of breast carcinomas (luminal A, luminal B, HER-2 overexpression, basal-like, and normal-like), each with unique recognizable phenotypes and clinical outcomes (McGrogan et al, 2008; Stickeler et al, 2009). By using classification to characterize each cancer patient, it may help select the suitable treatment strategies to achieve an optimal outcome and increase therapeutic efficacy.

2. Breast cancer metastasis

In the United States, about 178,480 new cases of invasive breast cancer were diagnosed in 2007 and approximately 40,460 women died (Jemal et al, 2007). In 2010, about 207,090 new breast cancer cases were diagnosed and 39,840 died (Jemal et al, 2010). The breast cancer incidence rate has been decreasing in the USA since 1999 and the majority of 40,000 women died each year were due to breast cancer metastasis (Giordano & Hortobagyi, 2003; Jemal et al, 2010). Cancer metastasis is a complex process that includes intercellular and intracellular signaling, activation, adhesion, migration and invasion (Im et al, 2004; Lee et al, 2006). Epithelial-to-mesenchymal transition (EMT) is also thought to be involved in cancer metastasis. EMT may promote cancer-cell progression and invasion into the surrounding microenvironment. Historically, epithelial and mesenchymal cells are distinct in their unique cellular appearance and the morphology of the multicellular structures they create (Shook & Keller, 2003). A typical morphology of epithelium is sheeted and thick with individual epithelial cells abutting each other in a uniform array. Cell-to-cell junctions and adhesions between neighboring epithelial cells hold cells tightly together and inhibit the movement of individual cells away from the epithelial monolayer. Mesenchymal cells, on the other hand, possess usually a more extended and elongated shape and do not exhibit either a regimented structure or tight intracellular adhesion. Mesenchymal cells are irregular in shape and not uniform in composition or density. Adhesions between mesenchymal cells are not as strong as those of their epithelial counterparts, allowing for increased migratory capacity. The transformation of an epithelial cell into a mesenchymal cell not only alters cellular morphology, architecture, adhesion capacity, and migration capacity but also enhances capability of the cell to metastasize (Shook & Keller, 2003). Conversely, the transformation of a mesenchymal cell into an epithelial cell (MET) may prevent cell invasion and suppress cell metastatic ability.

3. Breast cancer therapy

To date, adjuvant and neo-adjuvant therapies are commonly used in cancer metastasis therapy (McGrogan et al, 2008). Currently, there are three main groups of medications used for adjuvant breast cancer treatment: (1) hormone blocking therapy; (2) chemotherapy; and (3) monoclonal antibody therapy (McGrogan et al, 2008). The cell surfaces of some breast cancers are estrogen receptors positive (ER+) and/or progesterone receptors positive (PR+) and the cells require estrogen to continue growing. These cancers can be treated with drugs that block either the hormone receptors, such as tamoxifen or the production of estrogen, such as anastrozole (Arimidex) or letrozole (Femara). The drugs that inhibit estrogen production are only suitable for post-menopausal patients (Gonzalez-Angulo et al, 2007). Combination chemotherapy is predominately used for patients at stages 2-4, being particularly beneficial in ER-breast cancer. One of the most common treatments is cyclophosphamide plus doxorubicin (Adriamycin) which destroys rapidly growing or replicating cancer cells by causing DNA damage; however, these drugs also damage normal cells causing serious adverse effects. Damage to heart muscle is the most dangerous complication associated with doxorubicin. Taxane drugs such as paclitaxel, a microtubule-stabilizing agent that interferes with spindle microtubule dynamics causing cell-cycle arrest and apoptosis through interaction with β-tubulin (Bergstralh & Ting, 2006), is also used in the breast cancer metastasis therapy. However, resistance to paclitaxel is common and there is a need to identify patients most likely to respond to treatment (McGrogan et al, 2008). Other treatments like methotrexate and fluorouracil are also used in chemotherapy. Approximately 15-20% of breast cancers have an amplification of the HER-2/neu gene or overexpression of its protein product. This receptor is a marker for poor prognosis that is associated with increased disease recurrence during the period of cancer therapy (Brown et al, 2008). Trastuzumab (Herceptin), a humanized monoclonal antibody that specifically binds to the extracellular domain of the HER-2 receptor, has improved the 5-year disease free survival of stage 1-3 HER-2+ breast cancers to about 87%. However, about 2% of patients suffer significant heart damage after Herceptin treatment (Brown et al, 2008). Trastuzumab has also been used in combination with doxorubicin and proven to be highly effective for metastatic breast cancer patients with HER-2 over-expressing tumors. However, this regimen causes severe cardiac toxicity in 27% of treated patients when the two substances are given concurrently (Stickeler et al, 2009). Lapatinib (Tykerb, GlaxoSmithKline) is an orally active small molecule that inhibits the tyrosine kinases of HER-2 and epidermal growth factor receptor type 1 (EGFR). In preclinical studies, lapatinib showed no cross-resistance with trastuzumab (Jahanzeb, 2008).

Conventional radiotherapy is usually given after surgery to destroy remaining tumor cells that may have escaped surgery. Recently, radiotherapy has also been given at the time of surgery and found to reduce the risk of recurrence by 50-66% (Belletti et al, 2008). Despite such improvements in treatment modalities, there is still a high rate of failure among adjuvant interventions mainly due to tumor invasion and metastasis. Therefore, the search for new therapeutic targets and the development of new inhibitors of tumor cell resettlement and metastatic growth continues.

4. Surface membrane integrins as potential drug-discovery targets

It is well known that cell activation, migration, proliferation, and differentiation require direct contact between cells and the extracellular matrix (ECM). Cell-to-cell and cell-to-matrix interactions are mediated by the integrin, selectin, cadherin and/or immunoglobulin families and several studies have focused on investigating cancer therapies based on the integrin superfamily. Integrin expression on cancer cells is frequently associated with cancer progression and metastasis; therefore, targeting small-molecule antagonists of the integrin superfamily provides an opportunity to suppress cancer development and metastasis (Mullamitha et al, 2007). β1 integrin, which frequently aberrantly expressed in human breast carcinomas, has been verified to play a central role in metastasis and contribute to growth factor receptor signaling. Inhibition of the β1 integrin signaling pathway has been shown to abolish the formation of metastasis in breast and gastric cancer models. Additionally, the β1 integrin signaling pathway also plays a significant role in mediating resistance to cytotoxic chemotherapies by enhancing cell survival in hematologic malignancies, lung, and breast cancers (Lu et al, 2008). Recent studies have shown that α1β1, α2β1, and α3β1 integrins regulate hepatocarcinoma cell invasion, angiogenesis of human squamous cell carcinoma, and increase migration and invasion of malignant glioma, melanoma and mammary adenocarcinoma cells, respectively. Expression of α5β1 integrin in colon cancer cells decreases HER-2-mediated proliferation (Kuwada et al, 2005). Loss of the α7β1 integrin in melanoma increases highly tumorigenic and metastatic phenotypes (Ziober et al, 1999). Several preclinical and clinical trials have shown that some integrin targeting antibodies can effectively block tumor growth and metastasis. These antibodies include MEDI-522 (vitaxin) against αvβ3 integrin (Brooks et al, 1994), CNTO 95 against both αvβ3 and αvβ5 integrins (Mullamitha et al, 2007), 17E6 against αvβ3, αvβ5, and αvβ1 integrins (Mitjans et al, 2000), LM609 against αvβ3 integrin, and Tysabri (natalizumab) against α4 integrins (O'Connor, 2007). In addition, β1 integrins possess a RGD-binding region, therefore, based mainly on their RGD containing peptides and RGD peptidomimetics, some small molecule integrin antagonists have also shown potent inhibition of angiogenesis (Kumar et al, 2001). Both fibronectin and its receptor integrin α5β1 directly regulate angiogenesis (Kim et al., 2000). Thus, antagonist(s) of α5β1 integrin might be useful targets for the inhibition of angiogenesis associated with human tumor growth, and neovascular-related ocular and inflammatory diseases (Pasterkamp et al, 2003; Suzuki et al, 2007). Further, our own studies recently found that fibrillar bovine serum albumin (F-BSA) induced apoptosis in human breast duct carcinoma cell line T47D, and fibrillar fibronectin (F-FN) induced apoptosis in human breast cancer cell line MCF-7. F-BSA and F-FN induced BHK-21 cell (baby hamster kidney cell) apoptosis through negatively regulating the integrin/FAK/Akt/GSK-3β signaling pathway and activating SHP-2 and RhoA/ROCK (Huang et al, 2009; Huang et al, 2010). Together these results suggest that inhibition of the β1 integrin signaling pathway may provide a promising therapeutic approach to breast cancer metastasis.

5. Formation and purification of fibrillar human serum albumin

Some diseases like Alzheimer's disease, transmissible spongiform encephalopathies, pancreatic islet amyloidosis, and familial amyloidosis are caused primarily by amyloid-like fibrils aggregation in organs and in the circulation (Jackson & Clarke, 2000). Recently, it has been documented that amyloid-like fibrils are cytotoxic to neuronal cells, BHK-21 cells, SKOV-3, and MCF-7 cancer cells (Gharibyan et al, 2007; Su & Chang, 2001; Zamotin et al, 2006). Whether the fibrillar proteins may be used as anti-cancer drugs in the cancer therapies is largely unclear. We have developed a novel process to convert globular proteins, bovine serum albumin and fibronectin, to fibrillar forms using detergent assisted refolding chromatography (Huang et al, 2009; Huang et al, 2010). This procedure is easier to perform than other methods reported to convert proteins to fibrillar structures such as glycation, sonication, or high temperature incubation (Azakami et al, 2005; Taboada et al, 2006). Fibrillar protein F-BSA induced apoptosis in human breast duct carcinoma cell line T47D, and F-FN induced apoptosis in human breast cancer cell line MCF-7 suggesting that fibrillar proteins may have therapeutic effect in human breast cancer cells. We thus further investigated the effects of the fibrillar form of human serum albumin (F-HSA) on the malignant breast cancer cell lines, TS/A and MDA-MB-231. We chose F-HSA for further study for two reasons: first, because F-HSA is less likely to provoke an immune response in the human body; and second, because HSA is easier to obtain and less costly than FN. We produced F-HSA using the same process as was used to produce F-BSA. In brief, 20 mg of HSA from human serum was dissolved in 10 ml of PBS with 1% SDS (w/v). The HSA solution was sonicated for 5 minutes and subsequently applied to a Superdex-200 column previously equilibrated with the eluting buffer (25 mM Tris-HCl, pH 8.0, 1 mM EDTA, 0.1 M NaCl, and 0.05% SDS). The fractions that contained HSA were pooled and dialysed against PBS to remove SDS. The yield of the F-HSA was about 67% (Fig. 1). The F-HSA produced was then tested for fibrillar structure by transmission electron microscopy (TEM). For TEM analysis of F-HSA, 2 mg/ml of protein was applied to a 300-mesh carbon-coated copper grid. Excess samples were removed, and the grid was air dried. The protein-bearing grid was negatively stained with 1% (w/v) phosphotungstic acid for 1 minute. Transmission electron micrographs were observed at 20,000–150,000× magnification at 75 kV on a Hitachi H-7000 electron microscope. TEM analysis showed that F-HSA did indeed have a fibril structure (Fig. 2).

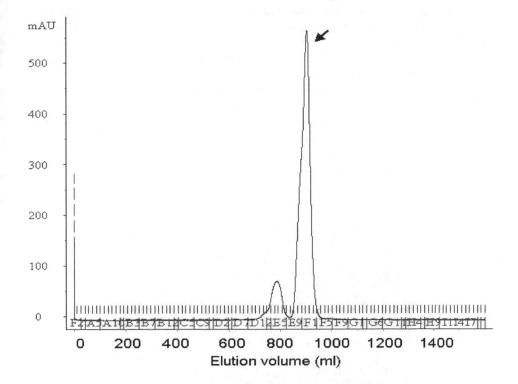

Fig. 1. Elution profile of F-HSA from a Superdex-200 column. HSA (2 mg/ml dissolved in PBS containing 1% SDS) was applied to a Superdex-200 column and eluted at a rate of 1 ml/min with a buffer solution containing 0.05% SDS. Arrow shows F-HSA.

Specific binding to Thioflavin T (ThT) is one of the characteristics of amyloid-like proteins. ThT fluorescence assay was, thus, used to identify amyloid-like fibrils (LeVine, 1999). Like Aβ (1-42), which is known to have fibrillar structure and was used as a positive control, F-HSA obtained from the Superdex-200 column exhibited a gradual dose-dependent increase in ThT fluorescence level (Fig. 3).

6. Effects of F-HSA on cell viability

Previously, we demonstrated that F-BSA and F-FN induced apoptosis in the less malignant T47D and MCF-7 breast cancer cell lines, respectively (Huang et al, 2009; Huang et al, 2010). In this study, we examine whether F-HSA induced cytotoxicity in the more malignant breast cancer cell lines, TS/A and MDA-MB-231, using a 3-(4,5-cimethylthiazol-2-yl)-2,5-diphenyl tetrazolium bromide (MTT)-colorimetry assay to measure the cell viability (MERCK, Darmstadt, Germany). TS/A, a murine mammary adenocarcinoma cell line that is estrogen dependent, was cultured in Dulbecco's modified Eagle's medium (DMEM; GIBCO®); and MDA-MB-231 (ATCC **HTB-26™**), a metastatic human breast cancer cell line that is estrogen independent, was cultured in DMEM/F12 medium (GIBCO®). In brief, 2×10^4 breast cancer cells were incubated in serum-free medium and treated with serial dilutions of F-HSA. After incubation for 24 hours to allow the drug to take effect, 10 μl MTT solution was added to each well. After incubation at 37°C in 5% CO_2 for another 2 hours to allow the MTT solution to be metabolized, formazan (MTT metabolic product) was resuspended in 200 ul DMSO. Finally, the proportions of surviving cells were determined by optical density (570 nm test wavelength, 630 nm reference wavelength). The percentage of surviving cells was calculated as (O.D.$_{treatment}$/O.D.$_{control}$) × 100%, and the percentage of growth inhibition was calculated as [1 - (O.D.$_{treatment}$/O.D.$_{control}$)] × 100%. IC$_{50}$ value is the concentration at which the reagent produces 50% inhibition of cellular viability. F-HSA inhibited growth of the breast cancer cell lines TS/A and MDA-MB-231 in a dose dependent manner with IC$_{50}$ values of 0.15 and 0.48 μM, respectively (Fig. 4). F-HSA at concentrations over 0.4 μM induced dose-dependent cytotoxicity in both TS/A cells and MDA-MB-231 cells, whereas concentrations of 0.1-0.2 μM did not affect cell viability significantly.

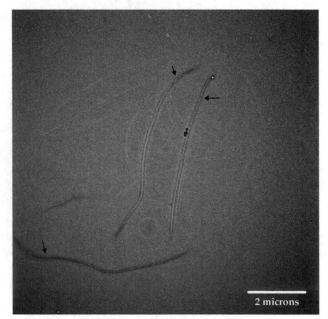

2 microns

Fig. 2. Ultra-structures of F-HSA were observed by TEM. F-HSA was applied to a 300-mesh carbon-coated copper grid then the grid was air-dried. The F-HSA-bearing grid was negatively stained with 1% (w/v) phosphotungstic acid. Finally, transmission electron micrographs were observed at 20,000–150,000× magnification at 75 kV on a Hitachi H-7000 electron microscope. Arrows show F-HSA.

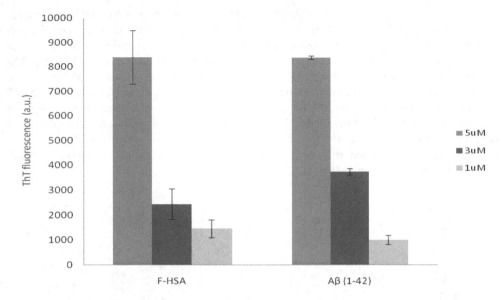

Fig. 3. ThT fluorescence assay of F-HSA. For fluorescence measurements, increasing concentrations of proteins were incubated with 20 μM ThT for 1 h at room temperature, and fluorescence was measured in triplicate on a Wallac Victor² 1420 Multilabel Counter (Perkin Elmer Life Science, Waltham, MA, USA). Excitation and emission wavelengths were 430 nm and 486 nm, respectively. ThT background signal from buffer solution was subtracted from the corresponding measurements. Aβ (1-42) was used as a positive control.

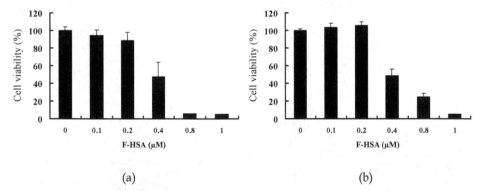

(a)   (b)

Fig. 4. Effect of F-HSA on viability of TS/A (A) and MDA-MB-231 cells (B).

To understand the effects of F-HSA on cell morphology and MET in TS/A cells and MDA-MB-231 cells, breast cancer cells were treated low concentrations of F-HSA and cell morphology was observed under light microscopy. F-HSA induced a morphological alteration in cells, from a fibroblast-like shape to a round shape (Fig. 5). We also examined whether F-HSA suppressed breast cancer-cell migration at non-cytotoxic concentrations by wound-healing assay. TS/A and MDA-MB-231 cells were plated onto six-well tissue culture dishes in complete tissue culture medium until they formed a confluent monolayer. The cell monolayer was scratched with a sterile pipette tip to generate a wound (width 2 mm). The remaining cells were washed three times with culture medium to remove cell debris. The medium was immediately replaced with serum-free medium with 0.1 or 0.2 μM of F-HSA, and cultured at 37°C for 24 hours. Spontaneous cellular migration was then monitored at 0 hours (immediately after wounding) and 24 hours (the end of F-HSA treatment) using and inverted microscope (Axiovert 200M; Zeiss) at 100× original magnification. The extent of wound healing was determined by the distance (migrating distance) traversed by cells migrating into the denuded area. F-HSA at concentrations of 0.1 to 0.2 μM suppressed cell migration of both TS/A and MDA-MB-231 cells (Figs. 6-7).

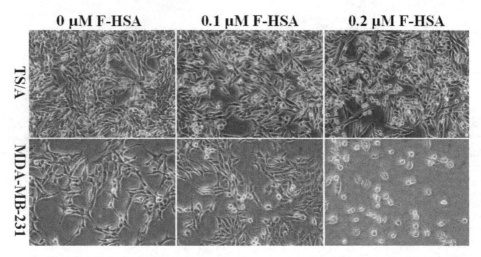

Fig. 5. F-HSA induced morphological alterations and mesenchymal-to-epithelial transition in breast cancer cells. After 0.1 μM and 0.2 μM of F-HSA treatment at 37°C for 24 h, cell morphology was observed under light microscopy. Scale bar, 5 μm

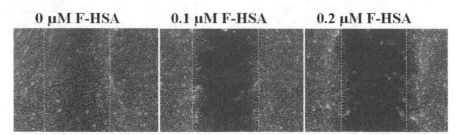

Fig. 6. F-HSA suppressed TS/A cell migration in a breast cancer cell wound-healing assay. After 0.1 μM and 0.2 μM of F-HSA treatment at 37°C for 24 h, cell migration was observed under light microscopy.

Fig. 7. F-HSA suppressed MDA-MB-231 cell migration in a wound-healing assay. After 0.1 µM and 0.2 µM of F-HSA treatment at 37°C for 24 h, cell migration was observed under light microscopy.

7. F-HSA suppresses breast cancer cell migration via β1 integrin signaling pathway

Cell surface receptors mediate cell-to-matrix and cell-to-cell interactions. Integrins are a large family of heterodimeric transmembrane receptors that mediate cell-ECM interactions. In eukayotic cells, integrins consist of 18 α subunits and 8 β subunits that form 24 different αβ integrins. The particular combination of α and β subunits in integrin dimers determines their specificity for ligands, which include most of the ECM proteins such as FN and collagen (Plow et al, 2000). Upon activation by ECM proteins, integrins mediate cellular adhesion, migration, survival, and proliferation (Ginsberg et al, 2005). Integrin signaling is activated by ECM proteins or growth factors through focal adhesion kinase (FAK), PI3K, and Akt, a major downstream target of PI3K signaling, known to be involved in various cellular processes such as cell survival, cell cycle, metabolism, protein synthesis, and transcriptional regulation (Mitra & Schlaepfer, 2006). We showed that fibrillar proteins induced cellular apoptosis (Huang et al, 2009; Huang et al, 2010). The mechanism of the cytotoxic effects of F-BSA in BHK-21 cells (baby hamster kidney cell) was due to modulation of the α5β1 integrin/FAK/Akt/GSK-3β/caspase-3 signaling pathway. Furthermore, F-FN induced cytotoxicity via activating SHP-2 and RhoA/ROCK, and deactivation of Akt/GSK-3β. Taken together these findings suggested that β1 integrin may play a critical role in mediating cancer growth and metastasis. Therefore, we measured the proportion of α5 integrin+ cells or β1 integrin+ cells in TS/A and MDA-MB-231 cells by flow cytometry. First, TS/A or MDA-MB-231 cells were collected and washed with 1× PBS three times. Then, specific monoclonal antibodies for α5 integrin-FITC and β1 integrin-FITC were added and co-incubated with cells (1×10^5/ml) at 4°C for 30 minutes. Cells were then washed three times using 1× PBS and finally stained with 5 µg/ml propidium iodide (PI) at 4°C for 10 minutes to exclude dead cells. Cell viability was determined using a flow cytometer (FACSCalibur; BD Bioscience) and CellQuest software. Data showed that 58.67% and 66.19% of TS/A cells were α5 integrin+ and β1 integrin+, respectively. 42.99% and 97.65% of MDA-MB-231 cells were α5 integrin+ and β1 integrin+, respectively (Table 1). Blocking β1 integrin signaling pathway with a specific mAb (mouse anti-human integrin beta1 monoclonal antibody; Millipore) could reverse F-HSA's effect on TS/A and MDA-MB-231 breast cancer cell migration (Fig. 8). Taken together, these results indicated that the suppression of breast cancer migration by F-HSA may be mediated by binding of β1 integrin.

	α5 integrin	β1 integrin
TS/A	58.67 (%)	66.19 (%)
MDA-MB-231	42.99 (%)	97.65 (%)

Table 1. Percentages of α5 integrin⁺ cells and β1 integrin⁺ cells in TS/A and MDA-MB-231 cells.

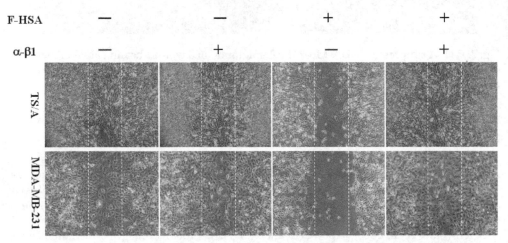

Fig. 8. Blocking the β1 integrin signaling pathway with a specific mAb (mouse anti-human integrin beta1 monoclonal antibody) reversed the effect of 0.2 μM F-HSA on TS/A and MDA-MB-231 breast cancer cell migration.

8. Conclusion

The search for novel therapeutic targets and the development of inhibitors of cancer metastasis is an ongoing challenge. Herein, we used a detergent assisted refolding chromatography process to convert globular HSA into fibrillar F-HSA. Unlike globular HSA, this novel F-HSA caused cell death, reversed EMT, and suppressed breast cancer cell migration through targeting β1 integrin signaling pathway. These important findings may be useful for the development of better therapeutics for the intervention of breast cancer metastasis.

9. Acknowledgments

Grant support: National Science Council, Taiwan (NSC 96-2313-B-001-005-MY3 to S.-M.L) and Academia Sinica (to S.-M.L.). We thank Miss Miranda Loney (Institute of Molecular Biology, Academia Sinica, Taiwan) for English editorial assistance.

10. References

Azakami H, Mukai A, Kato A (2005) Role of amyloid type cross beta-structure in the formation of soluble aggregate and gel in heat-induced ovalbumin. *J Agric Food Chem* 53(4): 1254-1257

Belletti B, Vaidya JS, D'Andrea S, Entschladen F, Roncadin M, Lovat F, Berton S, Perin T, Candiani E, Reccanello S, Veronesi A, Canzonieri V, Trovo MG, Zaenker KS, Colombatti A, Baldassarre G, Massarut S (2008) Targeted intraoperative radiotherapy impairs the stimulation of breast cancer cell proliferation and invasion caused by surgical wounding. *Clin Cancer Res* 14(5): 1325-1332

Bergstralh DT, Ting JP (2006) Microtubule stabilizing agents: their molecular signaling consequences and the potential for enhancement by drug combination. *Cancer Treat Rev* 32(3): 166-179

Brooks PC, Montgomery AM, Rosenfeld M, Reisfeld RA, Hu T, Klier G, Cheresh DA (1994) Integrin alpha v beta 3 antagonists promote tumor regression by inducing apoptosis of angiogenic blood vessels. *Cell* 79(7): 1157-1164

Brown PH, Subbaramaiah K, Salmon AP, Baker R, Newman RA, Yang P, Zhou XK, Bissonnette RP, Dannenberg AJ, Howe LR (2008) Combination chemoprevention of HER2/neu-induced breast cancer using a cyclooxygenase-2 inhibitor and a retinoid X receptor-selective retinoid. *Cancer Prev Res (Phila)* 1(3): 208-214

Gharibyan AL, Zamotin V, Yanamandra K, Moskaleva OS, Margulis BA, Kostanyan IA, Morozova-Roche LA (2007) Lysozyme amyloid oligomers and fibrils induce cellular death via different apoptotic/necrotic pathways. *J Mol Biol* 365(5): 1337-1349

Ginsberg MH, Partridge A, Shattil SJ (2005) Integrin regulation. *Curr Opin Cell Biol* 17(5): 509-516

Giordano SH, Hortobagyi GN (2003) Inflammatory breast cancer: clinical progress and the main problems that must be addressed. *Breast Cancer Res* 5(6): 284-288

Gonzalez-Angulo AM, Morales-Vasquez F, Hortobagyi GN (2007) Overview of resistance to systemic therapy in patients with breast cancer. *Adv Exp Med Biol* 608: 1-22

Huang CY, Liang CM, Chu CL, Liang SM (2009) Albumin fibrillization induces apoptosis via integrin/FAK/Akt pathway. *BMC Biotechnol* 9: 2

Huang CY, Liang CM, Chu CL, Peng JM, Liang SM (2010) A fibrillar form of fibronectin induces apoptosis by activating SHP-2 and stress fiber formation. *Apoptosis* 15(8): 915-926

Im JH, Fu W, Wang H, Bhatia SK, Hammer DA, Kowalska MA, Muschel RJ (2004) Coagulation facilitates tumor cell spreading in the pulmonary vasculature during early metastatic colony formation. *Cancer Res* 64(23): 8613-8619

Jackson GS, Clarke AR (2000) Mammalian prion proteins. *Curr Opin Struct Biol* 10(1): 69-74

Jahanzeb M (2008) Adjuvant trastuzumab therapy for HER2-positive breast cancer. *Clin Breast Cancer* 8(4): 324-333

Jemal A, Siegel R, Ward E, Murray T, Xu J, Thun MJ (2007) Cancer statistics, 2007. *CA Cancer J Clin* 57(1): 43-66

Jemal A, Siegel R, Xu J, Ward E (2010) Cancer statistics, 2010. *CA Cancer J Clin* 60(5): 277-300

Kim S, Bell K, Mousa SA, Varner JA (2000) Regulation of angiogenesis *in vivo* by ligation of integrin alpha5beta1 with the central cell-binding domain of fibronectin. *Am J Pathol* 156(4): 1345-1362

Kumar CC, Malkowski M, Yin Z, Tanghetti E, Yaremko B, Nechuta T, Varner J, Liu M, Smith EM, Neustadt B, Presta M, Armstrong L (2001) Inhibition of angiogenesis and tumor growth by SCH221153, a dual alpha(v)beta3 and alpha(v)beta5 integrin receptor antagonist. *Cancer Res* 61(5): 2232-2238

Kuwada SK, Kuang J, Li X (2005) Integrin alpha5/beta1 expression mediates HER-2 down-regulation in colon cancer cells. *J Biol Chem* 280(19): 19027-19035

Lee JM, Dedhar S, Kalluri R, Thompson EW (2006) The epithelial-mesenchymal transition: new insights in signaling, development, and disease. *J Cell Biol* 172(7): 973-981

LeVine H, 3rd (1999) Quantification of beta-sheet amyloid fibril structures with thioflavin T. *Methods Enzymol* 309: 274-284

Lu X, Lu D, Scully M, Kakkar V (2008) The role of integrins in cancer and the development of anti-integrin therapeutic agents for cancer therapy. *Perspect Medicin Chem* 2: 57-73

McGrogan BT, Gilmartin B, Carney DN, McCann A (2008) Taxanes, microtubules and chemoresistant breast cancer. *Biochim Biophys Acta* 1785(2): 96-132

McSherry EA, Donatello S, Hopkins AM, McDonnell S (2007) Molecular basis of invasion in breast cancer. *Cell Mol Life Sci* 64(24): 3201-3218

Mitjans F, Meyer T, Fittschen C, Goodman S, Jonczyk A, Marshall JF, Reyes G, Piulats J (2000) In vivo therapy of malignant melanoma by means of antagonists of alphav integrins. *Int J Cancer* 87(5): 716-723

Mitra SK, Schlaepfer DD (2006) Integrin-regulated FAK-Src signaling in normal and cancer cells. *Curr Opin Cell Biol* 18(5): 516-523

Mullamitha SA, Ton NC, Parker GJ, Jackson A, Julyan PJ, Roberts C, Buonaccorsi GA, Watson Y, Davies K, Cheung S, Hope L, Valle JW, Radford JA, Lawrance J, Saunders MP, Munteanu MC, Nakada MT, Nemeth JA, Davis HM, Jiao Q, Prabhakar U, Lang Z, Corringham RE, Beckman RA, Jayson GC (2007) Phase I evaluation of a fully human anti-alphav integrin monoclonal antibody (CNTO 95) in patients with advanced solid tumors. *Clin Cancer Res* 13(7): 2128-2135

O'Connor P (2007) Natalizumab and the role of alpha 4-integrin antagonism in the treatment of multiple sclerosis. *Expert Opin Biol Ther* 7(1): 123-136

Pasterkamp RJ, Peschon JJ, Spriggs MK, Kolodkin AL (2003) Semaphorin 7A promotes axon outgrowth through integrins and MAPKs. *Nature* 424(6947): 398-405

Plow EF, Haas TA, Zhang L, Loftus J, Smith JW (2000) Ligand binding to integrins. *J Biol Chem* 275(29): 21785-21788

Shook D, Keller R (2003) Mechanisms, mechanics and function of epithelial-mesenchymal transitions in early development. *Mech Dev* 120(11): 1351-1383

Stickeler E, Klar M, Watermann D, Geibel A, Foldi M, Hasenburg A, Gitsch G (2009) Pegylated liposomal doxorubicin and trastuzumab as 1st and 2nd line therapy in her2/neu positive metastatic breast cancer: a multicenter phase II trial. *Breast Cancer Res Treat* 117(3): 591-598

Su Y, Chang PT (2001) Acidic pH promotes the formation of toxic fibrils from beta-amyloid peptide. *Brain Res* 893(1-2): 287-291

Suzuki K, Okuno T, Yamamoto M, Pasterkamp RJ, Takegahara N, Takamatsu H, Kitao T, Takagi J, Rennert PD, Kolodkin AL, Kumanogoh A, Kikutani H (2007) Semaphorin 7A initiates T-cell-mediated inflammatory responses through alpha1beta1 integrin. *Nature* 446(7136): 680-684

Taboada P, Barbosa S, Castro E, Mosquera V (2006) Amyloid fibril formation and other aggregate species formed by human serum albumin association. *J Phys Chem B* 110(42): 20733-20736

Zamotin V, Gharibyan A, Gibanova NV, Lavrikova MA, Dolgikh DA, Kirpichnikov MP, Kostanyan IA, Morozova-Roche LA (2006) Cytotoxicity of albebetin oligomers depends on cross-beta-sheet formation. *FEBS Lett* 580(10): 2451-2457

Ziober BL, Chen YQ, Ramos DM, Waleh N, Kramer RH (1999) Expression of the alpha7beta1 laminin receptor suppresses melanoma growth and metastatic potential. *Cell Growth Differ* 10(7): 479-490

6

On the Role of Cell Surface Chondroitin Sulfates and Their Core Proteins in Breast Cancer Metastasis

Ann Marie Kieber-Emmons, Fariba Jousheghany
and Behjatolah Monzavi-Karbassi
Department of Pathology and Winthrop P. Rockefeller Cancer institute
University of Arkansas for Medical Sciences
Little Rock
USA

1. Introduction

Breast cancer is the most common cancer diagnosis among women worldwide (Jemal et al., 2011). Significant numbers of women present with advanced metastatic breast cancer despite major improvements in population screening and health awareness (Breast Cancer Facts & Figures 2009-2010, 2009; Autier et al., 2011). Metastatic spread leads to the poor prognosis and incurring low survival rates of patients presenting with advanced stage breast cancer or tumor recurrence. Therefore, effective therapies targeting metastatic spread should be designed to prevent the devastating consequences of breast cancer progression. In this regard, novel pro-metastatic molecules must be identified and their functional roles in the progression of the disease need to be addressed.

Cell–cell and cell–matrix adhesions have a profound role in the hematogenous phase of cancer metastasis. Tumor-associated glycans participate in these cell–cell and cell–matrix adhesions and their expression is associated with the metastatic potential of tumor cells and the prognosis of cancer patients (Hakomori, 1996; Couldrey and Green, 2000; Gorelik et al., 2001; Kawaguchi, 2005; Korourian et al., 2008).

We have been studying the role carbohydrates play in breast cancer metastasis (Monzavi-Karbassi et al., 2005; Carcel-Trullols et al., 2006; Monzavi-Karbassi et al., 2007). A large body of evidence indicates that P-selectin expressed on endothelial cells and platelets plays a crucial role during hematogenous metastasis (Borsig et al., 2001; Kohler et al., 2010). In a murine model of breast cancer we observed that the expression of carbohydrates that react with the P-selectin receptor plays a major role in metastasis (Monzavi-Karbassi et al., 2005). This evidence indicates that P-selectin-mediated interaction of breast cancer cells with platelets is a relevant cellular adhesion mechanism that participates in establishing distant metastases. A novel finding in our work is the observation that chondroitin sulfate glycosaminoglycans (CS-GAGs) can serve as P-selectin ligands on breast cancer cells. This observation links CS-GAGs to P-selectin binding in defining the metastatic phenotype dependent on the interaction of cancer cells with platelets (Monzavi-Karbassi et al., 2007). Therefore, CS-GAGs can be targeted for development of novel anti-metastatic therapies.

Large variation exists in CS-GAG sequences and in proteoglycans (PGs) presenting them. The prevalence of a presenting core protein may predict the functional outcomes of P-selectin-mediated adhesion of tumor cells. To use these molecules as targets for diagnostic or therapeutic purposes, a thorough understanding of their presentation and expression is necessary. This chapter reviews the biological roles of chondroitin sulfates (CS) in tumor development and metastasis and the role of different types of CS and the core protein carrying these polysaccharides.

2. Chondroitin sulfate biosynthesis and presentation

A relative variation in the composition of CS/DS has been reported in neoplastic tissues (Chiarugi and Dietrich, 1979; Bumol et al., 1982; Reisfeld and Cheresh, 1987; Olsen et al., 1988; Alini and Losa, 1991; Vijayagopal et al., 1998; Vynios et al., 2008).

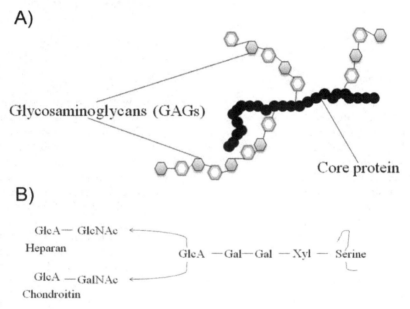

Fig. 1. **A)** Proteoglycans consist of a core protein and covalently attached GAG chains. **B)** Biosynthesis of chondroitin and heparan sulfate building blocks initiates by the formation of a linkage tetrasaccharide attached to serine residue on the core protein. GlcA: Glucuronic acid; GlcNAc: N-acetyl-D-glucosamine; GalNAc: N-acetyl-D-galactosamine; Gal: Galactose; Xyl: xylose.

Chondroitin sulfate (CS)/ dermatan sulfate (DS) polysaccharides are widely distributed in extracellular matrices and at cell surfaces as PGs, in which glycosaminoglycan (GAG) chains are covalently attached to a variety of core proteins (**Figure 1A**) (Esko et al., 1999). Chondroitin or heparan backbone is synthesized on the common GAG-protein linkage region tetrasaccharide (GlcUA-Galactose-Galactose-Xlylose) (**Figure 1B**), which is attached to specific serine residues in the respective core protein (Silbert and Sugumaran, 2002; Sugahara et al., 2003).

The Chondroitin chain backbone consists of repetitive disaccharide units containing D-glucuronic acid (GlcUA) and *N*-acetyl-D-galactosamine (GalNAc) residues. They further differentiate into variable chains with distinct structures and functions after various modifications. Sulfation and epimerization will further generate CS/DS isomers (**Table 1**). DS or CS-B is a stereoisomeric variant of CS with varying proportions of L-iduronic acid (IdoUA) in place of GlcUA, which forms by epimerization of GlcUA to IdoUA (**Table 1**).

Chondroitin type	Disaccharide repeat	Modifying enzymes	
		Sulfotransferase	Epimerase
A	[GlcUAβ1-3GalNAc(4S)]	Carbohydrate (chondroitin-4) sulfotransferase 11, 12 and 13 (CHST11, CHST12 and CHST13)	-
B	[IdoUA(2s)α1-3GalNAc(4S)]	Uronyl-2-O-sulfotransferase (UST) and CHST11, CHST12 and Carbohydrate (N-acetylgalactosamine 4-O) Sulfotransferase 14 (CHST14)	Dermatan-sulfate 5-epimerase
C	[GlcUAβ1-3GalNAc(6S)]	Carbohydrate (chondroitin 6) sulfotransferase 3 (CHST3) and Carbohydrate (N-acetylglucosamine 6-O) sulfotransferase 7 (CHST7)	-
D	[GlcUA(2S)β1-3GalNAc(6S)]	UST, CHST3 and CHST7	-
E	[GlcUAβ1-3GalNAc(4S,6S)]	CHST11, CHST12, CHST13 and CHST15 (N-acetylgalactosamine 4-sulfate 6-O-sulfotransferase)	-
iE	[IdoUAα1-3GalNAc(4S,6S)]	CHST11, CHST12, CHST14 and CHST15	Dermatan-sulfate 5-epimerase

Table 1. Chondroitin sulfate types

The monosulfated disaccharide A-unit [GlcUA-GalNAc(4S)] and C-unit [GlcUA-GalNAc(6S)] are common and major components of mammalian CS chains. Disulfated disaccharide D-unit [GlcUA(2S)-GalNAc(6S)] and E-unit [GlcUA-GalNAc(4S,6S)] also exist that are based on further sulfation of monosulfated C and A units, respectively.

CS/DS chains that often found as CS/DS hybrid structures have the potential to display an enormous structural diversity by embedding multiple overlapping sequences constructed with distinct disaccharide blocks modified by different patterns of sulfation (Kusche-Gullberg and Kjellen, 2003; Sugahara et al., 2003). Given the complexity of these structures, the expression of modifying enzymes may correlate better with an aggressive tumor phenotype. Therefore, linking the expression of these enzymes with a functional role of cell surface CS glycans is highly significant

2.1 Biological functions of CS/DS chains

CS/DS chains specifically interact with heparin binding proteins. The interaction of DS chains with fibroblast growth factor (FGF) activates FGF-2 to signal cell proliferation (Penc et al., 1998). DS also acts as a cofactor for FGF-7 (Trowbridge et al., 2002). In addition, DS has been shown to bind and activate hepatocyte growth factor/scatter factor (HGF/SF), a paracrine growth factor whose receptor, c-met (previously characterized as a proto-oncogene), is also a transmembrane tyrosine kinase.

The CS/DS chains of the PG versican, which is expressed in many tissues including kidney, skin, aorta, and brain, bind the adhesion molecules L- and P-selectin (Kawashima et al., 2002), molecules that have been implicated in leukocyte trafficking, inflammatory disease, and tumor dissemination. Interestingly, these interactions are specifically inhibited by CS or DS containing the 'E' disaccharide unit GlcUA-GalNAc (4S, 6S) or the 'iE' unit IdoUA-GalNAc (4S, 6S), respectively.

In previous studies we found that CS/DS-GAGs are expressed on the cell surface of murine and human breast cancer cell lines with high metastatic capacity. This suggests that CS/DS-GAGs can mediate P-selectin binding and P-selectin-mediated adhesion of cancer cells to platelets and endothelial cells (Monzavi-Karbassi et al., 2007). In inhibition assays performed in vitro, we showed that among the CS types only CS-B (DS), and CS-E can efficiently block P-selectin binding to tumor cells (Monzavi-Karbassi et al., 2007). Other studies have also suggested important interactions mediated by CS-A and CS-E in tumor progression and metastasis (Iida et al., 2007; Li et al., 2008; Basappa et al., 2009). Therefore, enzymes involved in sulfation (sulfotransferases) or epimerization (DS epimerase) of CS chains may play a fundamental role in defining the malignant phenotype of breast tumors.

The expression of several sulfotransferases including CHST11 and CHST15 appears to be greater in human breast carcinoma compared to normal breast tissue (Potapenko et al., 2010). An increase in CHST11 expression is observed in malignant plasma cells from myeloma patients compared to normal bone-marrow plasma cells (Bret et al., 2009). In searches for genes involved in the transition of DCIS to IDC, Schuetz et al. (Schuetz et al., 2006) found a significant increase in DS epimerase (Maccarana et al., 2006).

Collectively, the evidence implicates CS/DS GAGs in a wide array of molecular and cellular interactions resulting in tumorigenesis and metastasis.

3. Potential cell membrane CS/DS-carrying PGs of breast carcinoma

Malignant neoplasms exhibit changes in production of PGs (Bumol and Reisfeld, 1982; Iozzo, 1985; Iozzo, 1988; Stylianou et al., 2008). The variation, abundance and function of CS/DS-GAGs are also affected by the expression of the PG core protein presenting them. Therefore, it is imperative to study these polysaccharides in the context of their carrying PG. PG are involved in signaling and tumorigenicity and their attached GAG contributes to their functions. There is a growing list of PGs that have been implicated as possessing CS/DS side chains (Esko et al., 1999; Taylor and Gallo, 2006). PGs that may be modified by CS/DS chains include aggrecan, neurocan, brevican, bamacan, a CD44 isoform, chondroitin sulfate proteoglycan 4 (CSPG4), syndecans, betaglycan, serglycin, versican, decorin, biglycan, and endocan, most of which are extracellular matrix PGs. Our focus is on the cell membrane PGs that are able to bind to P-selectin (Monzavi-Karbassi et al., 2007). CD44 variants (CD44v), CSPG4, syndecan-1 (SDC-1) and syndecan-4 (SDC-4) are among the cell surface candidates (Faassen et al., 1992; Jackson et al., 1995; Barbareschi et al., 2003; Burbach et al., 2003; Baba et al., 2006; Gotte et al., 2007; Wang et al., 2010). Recently, It has been demonstrated that substantial fraction of neuropilin-1 (NRP-1), a membrane glycoprotein, is a PG modified with either HS or CS-GAG chains (Shintani et al., 2006).

Many articles are now devoted to CD44 in cancer stem cells and its role in cancer progression and metastasis (Lesley et al., 1997; Naor et al., 1997; Lesley and Hyman, 1998; Kalish et al., 1999; Toole, 2009). Here we focus on SDC-1, SDC-4, CSPG4 and NRP-1 as potential CS-carrying PGs on the surface of breast tumor cells.

3.1 Role of CS-carrying PGs in tumor progression and metastasis

Alteration in the production and structure of GAG chains and the functional consequences of such alterations is dependent on the PG carrying the GAG chain. PGs isolated from carcinomas contained 32.2% more CS, 18% less DS, and 30% less HS than PGs of normal breast tissue (Vijayagopal et al., 1998). Chondroitin sulfate proteoglycans (CSPGs) were expressed significantly more often in metastases than in primary tumors of uveal melanoma (Kiewe et al., 2006). We have recently found that CSPGs on breast cancer cells also bind to P-selectin receptors, and interruption of this interaction leads to significant reduction in hematogenous metastasis (Monzavi-Karbassi et al., 2007).

Selectin-mediated binding of tumor cells to platelets, leukocytes, and vascular endothelium may regulate their hematogenous spread in the microvasculature (Krause and Turner, 1999). Among selectin molecules, evidence strongly supports P-selectin involvement in tumor metastasis (Kim et al., 1998; Stevenson et al., 2005). Our data suggest that inhibition of P-selectin interaction with CS-GAGs significantly attenuates hematogenous lung metastasis (Monzavi-Karbassi et al., 2007). We have demonstrated that P-selectin binding to the surface of the aggressive breast cancer cell line MDA-MB-231 and MDA-MET is also CS-dependent, suggesting a role for CSPGs in metastatic behavior of human cancer cells. Because of the role of some of these PGs in signaling and tumor phenotype, we speculate that P-selectin interaction with a particular PG may lead to an exclusive tumor cell activation, and consequently survival in circulation. Here, we review the role of the surface PGs able to present CS-GAGs in malignancy.

3.1.1 CSPG4

CSPG4 is a human homolog of Rat neuroglycan 2 (NG2), which is also known as High Molecular Weight Melanoma Associated Antigen and Melanoma Chondroitin Sulfate Proteoglycan (Stallcup, 1981; Bumol and Reisfeld, 1982; Pluschke et al., 1996) and exclusively carries CS chains (Bumol and Reisfeld, 1982; Nishiyama et al., 1991). This tumor-associated cell surface PG potentiates cell motility, promotes invasiveness and the metastatic potential of tumor cells in melanoma (Burg et al., 1998; Campoli et al., 2004; Iida et al., 2007; Wang et al., 2010), and modulates responses to growth factors (Grako and Stallcup, 1995; Yang et al., 2009), processes that are critical for the proliferation and migration of tumor cells. It is suggested that CSPG4 facilitates the invasion of aggressive primary tumors within the dermis by enhancing the local concentration and/or activation of specific matrix metalloproteinases (MMPs) at sites of contact between melanoma cells and the underlying ECM (Iida et al., 2001). The authors demonstrated that CSPG4 on WM1341D cells, interacts with membrane-type matrix metalloproteinase (MT3-MMP), facilitating invasion, and that the interaction is CS-dependent. Inhibiting CS presentation by treating cells with p-nitrophenyl beta-D-xylopyranoside (beta-D-xyloside or βDX), a compound that uncouples the CS chain from the PG, led to a decrease in melanoma cell invasion into type I collagen (Faassen et al., 1992). CSPG4 is highly expressed on aggressive breast cancer cell lines **(Figure 2)** and is considered as a major CS-carrying PG.

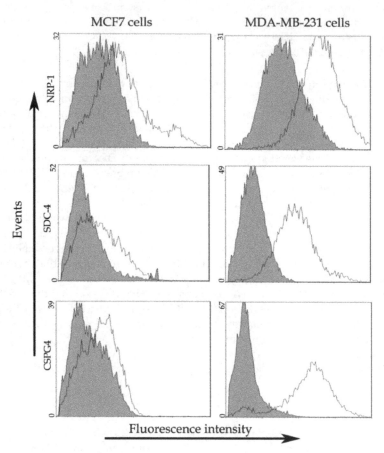

Fig. 2. Expression of NRP-1, SDC-4 and CSPG4 in breast cancer cells. Cells were grown in standard medium, harvested and then stained with monoclonal antibodies against the indicated targets. Stained cells were then analyzed by flow cytometry.

3.1.2 NRP-1

NRP-1 is a 120-130 kDa transmembrane glycoprotein, initially characterized as a neuronal receptor for specific secreted members of the semaphorin family involved in exon repulsation (Kolodkin et al., 1997). A substantial fraction of NRP-1 is a PG with a GAG chain attached (Shintani et al., 2006). In addition to being a receptor for a number of class 3 semaphorins, NRP-1 also serves as a receptor for some members of vascular endothelial growth factor (VEGF), and placental growth factor (PlGF) (Migdal et al., 1998; Soker et al., 1998; Makinen et al., 1999; Wise et al., 1999; Klagsbrun et al., 2002).

Considerable data support a functional role for NRP-1 in regulating VEGF activities in endothelium. It has been shown that semaphorin-3A competes with $VEGF_{165}$ binding to NRP-1 and inhibits angiogenesis *in vitro* (Miao et al., 1999). NRP-1 knock-out mice, in addition to neural defects, exhibit transposition of large vessels, disorganized and insufficient capillary formation, and defects in heart development (Kawasaki et al., 1999). In contrast, over-expression of NRP-1 leads to over-stimulation of blood vessel formation (Kitsukawa et al., 1995). Studies have shown that NRP-1interacts with a subset of heparin binding proteins like FGF-1, FGF-2, FGF-4, FGF-7, FGF receptor-1, and HGF/SF (West et al., 2005). Investigation of the role of NRP-1 in human glioma progression, Hu et al. (Hu et al., 2007) have shown that NRP-1 expression correlates with tumor progression in clinical setting, and that NRP-1 expression promotes tumor growth and survival through an autocrine HGF/SF/c-met signaling pathway. We observed an overexpression of NRP-1 in aggressive human breast cancer cell line MDA-MB-231 compare to MCF-7 cells (**Figure 2**). This PG is also considered as a potential CS-carrying PG that can present CS-GAGs to P-selectin.

3.1.3 SDC-1 and SDC-4

SDC-1 is mainly expressed by epithelia and plasma cells. Although there are inconsistent reports (Barbareschi et al., 2003; Tsanou et al., 2004), the expression of SDC-1 is generally down-regulated in malignant tumors, and lower levels of expression have been associated with high metastatic/aggressive potential in many tumors (Nackaerts et al., 1997; Kumar-Singh et al., 1998; Mikami et al., 2001; Numa et al., 2002). SDC-1 has also been shown to act as a tumor suppressor molecule by inhibiting cell growth and inducing apoptosis (Mali et al., 1994; Dhodapkar et al., 1998). Therefore, during tumor development the decrease of SDC-1 expression may be an important step from tumorigenesis to a metastatic phenotype. However, there are conflicting data on the role of SDC-1; both its loss and over-expression in carcinoma cells have been associated with malignant progression (Baba et al., 2006).

SDC-4 is more ubiquitously expressed by most cell types, and little is known about its role in malignancy. Among the four members of the syndecan family, SDC-4 is the only one involved in the formation of fibronectin-induced focal adhesions, in cooperation with β1-integrin receptors (Woods and Couchman, 1994; Woods et al., 2000). SDC-4 has been implicated in cytoskeletal organization and regulation of cell adhesiveness. The migratory capacity of lymphocytes and dendritic cells has been reported to be mediated by SDC-4 (Kaneider et al., 2002; Greene et al., 2003; Feistritzer et al., 2004; Averbeck et al., 2007). Our data suggest a role for relative expression of SDC-1 and SDC-4, low SDC-1 and high SDC-4 expression, in metastatic breast cancer cells (**Figure 3**).

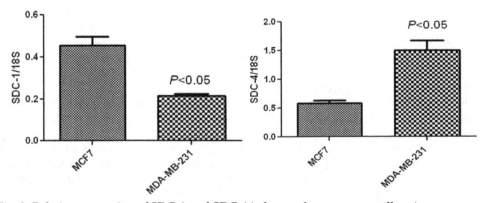

Fig. 3. Relative expression of SDC-1 and SDC-4 in human breast cancer cells using quantitative real-time PCR. Means of three independent experiments (±SD) are shown.

Therefore, relative expression of certain PGs or modification in their GAG chains may affect tumor aggressive phenotype through promoting survival, growth, and the metastatic capability of tumor cells. P-selectin can bind to CS-GAGs of these PGs and binding to each PG can have different functional consequences. These molecules has been linked to motility, invasion, angiogenesis, and cancer stem cell properties. Therefore, depending on the setting and expression of other molecules, P-selectin interaction may lead to various tumor promoting outcomes.

In studying the role of P-selectin in tumor growth and metastasis in a P-selectin-deficient Rag2-/- background, it was demonstrated that growth of subcutaneously challenged tumor cells were reduced significantly in the absence of P-selectin (Kim et al., 1998). This significantly slower growth rate in P-selectin deficient mice was unexpected because P-selectin is assumed to play a role in leukocytic infiltrates within tumors, which are generally inversely associated with tumor growth (Kreider et al., 1984). These findings, consistent with our hypothesis, demonstrate that the presence of P-selectin ligands on tumor cells and P-selectin-mediated interactions with stroma leads to tumorigenesis and tumor growth promotion.

4. Diagnostic and therapeutic values

Overexpression of particular CS chains can be used to develop diagnostic tests predicting tumor behavior or for prognostic purposes. In this regard, further attempts should be made to link the expression of a combination of genes that define GAG remodeling to the initiation and outcome of the disease in clinical setting.

Expression of CS can also be used for drug delivery purposes. Polyethylene glycol coated liposomes, containing a cationic lipid with CS specificity were used to deliver cisplatin to metastatic tumor cells (Lee et al., 2002). The cisplatin loaded CS-reactive liposomes suppressed metastatic spread of the murine osteosarcoma cells to the liver.

We have shown CS interactions with P-selectin and the significance of P-selectin binding in metastasis of a murine mammary cell line (Monzavi-Karbassi et al., 2007). Our findings support the concept that CS chains promote survival in the circulation, and tumor cell extravasation via P-selectin-mediated binding to platelets and endothelial cells. Using heparin to block P-selectin binding to tumor cells as anti-metastatic therapy has been the subject of many studies (Borsig et al., 2001; Stevenson et al., 2005). However, blocking P-selectin action through the inhibition of binding to its many ligands may affect cellular immunity that could be a tumor friendly side effect of a potential treatment. To avoid unfavorable impact of such a treatment on lymphocyte trafficking and infiltration, targeting relevant tumor-specific P-selectin ligands should be prioritized as an alternative long-term therapeutic strategy for aggressive breast cancer.

To develop therapeutics targeting CS entity we envision three major strategies. 1) Targeting particular CS types through blocking the expression of particular CS structures or the usage of small molecules, is supposed to attenuate metastasis efficiency. In this category, blocking the expression of a key sulfotransferase with siRNA may be considered a potential therapeutic approach at this point. Development of small molecules with fine specificity can also be proposed for blocking particular isomers of CS with reactive molecules. 2) Specific targeting of a prominent CS-carrying PG with definite impact on tumor progression and metastasis. CSPG4 is considered a prominent CSPG with a tumor promoting role. MAb targeting CSPG4 have been developed in melanoma and testing them for treatment of patients with aggressive breast cancer falls in line with our data (Wang et al., 2010a; Wang et al., 2010b). However, targeting a core protein may bring in specificity issues as these PGs are also expressed in stroma. Additionally, tumor cells can escape treatment by immune editing and replacing a PG with another one. 3) Targeting a combination of sugar and PG that can be accomplished by simultaneous targeting of the core protein and the polysaccharide, or by developing reagents like mAb specific for the whole entity (polysaccharide and the core protein).

5. Conclusion

Breast cancer cell surface CS-GAGs and their interaction with P-selectin should be considered as viable targets for the development of novel diagnostic or therapeutic strategies. Our studies suggest that CS-GAGs, their biosynthetic pathway, or the core protein carrying them, can be potential targets in dealing with aggressive breast tumors. However, in order to efficiently block tumor cell dissemination by interrupting P-selectin/CS interaction, targeting any single PG does not seem to be enough, as other PGs can probably compensate and support metastatic processes. In this regard, global targeting of specific CS isomers, or combined targeting of the glycan and the PG, may be effective approaches.

6. Acknowledgement

The study was supported in part by a pilot project grant through the UAMS Center for Clinical and Translational Research, Award Number 1UL1RR029884 from the National Center for Research Resources, and in part by a UAMS College of Medicine grant (both to BMK). The funders had no role in the study design, data collection and analysis, decision to publish, or preparation of the manuscript. We thank Dr. Thomas Kieber-Emmons for useful discussions regarding directions for these studies.

7. References

Alini, M & Losa, G A (1991). Partial characterization of proteoglycans isolated from neoplastic and nonneoplastic human breast tissues. *Cancer Res,* Vol. 51, No. 5, pp, 1443-1447.

Autier, P, Boniol, M, Middleton, R, Dore, J F, Hery, C, Zheng, T & Gavin, A (2011). Advanced breast cancer incidence following population-based mammographic screening. *Ann Oncol,* Vol., No., pp.

Averbeck, M, Gebhardt, C, Anderegg, U, Termeer, C, Sleeman, J P & Simon, J C (2007). Switch in syndecan-1 and syndecan-4 expression controls maturation associated dendritic cell motility. *Exp Dermatol,* Vol. 16, No. 7, pp, 580-589.

Baba, F, Swartz, K, van Buren, R, Eickhoff, J, Zhang, Y, Wolberg, W & Friedl, A (2006). Syndecan-1 and syndecan-4 are overexpressed in an estrogen receptor-negative, highly proliferative breast carcinoma subtype. *Breast Cancer Res Treat,* Vol. 98, No. 1, pp, 91-98.

Barbareschi, M, Maisonneuve, P, Aldovini, D, Cangi, M G, Pecciarini, L, Angelo Mauri, F, Veronese, S, Caffo, O, Lucenti, A, Palma, P D, Galligioni, E & Doglioni, C (2003).

High syndecan-1 expression in breast carcinoma is related to an aggressive phenotype and to poorer prognosis. *Cancer*, Vol. 98, No. 3, pp, 474-483.

Basappa, Murugan, S, Sugahara, K N, Lee, C M, ten Dam, G B, van Kuppevelt, T H, Miyasaka, M, Yamada, S & Sugahara, K (2009). Involvement of chondroitin sulfate E in the liver tumor focal formation of murine osteosarcoma cells. *Glycobiology*, Vol. 19, No. 7, pp, 735-742.

Borsig L, Wong R, Feramisco J, Nadeau DR, Varki NM, Varki A (2001). Heparin and cancer revisited: mechanistic connections involving platelets, P-selectin, carcinoma mucins, and tumor metastasis. *Proc Natl Acad Sci U S A*, 98(6):3352-3357.

American cancer Society (2009) "Breast Cancer Facts & Figures 2009-2010."American cancer society, pp, 1-38.

Bret, C, Hose, D, Reme, T, Sprynski, A C, Mahtouk, K, Schved, J F, Quittet, P, Rossi, J F, Goldschmidt, H & Klein, B (2009). Expression of genes encoding for proteins involved in heparan sulphate and chondroitin sulphate chain synthesis and modification in normal and malignant plasma cells. *Br J Haematol*, Vol. 145, No. 3, pp, 350-368.

Bumol, T F, Chee, D O & Reisfeld, R A (1982). Immunochemical and biosynthetic analysis of monoclonal antibody-defined melanoma-associated antigen. *Hybridoma*, Vol. 1, No. 3, pp, 283-292.

Bumol, T F & Reisfeld, R A (1982). Unique glycoprotein-proteoglycan complex defined by monoclonal antibody on human melanoma cells. *Proc Natl Acad Sci U S A*, Vol. 79, No. 4, pp, 1245-1249.

Burbach, B J, Friedl, A, Mundhenke, C & Rapraeger, A C (2003). Syndecan-1 accumulates in lysosomes of poorly differentiated breast carcinoma cells. *Matrix Biol*, Vol. 22, No. 2, pp, 163-177.

Burg, M A, Grako, K A & Stallcup, W B (1998). Expression of the NG2 proteoglycan enhances the growth and metastatic properties of melanoma cells. *J Cell Physiol*, Vol. 177, No. 2, pp, 299-312.

Campoli, M R, Chang, C C, Kageshita, T, Wang, X, McCarthy, J B & Ferrone, S (2004). Human high molecular weight-melanoma-associated antigen (HMW-MAA): a melanoma cell surface chondroitin sulfate proteoglycan (MSCP) with biological and clinical significance. *Crit Rev Immunol*, Vol. 24, No. 4, pp, 267-296.

Carcel-Trullols, J, Stanley, J S, Saha, R, Shaaf, S, Bendre, M S, Monzavi-Karbassi, B, Suva, L J & Kieber-Emmons, T (2006). Characterization of the glycosylation profile of the human breast cancer cell line, MDA-231, and a bone colonizing variant. *Int J Oncol*, Vol. 28, No. 5, pp, 1173-1183.

Chiarugi, V P & Dietrich, C P (1979). Sulfated mucopolysaccharides from normal and virus transformed rodent fibroblasts. *J Cell Physiol*, Vol. 99, No. 2, pp, 201-206.

Couldrey, C & Green, J E (2000). Metastases: the glycan connection. *Breast Cancer Res*, Vol. 2, No. 5, pp, 321-323.

Dhodapkar, M V, Abe, E, Theus, A, Lacy, M, Langford, J K, Barlogie, B & Sanderson, R D (1998). Syndecan-1 is a multifunctional regulator of myeloma pathobiology: control of tumor cell survival, growth, and bone cell differentiation. *Blood*, Vol. 91, No. 8, pp, 2679-2688.

Esko, J D, Kimata, K & Lindahl, U (1999). Proteoglycans and Sulfated Glycosaminoglycans.Im: *Essentials of Glycobiology*. A. Varki, R. D. Cummings, J. D. Eskoet al. Cold spring harbor, NY, Cold Sprin Harbor Laboratory press, Cold spring harbor, NY

Faassen, A E, Schrager, J A, Klein, D J, Oegema, T R, Couchman, J R & McCarthy, J B (1992). A cell surface chondroitin sulfate proteoglycan, immunologically related to CD44, is involved in type I collagen-mediated melanoma cell motility and invasion. *J Cell Biol*, Vol. 116, No. 2, pp, 521-531.

Feistritzer, C, Kaneider, N C, Sturn, D H & Wiedermann, C J (2004). Syndecan-4-dependent migration of human eosinophils. *Clin Exp Allergy*, Vol. 34, No. 5, pp, 696-703.

Gorelik, E, Galili, U & Raz, A (2001). On the role of cell surface carbohydrates and their binding proteins (lectins) in tumor metastasis. *Cancer Metastasis Rev*, Vol. 20, No. 3-4, pp, 245-277.

Gotte, M, Kersting, C, Radke, I, Kiesel, L & Wulfing, P (2007). An expression signature of syndecan-1 (CD138), E-cadherin and c-met is associated with factors of angiogenesis and lymphangiogenesis in ductal breast carcinoma in situ. *Breast Cancer Res*, Vol. 9, No. 1, pp, R8.

Grako, K A & Stallcup, W B (1995). Participation of the NG2 proteoglycan in rat aortic smooth muscle cell responses to platelet-derived growth factor. *Exp Cell Res*, Vol. 221, No. 1, pp, 231-240.

Greene, D K, Tumova, S, Couchman, J R & Woods, A (2003). Syndecan-4 associates with alpha-actinin. *J Biol Chem*, Vol. 278, No. 9, pp, 7617-7623.

Hakomori, S (1996). Tumor malignancy defined by aberrant glycosylation and sphingo(glyco)lipid metabolism. *Cancer Res*, Vol. 56, No. 23, pp, 5309-5318.

Hu, B, Guo, P, Bar-Joseph, I, Imanishi, Y, Jarzynka, M J, Bogler, O, Mikkelsen, T, Hirose, T, Nishikawa, R & Cheng, S Y (2007). Neuropilin-1 promotes human glioma progression through potentiating the activity of the HGF/SF autocrine pathway. *Oncogene*, Vol., No., pp.

Iida, J, Pei, D, Kang, T, Simpson, M A, Herlyn, M, Furcht, L T & McCarthy, J B (2001). Melanoma chondroitin sulfate proteoglycan regulates matrix metalloproteinase-dependent human melanoma invasion into type I collagen. *J Biol Chem*, Vol. 276, No. 22, pp, 18786-18794.

Iida, J, Wilhelmson, K L, Ng, J, Lee, P, Morrison, C, Tam, E, Overall, C M & McCarthy, J B (2007). Cell surface chondroitin sulfate glycosaminoglycan in melanoma: role in the activation of pro-MMP-2 (pro-gelatinase A). *Biochem J*, Vol. 403, No. 3, pp, 553-563.

Iozzo, R V (1985). Neoplastic modulation of extracellular matrix. Colon carcinoma cells release polypeptides that alter proteoglycan metabolism in colon fibroblasts. *J Biol Chem*, Vol. 260, No. 12, pp, 7464-7473.

Iozzo, R V (1988). Proteoglycans and neoplasia. *Cancer Metastasis Rev*, Vol. 7, No. 1, pp, 39-50.

Jackson, D G, Bell, J I, Dickinson, R, Timans, J, Shields, J & Whittle, N (1995). Proteoglycan forms of the lymphocyte homing receptor CD44 are alternatively spliced variants containing the v3 exon. *J Cell Biol*, Vol. 128, No. 4, pp, 673-685.

Jemal, A, Bray, F, Center, M M, Ferlay, J, Ward, E & Forman, D (2011). Global cancer statistics. *CA Cancer J Clin*, Vol. 61, No. 2, pp, 69-90.

Kalish, E D, Iida, N, Moffat, F L & Bourguignon, L Y (1999). A new CD44V3-containing isoform is involved in tumor cell growth and migration during human breast carcinoma progression. *Front Biosci*, Vol. 4, No., pp, A1-8.

Kaneider, N C, Reinisch, C M, Dunzendorfer, S, Romisch, J & Wiedermann, C J (2002). Syndecan-4 mediates antithrombin-induced chemotaxis of human peripheral blood lymphocytes and monocytes. *J Cell Sci*, Vol. 115, No. Pt 1, pp, 227-236.

Kawaguchi, T (2005). Cancer metastasis: characterization and identification of the behavior of metastatic tumor cells and the cell adhesion molecules, including carbohydrates. *Curr Drug Targets Cardiovasc Haematol Disord*, Vol. 5, No. 1, pp, 39-64.

Kawasaki, T, Kitsukawa, T, Bekku, Y, Matsuda, Y, Sanbo, M, Yagi, T & Fujisawa, H (1999). A requirement for neuropilin-1 in embryonic vessel formation. *Development*, Vol. 126, No. 21, pp, 4895-4902.

Kawashima, H, Atarashi, K, Hirose, M, Hirose, J, Yamada, S, Sugahara, K & Miyasaka, M (2002). Oversulfated chondroitin/dermatan sulfates containing GlcAbeta1/IdoAalpha1-3GalNAc(4,6-O-disulfate) interact with L- and P-selectin and chemokines. *J Biol Chem*, Vol. 277, No. 15, pp, 12921-12930.

Kiewe, P, Bechrakis, N E, Schmittel, A, Ruf, P, Lindhofer, H, Thiel, E & Nagorsen, D (2006). Increased chondroitin sulphate proteoglycan expression (B5 immunoreactivity) in metastases of uveal melanoma. *Ann Oncol*, Vol. 17, No. 12, pp, 1830-1834.

Kim, Y J, Borsig, L, Varki, N M & Varki, A (1998). P-selectin deficiency attenuates tumor growth and metastasis. *Proc Natl Acad Sci U S A*, Vol. 95, No. 16, pp, 9325-9330.

Kitsukawa, T, Shimono, A, Kawakami, A, Kondoh, H & Fujisawa, H (1995). Overexpression of a membrane protein, neuropilin, in chimeric mice causes anomalies in the cardiovascular system, nervous system and limbs. *Development*, Vol. 121, No. 12, pp, 4309-4318.

Klagsbrun, M, Takashima, S & Mamluk, R (2002). The role of neuropilin in vascular and tumor biology. *Adv Exp Med Biol*, Vol. 515, No., pp, 33-48.

Kohler, S, Ullrich, S, Richter, U & Schumacher, U (2010). E-/P-selectins and colon carcinoma metastasis: first in vivo evidence for their crucial role in a clinically relevant model of spontaneous metastasis formation in the lung. *Br J Cancer*, Vol. 102, No. 3, pp, 602-609.

Kolodkin, A L, Levengood, D V, Rowe, E G, Tai, Y T, Giger, R J & Ginty, D D (1997). Neuropilin is a semaphorin III receptor. *Cell*, Vol. 90, No. 4, pp, 753-762.

Korourian, S, Siegel, E, Kieber-Emmons, T & Monzavi-Karbassi, B (2008). Expression analysis of carbohydrate antigens in ductal carcinoma in situ of the breast by lectin histochemistry. *BMC Cancer*, Vol. 8, No., pp, 136.

Krause, T & Turner, G A (1999). Are selectins involved in metastasis? *Clin Exp Metastasis*, Vol. 17, No. 3, pp, 183-192.

Kreider, J W, Bartlett, G L & Butkiewicz, B L (1984). Relationship of tumor leucocytic infiltration to host defense mechanisms and prognosis. *Cancer Metastasis Rev*, Vol. 3, No. 1, pp, 53-74.

Kumar-Singh, S, Jacobs, W, Dhaene, K, Weyn, B, Bogers, J, Weyler, J & Van Marck, E (1998). Syndecan-1 expression in malignant mesothelioma: correlation with cell differentiation, WT1 expression, and clinical outcome. *J Pathol*, Vol. 186, No. 3, pp, 300-305.

Kusche-Gullberg, M & Kjellen, L (2003). Sulfotransferases in glycosaminoglycan biosynthesis. *Curr Opin Struct Biol*, Vol. 13, No. 5, pp, 605-611.

Lee, C M, Tanaka, T, Murai, T, Kondo, M, Kimura, J, Su, W, Kitagawa, T, Ito, T, Matsuda, H & Miyasaka, M (2002). Novel chondroitin sulfate-binding cationic liposomes loaded with cisplatin efficiently suppress the local growth and liver metastasis of tumor cells in vivo. *Cancer Res*, Vol. 62, No. 15, pp, 4282-4288.

Lesley, J & Hyman, R (1998). CD44 structure and function. *Front Biosci*, Vol. 3, No., pp, d616-630.

Lesley, J, Hyman, R, English, N, Catterall, J B & Turner, G A (1997). CD44 in inflammation and metastasis. *Glycoconj J*, Vol. 14, No. 5, pp, 611-622.

Li, F, Ten Dam, G B, Murugan, S, Yamada, S, Hashiguchi, T, Mizumoto, S, Oguri, K, Okayama, M, van Kuppevelt, T H & Sugahara, K (2008). Involvement of highly sulfated chondroitin sulfate in the metastasis of the Lewis lung carcinoma cells. *J Biol Chem*, Vol. 283, No. 49, pp, 34294-34304.

Maccarana, M, Olander, B, Malmstrom, J, Tiedemann, K, Aebersold, R, Lindahl, U, Li, J P & Malmstrom, A (2006). Biosynthesis of dermatan sulfate: chondroitin-glucuronate C5-epimerase is identical to SART2. *J Biol Chem*, Vol. 281, No. 17, pp, 11560-11568.

Makinen, T, Olofsson, B, Karpanen, T, Hellman, U, Soker, S, Klagsbrun, M, Eriksson, U & Alitalo, K (1999). Differential binding of vascular endothelial growth factor B splice and proteolytic isoforms to neuropilin-1. *J Biol Chem*, Vol. 274, No. 30, pp, 21217-21222.

Mali, M, Andtfolk, H, Miettinen, H M & Jalkanen, M (1994). Suppression of tumor cell growth by syndecan-1 ectodomain. *J Biol Chem*, Vol. 269, No. 45, pp, 27795-27798.

Miao, H Q, Soker, S, Feiner, L, Alonso, J L, Raper, J A & Klagsbrun, M (1999). Neuropilin-1 mediates collapsin-1/semaphorin III inhibition of endothelial cell motility: functional competition of collapsin-1 and vascular endothelial growth factor-165. *J Cell Biol*, Vol. 146, No. 1, pp, 233-242.

Migdal, M, Huppertz, B, Tessler, S, Comforti, A, Shibuya, M, Reich, R, Baumann, H & Neufeld, G (1998). Neuropilin-1 is a placenta growth factor-2 receptor. *J Biol Chem*, Vol. 273, No. 35, pp, 22272-22278.

Mikami, S, Ohashi, K, Usui, Y, Nemoto, T, Katsube, K, Yanagishita, M, Nakajima, M, Nakamura, K & Koike, M (2001). Loss of syndecan-1 and increased expression of heparanase in invasive esophageal carcinomas. *Jpn J Cancer Res*, Vol. 92, No. 10, pp, 1062-1073.

Monzavi-Karbassi, B, Stanley, J S, Hennings, L, Jousheghany, F, Artaud, C, Shaaf, S & Kieber-Emmons, T (2007). Chondroitin sulfate glycosaminoglycans as major P-selectin ligands on metastatic breast cancer cell lines. *Int J Cancer*, Vol. 120, No. 6, pp, 1179-1191.

Monzavi-Karbassi, B, Whitehead, T L, Jousheghany, F, Artaud, C, Hennings, L, Shaaf, S, Slaughter, A, Korourian, S, Kelly, T, Blaszczyk-Thurin, M & Kieber-Emmons, T

(2005). Deficiency in surface expression of E-selectin ligand promotes lung colonization in a mouse model of breast cancer. *Int J Cancer*, Vol. 117, No. 3, pp, 398-408.

Nackaerts, K, Verbeken, E, Deneffe, G, Vanderschueren, B, Demedts, M & David, G (1997). Heparan sulfate proteoglycan expression in human lung-cancer cells. *Int J Cancer*, Vol. 74, No. 3, pp, 335-345.

Naor, D, Sionov, R V & Ish-Shalom, D (1997). CD44: structure, function, and association with the malignant process. *Adv Cancer Res*, Vol. 71, No., pp, 241-319.

Nishiyama, A, Dahlin, K J, Prince, J T, Johnstone, S R & Stallcup, W B (1991). The primary structure of NG2, a novel membrane-spanning proteoglycan. *J Cell Biol*, Vol. 114, No. 2, pp, 359-371.

Numa, F, Hirabayashi, K, Kawasaki, K, Sakaguchi, Y, Sugino, N, Suehiro, Y, Suminami, Y, Hirakawa, H, Umayahara, K, Nawata, S, Ogata, H & Kato, H (2002). Syndecan-1 expression in cancer of the uterine cervix: association with lymph node metastasis. *Int J Oncol*, Vol. 20, No. 1, pp, 39-43.

Olsen, E B, Trier, K, Eldov, K & Ammitzboll, T (1988). Glycosaminoglycans in human breast cancer. *Acta Obstet Gynecol Scand*, Vol. 67, No. 6, pp, 539-542.

Penc, S F, Pomahac, B, Winkler, T, Dorschner, R A, Eriksson, E, Herndon, M & Gallo, R L (1998). Dermatan sulfate released after injury is a potent promoter of fibroblast growth factor-2 function. *J Biol Chem*, Vol. 273, No. 43, pp, 28116-28121.

Pluschke, G, Vanek, M, Evans, A, Dittmar, T, Schmid, P, Itin, P, Filardo, E J & Reisfeld, R A (1996). Molecular cloning of a human melanoma-associated chondroitin sulfate proteoglycan. *Proc Natl Acad Sci U S A*, Vol. 93, No. 18, pp, 9710-9715.

Potapenko, I O, Haakensen, V D, Luders, T, Helland, A, Bukholm, I, Sorlie, T, Kristensen, V N, Lingjaerde, O C & Borresen-Dale, A L (2010). Glycan gene expression signatures in normal and malignant breast tissue; possible role in diagnosis and progression. *Mol Oncol*, Vol. 4, No. 2, pp, 98-118.

Reisfeld, R A & Cheresh, D A (1987). Human tumor antigens. *Adv Immunol*, Vol. 40, No., pp, 323-377.

Schuetz, C S, Bonin, M, Clare, S E, Nieselt, K, Sotlar, K, Walter, M, Fehm, T, Solomayer, E, Riess, O, Wallwiener, D, Kurek, R & Neubauer, H J (2006). Progression-specific genes identified by expression profiling of matched ductal carcinomas in situ and invasive breast tumors, combining laser capture microdissection and oligonucleotide microarray analysis. *Cancer Res*, Vol. 66, No. 10, pp, 5278-5286.

Shintani, Y, Takashima, S, Asano, Y, Kato, H, Liao, Y, Yamazaki, S, Tsukamoto, O, Seguchi, O, Yamamoto, H, Fukushima, T, Sugahara, K, Kitakaze, M & Hori, M (2006). Glycosaminoglycan modification of neuropilin-1 modulates VEGFR2 signaling. *Embo J*, Vol. 25, No. 13, pp, 3045-3055.

Silbert, J E & Sugumaran, G (2002). Biosynthesis of chondroitin/dermatan sulfate. *IUBMB Life*, Vol. 54, No. 4, pp, 177-186.

Soker, S, Takashima, S, Miao, H Q, Neufeld, G & Klagsbrun, M (1998). Neuropilin-1 is expressed by endothelial and tumor cells as an isoform-specific receptor for vascular endothelial growth factor. *Cell*, Vol. 92, No. 6, pp, 735-745.

Stallcup, W B (1981). The NG2 antigen, a putative lineage marker: immunofluorescent localization in primary cultures of rat brain. *Dev Biol*, Vol. 83, No. 1, pp, 154-165.

Stevenson, J L, Choi, S H & Varki, A (2005). Differential metastasis inhibition by clinically relevant levels of heparins--correlation with selectin inhibition, not antithrombotic activity. *Clin Cancer Res*, Vol. 11, No. 19 Pt 1, pp, 7003-7011.

Stylianou, M, Skandalis, S S, Papadas, T A, Mastronikolis, N S, Theocharis, D A, Papageorgakopoulou, N & Vynios, D H (2008). Stage-related decorin and versican expression in human laryngeal cancer. *Anticancer Res*, Vol. 28, No. 1A, pp, 245-251.

Sugahara, K, Mikami, T, Uyama, T, Mizuguchi, S, Nomura, K & Kitagawa, H (2003). Recent advances in the structural biology of chondroitin sulfate and dermatan sulfate. *Curr Opin Struct Biol*, Vol. 13, No. 5, pp, 612-620.

Taylor, K R & Gallo, R L (2006). Glycosaminoglycans and their proteoglycans: host-associated molecular patterns for initiation and modulation of inflammation. *Faseb J*, Vol. 20, No. 1, pp, 9-22.

Toole, B P (2009). Hyaluronan-CD44 Interactions in Cancer: Paradoxes and Possibilities. *Clin Cancer Res*, Vol. 15, No. 24, pp, 7462-7468.

Trowbridge, J M, Rudisill, J A, Ron, D & Gallo, R L (2002). Dermatan sulfate binds and potentiates activity of keratinocyte growth factor (FGF-7). *J Biol Chem*, Vol. 277, No. 45, pp, 42815-42820.

Tsanou, E, Ioachim, E, Briasoulis, E, Charchanti, A, Damala, K, Karavasilis, V, Pavlidis, N & Agnantis, N J (2004). Clinicopathological study of the expression of syndecan-1 in invasive breast carcinomas. correlation with extracellular matrix components. *J Exp Clin Cancer Res*, Vol. 23, No. 4, pp, 641-650.

Vijayagopal, P, Figueroa, J E & Levine, E A (1998). Altered composition and increased endothelial cell proliferative activity of proteoglycans isolated from breast carcinoma. *J Surg Oncol*, Vol. 68, No. 4, pp, 250-254.

Vynios, D H, Theocharis, D A, Papageorgakopoulou, N, Papadas, T A, Mastronikolis, N S, Goumas, P D, Stylianou, M & Skandalis, S S (2008). Biochemical changes of extracellular proteoglycans in squamous cell laryngeal carcinoma. *Connect Tissue Res*, Vol. 49, No. 3, pp, 239-243.

Wang, X, Osada, T, Wang, Y, Yu, L, Sakakura, K, Katayama, A, McCarthy, J B, Brufsky, A, Chivukula, M, Khoury, T, Hsu, D S, Barry, W T, Lyerly, H K, Clay, T M & Ferrone, S (2010a). CSPG4 protein as a new target for the antibody-based immunotherapy of triple-negative breast cancer. *J Natl Cancer Inst*, Vol. 102, No. 19, pp, 1496-1512.

Wang, X, Wang, Y, Yu, L, Sakakura, K, Visus, C, Schwab, J H, Ferrone, C R, Favoino, E, Koya, Y, Campoli, M R, McCarthy, J B, DeLeo, A B & Ferrone, S (2010b). CSPG4 in cancer: multiple roles. *Curr Mol Med*, Vol. 10, No. 4, pp, 419-429.

West, D C, Rees, C G, Duchesne, L, Patey, S J, Terry, C J, Turnbull, J E, Delehedde, M, Heegaard, C W, Allain, F, Vanpouille, C, Ron, D & Fernig, D G (2005). Interactions of multiple heparin binding growth factors with neuropilin-1 and potentiation of the activity of fibroblast growth factor-2. *J Biol Chem*, Vol. 280, No. 14, pp, 13457-13464.

Wise, L M, Veikkola, T, Mercer, A A, Savory, L J, Fleming, S B, Caesar, C, Vitali, A, Makinen, T, Alitalo, K & Stacker, S A (1999). Vascular endothelial growth factor (VEGF)-like protein from orf virus NZ2 binds to VEGFR2 and neuropilin-1. *Proc Natl Acad Sci U S A*, Vol. 96, No. 6, pp, 3071-3076.

Woods, A & Couchman, J R (1994). Syndecan 4 heparan sulfate proteoglycan is a selectively enriched and widespread focal adhesion component. *Mol Biol Cell*, Vol. 5, No. 2, pp, 183-192.

Woods, A, Longley, R L, Tumova, S & Couchman, J R (2000). Syndecan-4 binding to the high affinity heparin-binding domain of fibronectin drives focal adhesion formation in fibroblasts. *Arch Biochem Biophys*, Vol. 374, No. 1, pp, 66-72.

Yang, J, Price, M A, Li, G Y, Bar-Eli, M, Salgia, R, Jagedeeswaran, R, Carlson, J H, Ferrone, S, Turley, E A & McCarthy, J B (2009). Melanoma proteoglycan modifies gene expression to stimulate tumor cell motility, growth, and epithelial-to-mesenchymal transition. *Cancer Res*, Vol. 69, No. 19, pp, 7538-7547.

7

The Mesenchymal-Like Phenotype
of the MDA-MB-231 Cell Line

Khoo Boon Yin

Institute for Research in Molecular Medicine (INFORMM),
Universiti Sains Malaysia, Penang,
Malaysia

1. Introduction

Mesenchymal stem cells (MSCs) are progenitor cells that can be isolated from all connective tissues such as bone, adipose, cartilage, blood and muscle (Wang *et al.*, 2009). MSCs have recently been described to localise within breast carcinomas where the stem cells integrate into tumour-associated stromal tissues whereby the MSCs promote breast cancer cell invasion and metastasis (Karnoub *et al.*, 2007). Previous studies have demonstrated that when combine with weakly metastatic human breast carcinoma cells, bone marrow-derived mesenchymal stem cells (BMSCs) increase the metastatic potency of the cancer cells greatly (Hombauer & Minguell, 2000). This phenomenon was significantly observed in MCF-7 cells where increase in cancer cell proliferation was observed when the cancer cells were co-cultured on the BMSCs feeder layer. Furthermore, light and epifluorescence microscopy studies revealed that the MCF-7 cluster grew in a dispersed fashion on the BMSCs feeder layer due to the decrease expression of adhesive molecules, such as E-cadherin and epithelial-specific antigen (ESA), in the cancer cells. The interaction between the MCF-7 cells and the BMSCs likely causes the loss of the adhesive molecules in the cancer cells. A phenomenon similar to this interaction was also observed in our recent study. Indeed, the study found that the growth of the MCF-7 cells was enhanced not only when the cancer cells were adhesively co-cultured with the BMSCs but also when they were co-cultured non-adhesively.

In the adhesive cell interaction, the growth or proliferation rate of the MCF-7 cells, which was measured by colony size, was observed to increase when the cancer cells were co-cultured on the BMSCs feeder layer (Fig. 1A and Fig. 1B). The non-adhesive interaction of the MCF-7 cells with BMSCs was also found to increase the growth of the cancer cells. When the cancer cells were incubated with the conditioned medium (culture supernatant) of the BMSCs, the proliferation rate of the MCF-7 cells increased approximately 16.6% when compared to the proliferation rate of the cancer cells incubated with growth medium only (Fig. 1C). This phenomenon indicates that the increase in the proliferation rate of the cancer cells due to the presence of the BMSCs must not be related to a direct physical cell–cell interaction, as similar findings are observed in both the adhesive and non-adhesive co-culture conditions.

Note: In this chapter, adhesive co-culture is defined as the growth of cancer cells on a non-tumorigenic cell monolayer where direct physical cell–cell interaction occurs. Non-adhesive co-culture is defined as the incubation of cancer cells with a conditioned medium that is withdrawn from the non-tumorigenic cells; here, the cells interact with one another *via* the culture medium.

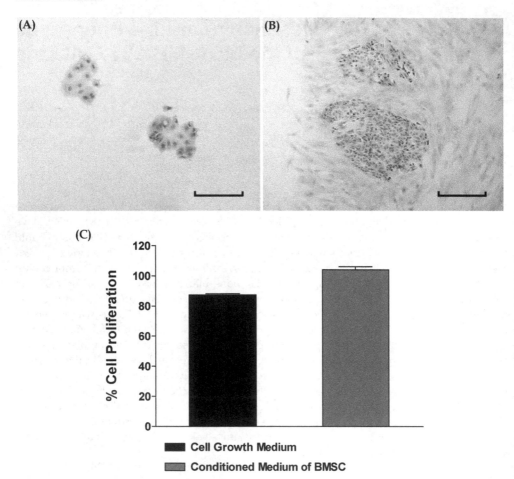

Fig. 1. Colony formation of the MCF-7 cells cultured with or without BMSCs. The pictures show Oil-Red-O staining of **(A)** the MCF-7 colonies alone and **(B)** the MCF-7 colonies grown on the BMSCs feeder layer for one week. The pictures were visualised under an inverted light microscope using same magnification. **(C)** The proliferation rate of the MCF-7 cells incubated with cell growth medium (control) and conditioned medium of BMSCs for one week. One hundred cells were used as the input prior to incubation. The values were expressed as mean±SD from three replicates, and the determination was carried out from three replicates each of three independent experiments.

The BMSCs likely secreted or influenced the MCF-7 cells to secrete certain soluble growth factors into the conditioned medium whereby the growth factors stimulated the MCF-7 cells in cluster and grow into single cell layer, after which the cells dispersed without any evidence of direct cell–cell contact (Fig. 2). Thus, the influence of the BMSCs on the changed of cell morphology and increased proliferation rate of the MCF-7 cells may be achieved *via* the culture medium without the need for any direct physical cell–cell interaction between the two cell lines. However, this phenomenon, in which the BMSCs increased the proliferation rate of the breast cancer cells, was not observed when the BMSCs were co-cultured with highly invasive and metastatic human breast cancer cells, such as MDA-MB-231 cells. The MDA-MB-231 cell line likely contains its own source that similar to the MSCs as progenitor factor in the cell population that is able to secrete a standard level of the soluble growth factors into the conditioned medium of the MDA-MB-231 cells. Therefore, the activity of the MDA-MB-231 cells was not influenced by their exposure to the MSCs-conditioned medium and few effects were observed when the cells were co-cultured with the MSCs (Sasser *et al.*, 2007a).

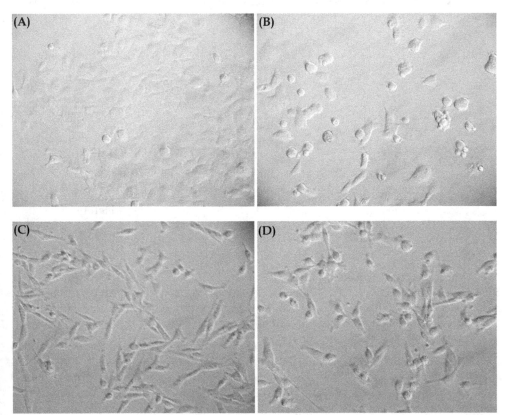

Fig. 2. Unstained MCF-7 and MDA-MB-231 cells as visualised under an inverted light microscope. Panels A and B show clustered and single cell layer of MCF-7 cells that were incubated with cell growth medium and BMSCs-conditioned medium, respectively, whereas panels **C** and **D** show few effects on cell morphology were observed when the MDA-MB-231 cells were incubated with cell growth medium and BMSCs-conditioned medium, respectively. The pictures were taken after one week of cell incubations.

2. Soluble growth factors in the conditioned medium of the MDA-MB-231 cells

2.1 Expression of MMPs in the conditioned medium

The MDA-MB-231 cell line is an estrogen receptor alpha (ERα)-negative human breast cancer cell line (Liu *et al.*, 2003). It was derived from a metastatic adenocarcinoma of the mammary gland of a 51-year-old Caucasian woman, according to the data sheet of the American Type Culture Collection (ATCC). This adherent epithelial cell line that likely contains more than one cell populations is a highly aggressive, invasive and poorly-differentiated human breast cancer cell line. Similar to other invasive cancer cell lines, the MDA-MB-231 cells display the invasiveness by mediating the proteolytic degradation of the extracellular matrix (ECM), including basement membrane and several mechanical barriers to the ECM, through the increased expression of matrix metalloproteinases (MMPs), including gelatinases, en route to their destinations (Fig. 3).

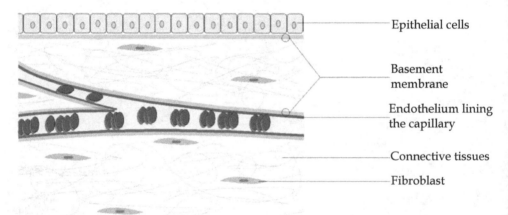

Fig. 3. Illustration depicts the ECM in relationship to the epithelium, endothelium and connective tissues. To reach their destination, the invasive cancer cells must penetrate the mechanical barriers of the ECM and basement membrane through proteolytic degradation. The figure was modified from the Wikimedia.

Type IV collagen, which is the main component of the basement membrane, is the first component that must be degraded to allow the invasion process (Boutaud *et al.*, 2000). The ability to degrade and penetrate the basement membrane is related with an increased potential of the cells for invasion and metastasis (Castro-Sanchez *et al.*, 2011). Tumour cells are able to produce MMPs that degrade the matrix barriers surrounding the tumour, including basement membrane, permitting invasion into connective tissues, entry and exit from blood and lymphatic vessels, and metastasis to distant organs. MMPs are family of zinc-dependent endopeptidases that collectively are capable of degrading all components of the ECM, including the basement membrane. Binding of breast cancer cells to type IV collagen in the basement membrane induces Discoidin domain receptor 1 (DDR1) activation and then it triggers signal transduction pathways and cellular processes that promotes secretion of MMPs which contributes to basement membrane degradation and cancer cell invasion. A previous study demonstrated that gelatinase B or MMP-9, which degrades the type IV collagen in the basement membrane, plays a crucial role in the invasion process of the MDA-MB-231 cells (Liu *et al.*, 2003). This phenomenon can be observed by determining the metastatic potential of the MDA-MB-231 cells in an experimental model that is closely correlated with the expression of the MMP-9 and the activities of the gelatinases in the conditioned medium of the MDA-MB-231 cells. According to the study, the invasion of the MDA-MB-231 cells was blocked by MMP-9-neutralising antibodies that reduced the gelatinolytic activities in the conditioned medium, as detected using Enzyme-linked immunosorbent assay (ELISA). This phenomenon also led to the significant inhibition of the invasive capacities of the MDA-MB-231 cells. This inhibition was induced by specific drugs e.g., peroxisome proliferator-activated receptor gamma ligands and all-trans-retinoic acid that were administered on a reconstituted basement membrane in a Matrigel® chamber *in vitro*. Therefore, MMP-9 was shown to play a crucial role in the invasion process of the MDA-MB-231 cells and it was shown to be absolutely required for the transmigration of this cell line.

Note: In this chapter, conditioned medium is denoted as culture supernatant that is withdrawn from feeder layer. To accomplish this, a culture of feeder layer e.g., BMSCs is maintained with fresh growth medium. After certain duration, the growth medium is withdrawn from the feeder layer as conditioned medium. The conditioned medium is believed to contain growth factors released by the feeder layer.

2.2 Activation of STAT3 and soluble IL-6 in the conditioned medium

In addition to MMP-9 in the conditioned medium, the MDA-MB-231 cells are also demonstrated to contain elevated level of signal transducer and activator of transcription 3 (STAT3) in the cells (Sasser *et al.*, 2007b). STAT3 is typically maintained in the cytoplasm as an inactive monomer. Once it is phosphorylated, the STAT3 forms homodimers and enters into nucleus where it activates the transcription of multiple genes associated with cell proliferation and survival (Heinrich *et al.*, 1998; Zinzalla *et al.*, 2010). The activation of STAT3 has been correlated with enhanced breast cancer cell growth, survival and immune evasion (Selander *et al.*, 2004; Ling *et al.*, 2005; Yu *et al.*, 2007). According to a previous study, exposure of MSCs-conditioned medium to MCF-7 and T-47D activated the levels of pTyr[705] STAT3 in the cells (Sasser *et al.*, 2007a). Correlatively, the enhancement of the cancer cell growth rates was observed in ERα-positive human breast cancer cell lines, including MCF-7 and T-47D, in the presence of the MSCs-conditioned medium. The growth rates of BT474 and ZR-75-1 cells were also observed to increase after the cancer cells were co-cultured with the MSCs-conditioned medium. All cancer cell growth rates were enhanced by approximately 2-3 fold, after the exposure to the conditioned medium (Fig. 4). The growth rate of an ERα-negative breast cancer cell line, MDA-MB-468, was also elevated in the presence of the MSCs-conditioned medium, albeit to a lesser extent than the other ERα-positive cell lines that were tested (Sasser *et al.*, 2007a; Sasser *et al.*, 2007b). However, this induction was not observed when the MDA-MB-231 cell line was exposed to the MSCs-conditioned medium.

Few effects were observed when the MDA-MB-231 cells were co-cultured with the MSCs-conditioned medium because the cell line likely contained a subpopulation in the cell population that secreted a standard level of soluble growth factors in the conditioned medium (Sasser *et al.*, 2007b). In this non-adhesive co-culture study, paracrine interleukin-6

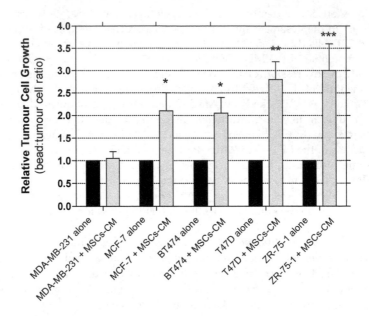

Fig. 4. Breast cancer cell growth in the presence or absence of MSCs-conditioned medium was assessed for MDA-MB-231, MCF-7, BT474, T47D and ZR-75-1 cells. The MDA-MB-231 cell growth was unaltered by MSCs-conditioned medium, whereas the growth of the four remaining ERα-positive cell lines in the presence of MSCs-conditioned medium was significantly elevated when compared to the cell lines growing alone for eight days (Sasser *et al.*, 2007b).

(IL-6) was found to be the principal mediator of the STAT3 phosphorylation in the cells. MSCs-induced STAT3 phosphorylation was lost when the IL-6 was depleted from the MSCs-conditioned medium. A similar phenomenon was observed when the IL-6 receptor in the cancer cells was blocked. This secretion of IL-6 from the MDA-MB-231 cells allowed for the activation and maintenance of the level of STAT3 as well as the growth in the MDA-MB-231 cells. Therefore, the conditioned medium of MDA-MB-231 cells has similar effect as the conditioned medium withdrawal from the MSCs, as evidenced by previous study, where the conditioned medium from the MDA-MB-231 cells with constitutively active STAT3 is sufficient to induce p-STAT3 levels in various recipients that do not possess elevated p-STAT3 levels, such as MCF-10A cells, a non-tumorigenic cell line (Lieblein *et al.*, 2008). This signalling occurs through the JAK/STAT3 pathway, leading to STAT3 phosphorylation as early as 30 minutes and was persistent for at least 24 hours, indicating that a correlation between elevated levels of IL-6 production and p-STAT3 in the cells, as confirmed by ELISA analysis. Neutralisation of the IL-6 ligand or gp130 was sufficient to block the increased levels of p-STAT3 (Y705) in the treated cells. These results demonstrate that the STAT3 phosphorylation in breast epithelial cells can be stimulated by paracrine signalling through soluble growth factors from both breast cancer cells and breast cancer associated fibroblasts with elevated STAT3 phosphorylation. The finding of growth factors within the MDA-MB-231 conditioned media was also sufficient to stimulate an increase in IL-6 production from

MCF-10A cells, as indicated in the previous study, may not correct as both MDA-MB-231 cells and MCF-10A cells secret IL-6 in the conditioned medium. Indeed, our study demonstrated that the conditioned media of the MDA-MB-231 cells and MCF-10A cells contained a high level of IL-6, although the level was not as high as in the MSCs-conditioned medium (Fig. 5).

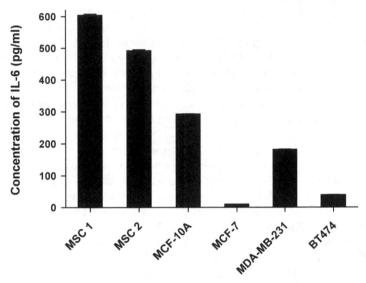

Fig. 5. The activity of IL-6 in the conditioned media of MSCs, non-tumorigenic cells and human breast cancer cells. The culture supernatants were withdrawn from one-week-old feeder layer of above cultures. The level of IL-6 in the conditioned medium was assayed using ELISA. The values were expressed as the mean±SD from three replicates, and the determination was carried out from three replicates each of three independent experiments.

Therefore, the finding indicates that the soluble growth factors within the MDA-MB-231 conditioned medium to stimulate an increase in IL-6 production from the MCF-10A cells might be due to combine of both conditioned media. Anyhow, this result indicates that the MDA-MB-231 cells may contain similar progenitor factor as MSCs in the cell population. This factor likely expresses the high level of IL-6 where it contributes to the induction of STAT3 phosphorylation and appears to be associated with cell proliferation of the MDA-MB-231 cells. Although the secretion of IL-6 allows for the activation and maintenance of the level of STAT3 as well as the growth in the MDA-MB-231 cells have been demonstrated, its role in invasiveness of the MDA-MB-231 remains unclear. Nevertheless, targeting the IL-6 in the conditioned medium can be an idea to diagnose patients with tumour that are ERα negative or express lower level of ERα.

2.3 CCL2 and CCL5 in the conditioned medium

Chemokines or chemotactic cytokines are small proteins that are classified into four conserved groups, CXC, CC, C and CX3C, based on the position of the first two cysteines that are adjacent to the amino acid (Balkwill, 2004; Lu & Kang, 2009). Among more than 50 identified human chemokines, chemokine (C-C motif) ligand 2 (CCL2 or MCP-1) and chemokine (C-C motif) ligand 5 (CCL5 or RANTES) are of particularly important. CCL2 is a potent chemoattractant for monocytes, memory T lymphocytes and natural killer cells whereas CCL5 is a potent inducer of leukocyte motility (Lu & Kang, 2009; Melgarejo et al., 2009; Yaal-Hahoshen et al., 2006). Both chemokines stimulate migration of leukocytes in response to inflammatory signals. The roles of CCL2 and CCL5 in breast malignancy have been extensively addressed in breast cancer studies (Goldberg-Bittman et al., 2004; Soria et al., 2008; Soria & Ben-Baruch, 2008; Wu et al., 2008; Fujimoto et al., 2009). Overexpression of the CCL2 and CCL5 are stimulated during breast cancer development and progression. They are also frequently associated with advanced tumour stage and metastatic relapse in breast cancer. Both chemokines act directly on the tumour cells to promote their pro-malignancy phenotype by increasing their migratory and invasion-related properties (Soria & Ben-Baruch, 2008). The chemokines are expressed by the cells of the tumour microenvironment osteoblasts and MSCs. In breast cells, the chemokines are highly expressed by breast tumour cells at primary tumour sites and minimally expressed by normal breast epithelial duct cells (Soria et al., 2008; Soria & Ben-Baruch, 2008). The chemokines are soluble growth factors that can be easily detected in serum and conditioned culture medium. Consistently, our recent study demonstrated that high levels of CCL2 and CCL5 were detected in the conditioned medium of the MDA-MB-231 cells, as determined by ELISA (Fig. 6). The results indicated that the CCL2 and CCL5 were present in the conditioned media of all of the tested cell lines. As expected, elevated levels of CCL2 and CCL5 were observed in the MSCs and MCF-10A cells. CCL2 was additionally more stably expressed in the non-tumorigenic cells, such as MCF-10A, than in the MDA-MB-231 cells. However, an opposite event was observed for CCL5 in the MCF-10A and MDA-MB-231 cells. Both CCL2 and CCL5 displayed relatively higher expression levels in the MDA-MB-231 cells than that in the weakly metastatic cells, such as MCF-7 and BT-474. However, the CCL2 level in the MDA-MB-231 cells was only slightly higher than in the MCF-7 and BT-474 cells.

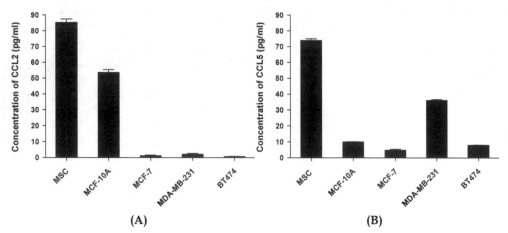

(A)   (B)

Fig. 6. The activities of **(A)** CCL2 and **(B)** CCL5 in the conditioned media of MSCs, human breast tumorigenic and non-tumorigenic cells. The levels of the soluble growth factors were assayed using ELISA. The values were expressed as mean±SD from three replicates, and the determination was carried out from three replicates each of three independent experiments.

The overexpression of chemokine decoy receptor proteins, such as D6 and Duffy antigen receptor for chemokines (DARC), have been demonstrated to inhibit the proliferation and invasion of the human breast cancer *in vitro*, tumorigenesis and lung metastasis *in vivo* (Wu et al., 2008). This inhibition is associated with decrease in chemokines, such as CCL2 and CCL5, vessel density and tumour-associated macrophage infiltration. The inhibition of CCL5 expression by short interfering RNA (siRNA) or by the use of neutralising antibodies against CCL5 impaired the tumour-supporting roles that were mediated by the CCL5-CCR5 loop; this significantly inhibited the metastatic potential of the MDA-MB-231 cells (Karnoub et al., 2007; Soria & Ben-Baruch, 2008). Moreover, CCL2-neutralizing antibodies inhibited bone resorption *in vitro* and bone metastasis *in vivo* as well as the tumour conditioned media-induced osteoclast formation *in vitro* and bone metastasis *in vivo*, indicating a role of the CCL2 and CCL5 in metastasis (Lu & Kang, 2009). The MDA-MB-231 cells are obviously having its own progenitor factor, which is in the cell population that produce the soluble growth factors in order to maintain the invasive and progressive phenotypes in the cells. Further identification and functional characterisation of CCL2 and CCL5, as well as MMP-9 and IL-6, would provide an effective treatment for systemic metastasis. Perhaps, the effects of certain inhibitors or drugs on the inhibition of proliferation and the reduction of invasion of breast cancer cell growth can be easily determined using these growth factors as they can be detected *via* serum and conditioned culture medium. Thus, all four molecules mentioned in this chapter could be considered as potential therapeutic targets for the development of a detection assay for human breast cancer.

3. The subpopulation in the MDA-MB-231 cells

Most of the cancer cell lines have recently been demonstrated by flow cytometry to contain a subpopulation of CD44+/CD24- where the MDA-MB-231 cells are found to contain a high percentage of the CD44+/CD24- subpopulation (85±5%) in the cells (Sheridan et al., 2006). Other cell lines that contain a high level of this subpopulation are MDA-MB-436 (72±5%), Hs578T (86±5%) and SUM1315 (97±3%) (Table 1). The subpopulation is shown to possess the capacity for self-renewal and the generation of heterogeneous progeny in the cells. Moreover, the subpopulation of the breast cancer cells has been reported to have stem/progenitor cell properties that contribute a unique ability to allow these cells to invade. Similar to the ability of the MSCs that was described above, the inherent properties of this subpopulation may impart their transformed counterparts with the ability to evade traditional antitumour therapies and to establish breast cancer metastasis (Reya et al., 2001; Behbod et al., 2005; Dean et al., 2005). Several studies suggested that this subpopulation of cells, as a subset of human breast cancer cells, possessed an enhanced ability to form tumour in immunocompromised mice (Al-Hajj et al., 2003; Ponti et al., 2005). However, the potential of this subpopulation to establish breast cancer metastasis in the cell line remains unclear.

The expression levels of pro-invasive genes, such as interleukin-1-alpha (IL-1α), IL-6, interleukin-8 (IL-8) and urokinase plasminogen activator (UPA), are higher in the cell lines that contained a significant CD44+/CD24- subpopulation (Sheridan et al., 2006). The results indicate that the cell lines with a significant number of CD44+/CD24- subpopulation are more invasive is consistent with the studies that demonstrate the metastatic process in breast cancer cells requires the following: (1) ECM degradation-associated proteins, including the

UPA/UPA receptor system and MMPs; (2) cytokines, including interleukin-1 (IL-1), IL-6, IL-8, interleukin-11 (IL-11), tumour necrosis factor (TNF) and transforming growth factor-beta 1 (TGF-β1); and (3) chemokines and their receptors, including stromal cell-derived factor-1-alpha (SDF-1α) and CXC chemokine receptor (CXCR4) (Edwards and Murphy, 1998; Dumont and Arteaga, 2003; Kang et al., 2003; Yodkeeree et al., 2010). In addition, a recent study described the role of nuclear factor-kappa B (NF-κB) and its ligand in the metastasis of breast cancer cells to the bone matrix (Jones et al., 2006). All of these factors may be directly related to breast cancer metastasis. However, the contribution of the subpopulation of CD44+/CD24- to the pro-invasive factors in breast cancer cells remains unclear.

No.	Cell Line	CD44+/CD24-	Cell Type Classification
a	MDA-MB-231	85±5	Mesenchymal
b	MDA-MB-436	72±5	Myoepithelial
c	Hs578T	86±5	Mesenchymal
d	MDA-MB-468	3±1	Basal
e	MCF-7	0	Luminal
f	T47-D	0	Luminal
g	ZR-75-1	0	Luminal
h	BT-474	0	Luminal/ErbB2+
i	SK-BR-3	0	Luminal/ErbB2+
j	MCF-10A	17±4	Basal

Table 1. Subpopulation of CD44+/CD24- in commonly used breast cancer cell lines. The CD44 and CD24 expression patterns in the subpopulation CD44+/CD24- were determined by flow cytometry. CD44 and CD24 were detected by a combination of fluorochrome-conjugated monoclonal antibodies against human CD44 (FITC) and CD24 (PE), respectively (Sheridan et al., 2006).

Demethoxycurcumin (DMC) is recently demonstrated to inhibit the adhesion, migration and invasion of the MDA-MB-231 cells (Yodkeeree et al., 2010). According to the study, the DMC-treated MDA-MB-231 cells contained decreasing levels of ECM degradation-associated proteins, which included MMP-9, membrane type-1 MMP (MT1-MMP), UPA and UPAR. DMC reduced also the expression of intercellular adhesion molecule-1 (ICAM-1) and CXCR4 in the MDA-MB-231 cells. These molecules are involved in the modulation of the tumour metastasis process. In addition, the study showed that treatment of the MDA-MB-231 cells with DMC inhibited the DNA binding activity of NF-κB, which is known to mediate the expression of MMPs, UPA, UPAR, ICAM-1 and CXCR4 in breast cancer cells. These results indicated also that NF-κB may play a role in the invasion process of the MDA-MB-231 cells. All of these findings suggest the presence of a correlation between the above molecules and the invasiveness of the MDA-MB-231 cells. However, the specific correlation between the above molecules and the subpopulation in the MDA-MB-231 cells has yet to be fully elucidated. The inhibition or depletion of the progenitor factor from the subpopulation is hypothesised to reduce the expression of the above molecules, thereby reducing the invasiveness of the MDA-MB-231 cells. Therefore, it is essential to identify more surface markers that can specifically be used to isolate the subpopulation. By targeting this subpopulation in the cells, the expression of the above molecules and the invasiveness of the MDA-MB-231 cells can be further elucidated.

4. Mesenchymal-like phenotype of the MDA-MB-231 cells

Before the subpopulation and invasiveness of the MDA-MB-231 cells can be further elucidated, hierarchy of the breast cancer stem cells in the breast cancer cell compartment should be understood. A breast cancer stem cell, as described in the cancer stem cell compartment hierarchy, is capable of undergoing an asymmetric cell division to generate one cell that is identical to itself (orange colour) and one that it is more committed towards a certain differentiation pattern (a breast cancer cell, grey colour) (Cariati & Purushotham, 2008; Fig. 7).

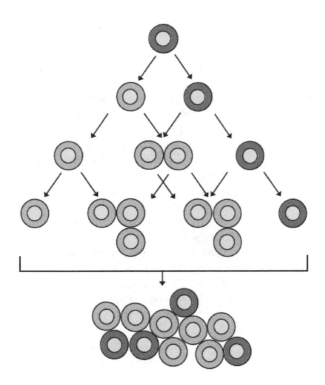

Fig. 7. A breast cancer stem cells-breast cancer cells compartment hierarchy. A breast cancer stem cell is capable of going through an asymmetric cell division to generate one cell that is identical to itself (orange colour) and one that tends toward a certain differentiation pattern (breast cancer cells, grey colour) (Modified from Cariati & Rurushotham, 2008).

The formation of the identical cell ensures that the cancer stem cell compartment is maintained throughout its time in the subpopulation. These distinct cells undergo series of divisions and differentiation steps that result in the generation of a terminally differentiated population of breast cancer stem cells and breast cancer cells. The existence of these cancer stem cells explains why only a small minority of cancer cells are capable of extensive proliferate and transfer to the tumour. Chemotherapy can remove breast cancer cells, but it fails to eliminate the cancer stem cells that can revive the breast cancer cells. This allows the regrowth of the breast cancer after the treatment has ended (Sanchez-Garcia *et al.*, 2008). This shortcoming explains the high recurrence of the disease. Therefore, the current strategy for the development of anti-breast cancer agents is to target both breast cancer stem cells and breast cancer cells. Moreover, the healthy breast cells transform into cancer cells *via* the formation of breast cancer stem cells is also a possibility, but, the precise mechanism of the transformation for this disease remains unclear. Therefore, study of the transformation remains warranted. By understanding the precise mechanism that transforms normal stem cells into cancer cells *via* the formation of the cancer stem cells, it would be possible to develop more effective tools for the ERα-negative human breast cancer prevention, detection and treatment.

The MDA-MB-231 cell line is a good example of a breast cancer cell line that consists of the above mentioned populations of breast cancer stem cells and breast cancer cells. As described above, the MDA-MB-231 cells have been demonstrated to contain a subpopulation of CD44+/CD24- that provides stem/progenitor cell properties to enhance the invasiveness of the cancer cells. Surprisingly, in our present study, we found that the MDA-MB-231 cells were positive for CD105 staining, while the weakly metastatic breast cancer cell lines, such as MCF-7 and T47D, were negative for the CD105 staining; the staining was visualised by fluorescent microscopy (Fig. 8A). CD105, also known as Endoglin, is a type I integral trans-membrane glycoprotein and is an accessory receptor for transforming growth factor-alpha (TGFβ) superfamily ligands (Barbara *et al.*, 1999). CD105 is found on activated monocytes, mesenchymal stromal cells and leukemic cells of lymphoid and myeloid lineages. The BMSCs, as well as other non-hematopoietic MSCs, are positive for the CD105 antibody staining, as visualised by fluorescent microscopy (Miao *et al.*, 2006; Bernacki *et al.*, 2008). Therefore, it is hypothesised that the MDA-MB-231 cells may have similar mesenchymal phenotypes as the progenitor factors that contribute to the metastatic potency of the cancer cells. Therefore, the cell line contains not only the stem/progenitor cell properties but also the mesenchymal-like stem/progenitor cell properties. This property likely contributes to the invasiveness of the cell line and causes the cell line to express high levels of MMP-9, IL-6, CCL2 and CCL5 in the conditioned medium. The Oil-Red-O-stained MDA-MB-231 cells were also observed to contain a mixture of epithelial cells and a mesenchymal-like subpopulation, as visualised by light microscopy (Fig. 8B).

These results focused our attention and research on the mesenchymal-like phenotype in the MDA-MB-231 cells. MDA-MB-231 and MCF-7 are cell lines that originate from pleural effusion metastatic cells in ductal invasive breast carcinomas (Burdall *et al.*, 2003; Lacroix & Leclercq, 2004). These cells are among the most commonly used breast cancer cell lines in medical research laboratories. MDA-MB-231 is a mesenchymal-like cell line that is highly aggressive and invasive, whereas MCF-7 is classified as a luminal (epithelial)-like cell line with a relatively low invasive phenotype and potential (Lacroix & Leclercq, 2004; Charafe-Jauffret *et al.*, 2006). A comparison of the two cell lines in terms of DNA copy number variation and gene expression profiles has been performed, and the expression levels of 2157 transcripts were shown to be significantly increased in the MDAMB-231 cells compared with the MCF-7 cells; the expression levels of 2345 transcripts were significantly increased in the MCF-7 cells compared with the MDA-MB-231 cells (Forozon *et al.*, 2000; Charafe-Jauffret *et al.*, 2006). Moreover, 387 of the above transcripts have been defined by the gene expression profile to be mesenchymal-like cellular subtypes (Charafe-Jauffret *et al.*, 2006). Recently, 31 mesenchymal-like and luminal-like subtype features of breast cancer cell lines were revealed in Charafe-Jauffret's study, which was based on the gene expression profiles. The study found that 680 transcripts were preferentially expressed in the group of mesenchymal-like cell lines, and 629 transcripts were expressed preferentially in the group of luminal-like breast cancer cell lines. In a recent expression study, 387 transcripts, which are also identified in the mesenchymal-like subtype gene list in Charafe-Jauffret's study, showed significantly higher expression levels in the MDA-MB-231 cells; and 328 transcripts, which were present on the luminal subtype gene list from Charafe-Jauffret's study, showed significantly higher expression levels in the MCF-7 cells (Li *et al.*, 2009). These data revealed the differential expression profiles of mesenchymal-like and luminal-like subtypes of the breast cancer cell lines. These expression profiles can be utilised to effectively overcome the invasion and metastasis of human breast cancer.

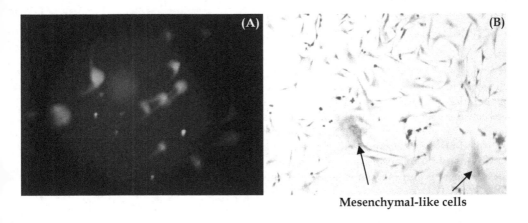

Mesenchymal-like cells

Fig. 8. **A:** The MDA-MB-231 cells, which were predicted to have a mesenchymal-like phenotype subpopulation, existed in the epithelial cell population. The cells were stained with Oil-red O and visualised using an inverted light microscope. **B:** The MDA-MB-231 cells were positive for the CD105 antibody staining as visualised using fluorescent microscope. These images were captured using a digital camera.

5. Future prospects

Our recent study proposes to isolate or withdraw the mesenchymal-like stem cells from the MDA-MB-231 population using CD105 and other known antibody-conjugated microbeads, thus allowing for a clearer understanding of the subpopulation of the cancer cells. Potential drugs will then be applied to the isolated CD105+ (mesenchymal-like stem cells) and CD105⁻ (epithelial cells) MDA-MB-231 cells. The invasion rate of the drug-treated CD105⁺ and CD105⁻ MDA-MB-231 will then be determined using the Matrigel invasion assay. The mRNA and protein expression levels of the ECM degradation-associated molecules in the drug-treated CD105⁺ and CD105⁻ MDA-MB-231 cells will also be assessed using real-time PCR and Western Blotting, respectively, and the gelatinase activities in the conditioned medium of drug-treated CD105⁺ and CD105⁻ MDA-MB-231 cells will be investigated using ELISA. The proposed project that will utilise cell separation and isolation techniques to study the breast cancer cell invasion is a new area of cancer research in the institute of my home country. The previous research projects regarding the MDA-MB-231 cell invasion and metastasis were related to drug treatments, the effects of herbal and plant extracts, and the understanding of a gene or protein activity in cancer cells and animal models. However, the approaches to study the cancer cell invasion and metastasis by isolating or withdrawing the mesenchymal-like breast cancer cells (CD105⁺) from the MDA-MB-231 cell population using cell separation or isolation have not been demonstrated. Therefore, this project may establish a new fundamental cancer research and new research topic in my institute. This study may also lay a research foundation that is focused on the inhibition of invasion for the ERα-negative human breast cancer cells. I also believe that, by targeting the mesenchymal-like phenotype in the MDA-MB-231 subpopulation, the invasion rate of the ERα-negative human breast cancer cells can be easily monitored and controlled.

6. Conclusion

All of the results mentioned above show that the MDA-MB-231 cells likely display a mesenchymal-like phenotype that facilitates the cells to be a highly metastatic breast cancer cell line. However, a deeper understanding of the cell morphology, gene expression and intracellular mechanisms and pathways of the cancer cells that can explain the interaction between mesenchymal-like and epithelial cells in the MDA-MB-231 cells is warranted. By targeting this phenotype, the metastatic potency and the growth of the cancer cells may be controlled or effectively reduced. A potential anticancer drug can also be identified to treat both human breast cancers and other malignancies. Perhaps, withdrawing the progenitor factor from a tumour may serve as a potential machinery target in cell-mediated therapy for human breast cancer.

7. Acknowledgements

This book chapter project was funded by a Fundamental Research Grant Scheme (FRGS) Fasa 2/2010 (203/CIPPM/6711162) from the Ministry of Higher Education (MoHE), Malaysia. The author also thanks the technical support of all members at the Division of Oncology and Hematology, Charité Campus Mitte, Humboldt University of Berlin, Germany.

8. References

Al-Hajj, M.; Wicha, M.S.; Benito-Hernandez, A.; Morrison, S.J. & Clarke, M.F. (2003) Prospective identification of tumorigenic breast cáncer cells. *Proc. Natl. Acad. Sci. USA*, 100, 3983-3988.

Balkwill, F. (2004) Cancer and the chemokine network. *Nat. Rev. Cancer*, 4, 540-550.

Barbara, N.P.; Wrana, J.L. & Letarte, M. (1999) Endoglin is an accessory protein that interacts with the signaling receptor complex of multiple members of the transforming growth factor-beta superfamily. *J. Biol. Chem.*, 274, 584-594.

Behbod, F. & Rosen, J.M. (2005) Will cancer stem cells provide new therapeutic targets? *Carcinogenesis*, 26, 703-711.

Bernacki, S.H.; Wall, M.E. & Loboa, E.G. (2008) Isolation of human mesenchymal stem cells from bone and adipose tissue. *Methods Cell Biol.*, 86, 257-278.

Boutaud, A.; Borza, D.B.; Bondar, O.; Gunwar, S.; Netzer, K.O.; Singh, N.; Ninomiya, Y.; Sado, Y.; Noelken, M.E. & Hudson, B.G. (2000) Type IV collagen of the glomerular basement membrane. Evidence that the chain specificity of network assembly is encoded by the noncollagenous NC1 domains. *J. Biol. Chem.*, 275, 30716-30724.

Burdall, S.E.; Hanby, A.M. & Lansdown, M.R. (2003) Speirs V: Breast cancer cell lines: friend or foe? *Breast Cancer Res.*, 5, 89-95.

Cariati, M. & Purushotham, A.D. (2008) Stem cells and breast cancer. *Histopathology*, 52, 99–107.

Castro-Sanchez, L.; Soto-Guzman, A.; Guaderrama-Diaz, M.; Cortes-Reynosa, P.; Salazar, E.P. (2011) Role of DDR1 in the gelatinases secretion induced by native type IV collagen in MDA-MB-231 breast cancer cells. *Clin. Exp. Metastasis*, 28(5): 463-77.

Charafe-Jauffret, E.; Ginestier, C.; Monville, F.; Finetti, P.; Adelaide, J.; Cervera, N.; Fekairi, S.; Xerri, L.; Jacquemier, J.; Birnbaum, D. & Bertucci, F. (2006) Gene expression profiling of breast cell lines identifies potential new basal markers. *Oncogene*, 25, 2273-2284.

Data sheet of ATCC for MDA-MB-231 cells, www.atcc.org/ATCCAdvancedCatalogSearch/ProductDetails/tabid/452/Default. aspx?ATCCNum=HTB-26&Template=cellBiology

Dean, M.; Fojo, T. & Bates, S. (2005) Tumour stem cells and drug resistance. *Nat. Rev. Cancer*, 5, 275-284.

Dumont, N. & Arteaga, C.L. (2003) Targeting the TGF beta signaling network in human neoplasia. *Cancer Cell*, 3, 531-536.

Edwards, D.R. & Murphy, G. (1998) Proteases: invasion and more. *Nature*, 394, 527-528.

Forozan, F.; Mahlamaki, E.H.; Monni, O.; Chen, Y.; Veldman, R.; Jiang, Y.; Gooden, G.C.; Ethier, S.P.; Kallioniemi, A. & Kallioniemi, O.P. (2000) Comparative genomic hybridization analysis of 38 breast cancer cell lines: a basis for interpreting complementary DNA microarray data. *Cancer Res.*, 60, 4519-4525.

Fujimoto, H.; Sangai, T.; Ishii, G.; Ikehara, A.; Nagashima, T.; Miyazaki, M. & Ochiai, A. (2009) Stromal MCP-1 in mammary tumors induces tumour-associated macrophage infiltration and contributes to tumour progression. *Int. J. Cancer*, 125, 1276-1284.

Goldberg-Bittman, L.; Neumark, E.; Sagi-Assif, O.; Azenshtein, E.; Meshel, T.; Witz, I.P. & Ben-Baruch, A. (2004) The expression of the chemokine receptor CXCR3 and its ligand, CXCL10, in human breast adenocarcinoma cell lines. *Immunol Lett.*, 92, 171-178.

Heinrich, P. C.; Behrmann, I.; Muller-Newen, G.; Schaper, F. & Graeve, L. (1998) Interleukin-6-type cytokine signaling through the gp130/Jak/STAT pathway. *Biochem. J.*, 334, 297-314.

Hombauer, H. & Minguell, J.J. (2000) Selective interactions between epithelial tumour cells and bone marrow mesenchymal stem cells. *Br. J. Cancer*, 82, 1290-1296.

Jones, D.H.; Nakashima, T.; Sanchez, O.H.; Kozieradzki, I.; Komarova, S.V.; Sarosi, I.; Morony, S.; Rubin, E.; Sarao, R.; Hojilla, C.V.; Komnenovic, V.; Kong, Y.Y.; Schreiber, M.; Dixon, S.J.; Sims, S.M.; Khokha, R.; Wada, T. & Penninger, J.M. (2006) Regulation of cancer cell migration and bone metastasis by RANKL. *Nature*, 440, 692-696.

Kang, Y.; Siegel, P.M.; Shu, W.; Drobnjak, M.; Kakonen, S.M.; Cordon-Cardo, C.; Guise, T.A. & Massague, J. (2003) A multigenic program mediating breast cancer metastasis to bone. *Cancer Cell*, 3, 537-549.

Karnoub, A.E.; Dash, A.B.; Vo, A.P.; Sullivan, A.; Brooks, M.W.; Bell, G.W.; Richardson, A.L.; Polyak, K.; Tubo, R. & Weinberg, R.A. (2007) Mesenchymal stem cells within tumour stroma promote breast cancer metastasis. *Nature*, 449, 557-563.

Lacroix, M. & Leclercq, G. (2004) Relevance of breast cancer cell lines as models for breast tumours: an update. *Breast Cancer Res. Treat.*, 83, 249-289.

Li, J.; Gao, F.; Li, N.; Li, S.; Yin, G.; Tian, G.; Jia, S.; Wang, K.; Zhang, X.; Yang, H.; Nielsen, A.L. & Bolund, L. (2009) An improved method for genome wide DNA methylation profiling correlated to transcription and genomic instability in two breast cancer cell lines. *BMC Genomics.* 10, 223.

Lieblein, J.C.; Ball, S.; Hutzen, B.; Sasser, A.K.; Lin, H.J.; Huang, T.H.; Hall, B.M. & Lin, J. (2008) STAT3 can be activated through paracrine signaling in breast epithelial cells. *BMC Cancer*, 8, 302-315.

Ling, X. & Arlinghaus, R. B. (2005) Knockdown of STAT3 expression by RNA interference inhibits the induction of breast tumors in immunocompetent mice. *Cancer Res.*, 65, 2532-2536.

Liu, H.; Zang, C.; Fenner, M.H.; Possinger, K. & Elstner, E. (2003) PPARgamma ligands and ATRA inhibit the invasion of human breast cancer cells in vitro. *Breast Cancer Res. Treat.*, 79, 63-74.

Lu, X. & Kang Y. (2009) Chemokine (C-C motif) ligand 2 engages CCR2+ stromal cells of monocytic origin to promote breast cancer metastasis to lung and bone. *J. Biol. Chem.*, 284, 29087-29096.

Melgarejo, E.; Medina, M.A.; Sa´nchez-Jime´nez, F.; & Urdiales, J.L. (2009) Monocyte chemoattractant protein-1: a key mediator in inflammatory processes. *Int. J. Biochem. Cell Biol.*, 41, 998-1001.

Miao, Z.; Jin, J.; Chen, L.; Zhu, J.; Huang, W.; Zhao, J.; Qian, H. & Zhang, X. (2006) Isolation of mesenchymal stem cells from human placenta: comparison with human bone marrow mesenchymal stem cells. *Cell Biol. Int.*, 30, 681-687.

Ponti, D.; Costa, A.; Zaffaroni, N.; Pratesi, G.; Petrangolini, G.; Coradini, D.; Pilotti, S.; Pierotti, M.A. & Daidone, M.G. (2005) Isolation and in vitro propagation of tumorigenic breast cancer cells with stem/progenitor cell properties. *Cancer Res*, 65, 5506-5511.

Reya, T.; Morrison, S.J.; Clarke, M.F. & Weissman, I.L. (2001) Stem cells, cancer, and cancer stem cells. *Nature*, 414, 105-111.

Sanchez-Garcia, Isidro, Cobaleda and Cesar. 2008. Cancer Stem Cells. *SciTopics*. Retrieved May 20, 2010, from www.scitopics.com/Cancer_Stem_Cells.html.

Sasser, A.K.; Mundy, B.L.; Smith, K.M.; Studebaker, A.W.; Axel, A.E.; Haidet, A.M.; Fernandez, S.A. & Hall, B.M. (2007a) Human bone marrow stromal cells enhance breast cancer cell growth rates in a cell line-dependent manner when evaluated in 3D tumour environments. *Cancer Lett.*, 254, 255-264.

Sasser, A.K.; Sullivan, N.J.; Studebaker, A.W.; Hendey, L.F.; Axel, A.E. & Hall, B.M. (2007b) Interleukin-6 is a potent growth factor for ER-alpha-positive human breast cancer. *Faseb J.*, 21, 3763-3770.

Selander, K.S.; Li, L.; Watson, L.; Merrell, M.; Dahmen, H.; Heinrich, P.C.; Muller-Newen, G. & Harris, K.W. (2004) Inhibition of gp130 signaling in breast cancer blocks constitutive activation of Stat3 and inhibits in vivo malignancy. *Cancer Res.*, 64, 6924–6933.

Sheridan, C.; Kishimoto, H.; Fuchs, R.K.; Mehrotra, S.; Bhat-Nakshatri, P.; Turner, C.H.; Goulet, R.Jr.; Badve, S. & Nakshatri, H. (2006) CD44+/CD24- breast cancer cells exhibit enhanced invasive properties: an early step necessary for metastasis. *Breast Cancer Res.*, 8, R59.

Soria, G. & Ben-Baruch, A. (2008) The inflammatory chemokines CCL2 and CCL5 in breast cancer. *Cancer Lett.*, 267, 271-285.

Soria, G.; Yaal-Hahoshen, N.; Azenshtein, E.; Shina, S.; Leider-Trejo, L.; Ryvo, L.; Cohen-Hillel, E.; Shtabsky, A.; Ehrlich, M.; Meshel, T.; Keydar, I. & Ben-Baruch, A. (2008) Concomitant expression of the chemokines RANTES and MCP-1 in human breast cancer: a basis for tumour-promoting interactions. *Cytokine*, 44, 191-200.

Wang, L.; Tran, I.; Seshareddy, K.; Weiss, M.L. & Detamore, M.S. (2009) A comparison of human bone marrow-derived mesenchymal stem cells and human umbilical cord-derived mesenchymal stromal cells for cartilage tissue engineering. *Tissue Eng. Part A*, 15, 2259-2266.

Wu, F.-Y.; Ou, Z.-L.; Feng, L.-Y.; Luo, J.-M.; Wang, L.-P.; Shen, Z.-Z. & Shao, Z.-M. (2008). Chemokine decoy receptor D6 plays a negative role in human breast cancer. *Molecular Cancer Research*, 6, 1276-1288.

Yaal-Hahoshen, N.; Shina, S.; Leider-Trejo, L.; Barnea, I.; Shabtai, E.L.; Azenshtein, E.; Greenberg, I.; Keydar, I. & Ben-Baruch, A. (2006) The Chemokine CCL5 as a Potential Prognostic Factor Predicting Disease Progression in Stage II Breast Cancer Patients. *Clin. Cancer Res.*, 12, 4474-4480.

Yodkeeree, S.; Ampasavate, C.; Sung, B.; Aggarwal, B.B. & Limtrakul, P. (2010) Demethoxycurcumin suppresses migration and invasion of MDA-MB-231 human breast cancer cell line. *Eur. J. Pharmacol.*, 627, 8-15.

Yu, H.; Kortylewski, M. & Pardoll, D. (2007) Crosstalk between cancer and immune cells: role of STAT3 in the tumour microenvironment. *Nat. Rev. Immunol.*, 7, 41–51.

Zinzalla, G.; Haque, M.R.; Basu, B.P.; Anderson, J.; Kaye, S.L.; Haider, S.; Hasan, F.; Antonow, D.; Essex, S.; Rahman, K.M.; Palmer, J.; Morgenstern, D.; Wilderspin, A.F.; Neidle, S. & Thurston, D.E. (2010) A novel small-molecule inhibitor of IL-6 signalling. *Bioorg. Med. Chem. Lett.*, 20, 7029-7032.

p130Cas and p140Cap as the Bad and Good Guys in Breast Cancer Cell Progression to an Invasive Phenotype

P. Di Stefano, M. del P. Camacho Leal, B. Bisaro, G. Tornillo, D. Repetto, A. Pincini, N. Sharma, S. Grasso, E. Turco, S. Cabodi and P. Defilippi
Molecular Biotechnology Center, Università di Torino, Torino
Italy

1. Introduction

Breast cancer is an aggressive malignancy affecting a large woman population. Even though important progress have been made in providing new therapies to treat this neoplasia, our knowledge on the mechanisms underlying the transformation of breast epithelial cells in tumor cells is still superficial. The neoplastic phenotype results from the alteration of multiple cellular signaling mechanisms controlling proliferation, survival and invasiveness. Moreover, the prognosis of breast cancer patients is tightly correlated with the degree of spread beyond the primary tumor. However the mechanisms by which epithelial tumor cells escape from the primary tumor and colonize a distant site are not entirely understood. In this chapter we will discuss recent data on the relevance of p130Cas and p140Cap adaptor molecules in breast cancer signalling related to the acquirement on invasive properties. Due to the presence of adaptor modules, these proteins create signalling platforms proximal to plasma membrane cell surface receptors, such as integrins and growth factor receptors. p130Cas and p140Cap exert opposite regulation on cell signalling. Indeed p130Cas has been shown to increase survival, proliferation and migration of normal and transformed cells either in response to cell matrix adhesion or to hormones and growth factors. Moreover, p130Cas has been recently linked to resistance to breast cancer treatments, revealing its potential use as a novel therapeutic target. Instead, p140Cap behaves as a potent negative regulator of signalling pathways leading to cancer cell proliferation and migration. In this chapter, we will discuss the increasing evidence that highlight the importance of these adaptor proteins in breast cancer.

It is well established that to migrate and to invade a cell needs to detach from its neighbors, i.e. adjacent cells in an epithelium, to extend lamellipodia and filopodia from the leading edge and to create new dynamic adhesions, which form and rapidly disassemble at the base of protrusions (Mitra *et al.*, 2005; Ridley *et al.*, 2003). Cell invasion also requires the release or activation of proteases that degrade the extracellular matrix (ECM) and allows cells to sort out from the basal lamina invading surrounding tissues (Eliceiri *et al.*, 2002). Under physiological conditions cell motility and invasion are tightly controlled by a complex interplay among cell-cell, cell matrix and growth factors receptors resulting in the maintenance of the architectural integrity of human tissues. This subtle regulation is lost in human tumours leading to uncontrolled dissemination of cancer cells into the body (Berx *et al.*, 2007; Cavallaro and Christofori, 2004; Giancotti, 2003; Guo and Giancotti, 2004),

At least three major classes of membrane proteins are involved in these events, namely, the E-cadherin, the Receptor tyrosine kinases (RPTKs), and the integrin receptors. The cell-cell adhesion receptor E-cadherin is the major membrane protein involved in binding between neighbouring cells in adherens junctions. As a practical consequence of its adhesive functions, E-cadherin has also been shown to prevent EGFR activation and downstream signalling, leading to negative regulation of proliferation (Berx and Van Roy, 2001; Gutkind, 2000; Perrais *et al.*, 2007; Qian *et al.*, 2004). E-cadherin is frequently down-regulated or lost in epithelial tumours, and its loss correlates with increased cancer cell invasiveness ((Peinado *et al.*, 2007; Reynolds and Carnahan, 2004);.

Integrins are cell surface heterodimeric receptors for the ECM formed by the non covalent association of alpha and beta subunits (Hynes, 2004). Integrins specifically localize to focal adhesions, which are sites of close apposition with the ECM where actin filaments are anchored to the plasma membrane. Integrins are catalytically inactive and translate positional cues into biochemical signals by direct and/or functional association with intracellular adaptors or growth factor and cytokine receptors, thus regulating integrin ability to transduce signals inside the cells, the so called "outside-in signalling" (Cabodi *et al.*, 2010). A growing body of evidence shows that integrins, RPTKs and cytokine receptors have no longer to be considered as individual receptors, but rather as joint modules in which attachment to the matrix confers positional control to respond to soluble growth factors (Cabodi *et al.*, 2010b; Cabodi *et al.*, 2008; Desgrosellier *et al.*, 2009; Streuli, 2009; Uberti *et al.*). In the case of the EGF receptor (EGFR), beta1 integrin is both sufficient to partially activate the receptor itself and required for the full activation of the EGFR in response to EGF (Morello *et al.*; Moro *et al.*, 1998)). Integrin-dependent EGFR trans-activation accounts for a specific repertoire of mechanisms, namely cell survival and actin cytoskeleton organization involved in cell migration.

In this chapter we will focus on p140Cap and p130Cas adaptors as major regulators of cell migration and invasion (Cabodi *et al.*). Owing to their modular structure, both proteins can undergo tyrosine phosphorylation and association with effector proteins, leading to the assembly of molecular platforms that regulate the variety of signalling events originating from the complex cross-talk among integrins, E-cadherin and RPTKs.

2. p130Cas adaptor protein

2.1 p130Cas adaptor features

p130Cas is coded in human by the BCAR-1 (Breast Cancer Anti-oestrogen Resistance 1) gene. This gene is conserved through many species and in humans is localized on Chromosome 16q23.1. Knock-out of the mouse gene results in embryonic lethality at 9.5 days, indicating that any other protein cannot fill in for its role during development. p130Cas is an ubiquitously expressed multi-site docking protein that consists of i) an N-terminal Src homology 3 (SH3) domain, ii) a substrate domain, which contains 15 repeats of a YXXP sequence (tyrosine-any two aminoacids-proline), iii) a serine rich region, and iv) a C-terminal domain (Figure 1A). The presence of these multiple conserved sequence motifs and extensive post-translational modification, mainly consisting of tyrosine and serine phosphorylation, allow the assembly of specific multi-protein complexes. In particular, the SH3 domain interacts with polyproline-rich sequences present in several proteins including

Fak, PYK2/RAFTK, phosphatases like PTP-PEST, PTP1B, and effectors as C3G and CIZ (Sakai *et al.*, 1994; Tikhmyanova *et al.*). The substrate domain, upon Src family kinases activation, is tyrosine phosphorylated and exposes additional binding sites for SH2 containing proteins such as the Crk adaptors (Salgia *et al.*, 1996), while the serine rich region represents a docking site for other partners such as 14-3-3 and Grb2. Lastly, the C-terminus contains a polyproline-rich region responsible for the binding of the Src family kinase, PI3K, Bcar3/AND-34, Chat-H and ubiquitin ligases such as AIP4, APC/C and CDH1, as well as a binding site for the adaptor protein p140Cap (Bouton *et al.*, 2001; Cabodi *et al.*, 2004; O'Neill *et al.*, 2000).

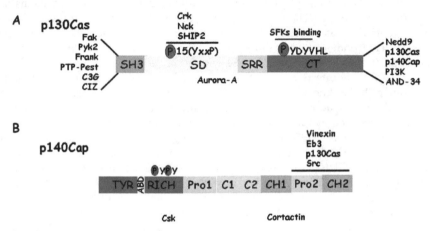

Fig. 1. p130Cas and p140Cap structure.
A) p130Cas consists of an N-terminal SH3 domain, a substrate domain (SD), a serine rich region (SRR), and a C-terminal domain (CT). The main interactors are indicated. In particular, many proteins associate to the N-terminal domain and the Src family kinases (SFKs) bind the CT domain. The 15 YxxP motifs are phosphorylated by Src family kinases to mediate Crk binding.
B) p140Cap consists of an N-terminal tyrosine–rich region (Tyr-rich), an actin binding domain (ABD), a proline rich domain (Pro1), a coil-coiled region (C1-C2), two domains rich in charged amino acids (CH1, CH2) and a C-terminal proline rich domain (Pro2). Src, p130Cas, EB3 and Vinexin bind to the Pro2 domain of p140Cap. The binding regions of Cortactin and Csk have yet to be defined.

2.2 p130Cas in human breast cancer
Although several reports highlight the relevance of p130Cas in tumour cell lines and animal models, investigation of its expression in biopsies of different human malignancies using immunohistochemistry, is still limited. However, it is noteworthy that a significant subset of human breast cancers where both ErbB2 and p130Cas are over-expressed are associated with increased proliferation and low prognosis (Cabodi *et al.*, 2006). In estrogen receptor (ER)-positive human breast tumours, p130Cas over-expression correlates with intrinsic resistance to tamoxifen treatment, high risk of relapse and loss of oestrogen-receptor in a large subset of human breast cancer samples, indicating that elevated BCAR1 might be a prognostic marker for breast tumours (Dorssers *et al.*, 2001; van der Flier *et al.*, 2001).

Therefore, at least in two classes of breast cancer that account for more than 90% of breast tumors, p130Cas over-expression is revealing its potential as prognostic factor in terms of therapy and disease progression.

2.3 p130Cas tyrosine phosphorylation in cell migration and invasion

p130Cas represents a nodal signalling platform on which integrin and RPTKs signalling convey. Integrins, RPTKs and oestrogen receptor (ER) are major upstream regulators of p130Cas, mainly through the activation of Src and Fak kinases, leading to p130Cas tyrosine phosphorylation on the C-terminal binding site YDYVHL (Figure 1) (Cabodi *et al.*). Moreover, physical stretching of p130Cas induces a conformational change that enables Src-family kinase-dependent p130Cas tyrosine phosphorylation. These findings point out a function for p130Cas as a sensor that integrates mechanical forces coming from the extracellular environment into intracellular signals leading to actin cytoskeleton reorganization (Kostic and Sheetz, 2006; Sawada *et al.*, 2006). The role of p130Cas in cell migration was initially inferred by studies performed on mouse embryo fibroblasts (MEFs) derived from p130Cas knock-out mice. p130Cas null MEFs show defects in stress fibre formation and cell spreading, impaired actin bundling and cell migration (Honda *et al.*, 1998), that were restored by full-length p130Cas expression. The tyrosine phosphorylation of the substrate domain of p130Cas provides binding sites for Crk proteins that in turn associates with DOCK180, a guanine nucleotide exchange factor that switches the small GTPase Rac1 from a GDP-bound inactive to a GTP-bound active state at lamellipodia and filopodia adhesion sites (Figure 2) (Kiyokawa *et al.*, 1998; Klemke *et al.*, 1998). This drives localized Rac activation, membrane ruffling and actin cytoskeleton remodelling, focal adhesion turnover, pseudopodia formation and extension. In addition, ARP2/3 and PAK kinase activation enhance cell migration (Heasman and Ridley, 2008). Uncoupling of p130Cas/Crk negatively regulates cell migration. Indeed, the non-receptor tyrosine kinase Abl phosphorylates Crk-II on tyrosine 221, inducing intramolecular folding that prevents binding of the C-terminal Crk-II SH2 domain to the phosphorylated p130Cas substrate domain, leading to decreased cell movement (Holcomb *et al.*, 2006; Kobashigawa *et al.*, 2007). Additional molecules that play important roles in modulating tyrosine phosphorylation of p130Cas leading to cell migration are the zyxin/Ajuba family of LIM proteins. These proteins bind to actin cytoskeleton and are implicated in cell motility. Ajuba allows p130Cas localization to nascent adhesive sites in migrating cells thereby leading to the activation of the small GTPase Rac, whereas Zyxin interacts with the SH3 domain of p130Cas and with a nucleocytoplasmic transcription factor, CIZ/NMP4/ZNF384 (Janssen and Marynen, 2006). Recent data also show that p130Cas activates several GTPases other than Rac. The association between p130Cas and And-34, an NSP family member, which acts as a GTP exchange factor for Ral, Rap1 and R-Ras enhances Src activation and cell migration, likely through a Rap1-dependent mechanism (Figure 2)(Riggins *et al.*, 2003). p130Cas tyrosine phosphorylation upon integrin or growth factor receptor activation has also been linked to cell invasion and it has been reported that the SH3 domain of p130Cas is also required for this process. Indeed, Focal adhesion kinase (Fak)-null cells are not invasive when transformed by v-Src, but they acquire invasive properties upon over-expression of p130Cas SH3 domain, indicating that this domain is required for rescue of v-Src cell invasion. In this context, the formation of Src/p130Cas/Crk/DOCK180 complex increases Rac1 and JNK activities and MMP-9 expression, leading to an invasive cell phenotype (Hsia *et al.*, 2003).

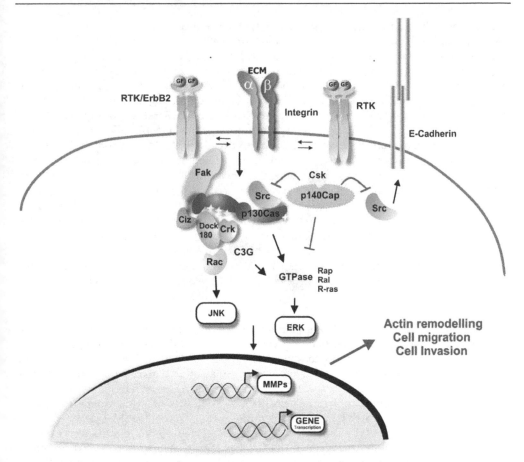

Fig. 2. p130Cas and p140Cap signalling involved in migration and invasion of breast cancer cells.

Upon extracellular matrix binding or growth factors stimulation, integrins and Receptor Protein Tyrosine Kinases (RPTK) represent the major upstream regulators of p130Cas and p140Cap, mainly through the regulation of Src kinase activity. Once tyrosine phosphorylated by Src, p130Cas recruits proteins that activate downstream pathways, resulting in actin cytoskeleton re-organization, increased cell motility and migration. p130Cas by acting on metalloproteinases (MMPs) promoter is also required for the invasive program. Upon cell matrix adhesion or mitogen stimulus, p140Cap inhibits Src kinase activity and p130Cas tyrosine phosphorylation and p130Cas/Crk complex formation. As a consequence, the effect of p130Cas on actin cytoskeleton re-organization is impaired and cell migration and invasion are inhibited. (Di Stefano et al., 2007) Moreover, by inactivating Src, p140Cap also regulates the epidermal growth factor receptor (EGFR) pathway through E-cadherin-dependent inactivation of EGFR signalling. p140Cap by interacting with E-cadherin and EGFR at the cell membrane, immobilizes E-Cadherin at the cell membrane thus preventing cell migration and invasion. (Damiano et al., 2010)

2.4 Role of p130Cas in c-Src dependent cell transformation

Hyper-phosphorylation or over-expression of p130Cas has been implicated in transformation induced by several oncogenes. For example, p130Cas involvement in c-Src-mediated tumourigenesis has been demonstrated by the inability of c-Src to transform p130Cas-null MEFs (Honda *et al.*, 1998). The C-terminal region of p130Cas containing the Src binding domain is sufficient to recover the ability of Src to promote anchorage-independent growth. In breast carcinoma cells p130Cas over-expression accelerates and up-regulates Src activity (Cabodi *et al.*, 2004) as well as increases tyrosine phosphorylation of multiple endogenous cellular proteins (Brabek *et al.*, 2004; Burnham *et al.*, 1996; Cabodi *et al.*, 2004). It was recently reported that bosutinib, a novel Src inhibitor, derived from breast cancer patients, inhibits cell spreading, migration, and invasion of human cancer cells, derived from breast cancer patients by stabilizing cell-to-cell adhesions and membrane localization of beta-catenin. These effects are dependent on the inhibition of the Src/Fak/p130Cas signaling pathway (Buettner *et al.*, 2008). It has been recently reported that Fak promotes mammary tumorigenesis by enabling Src-mediated phosphorylation of p130Cas. Consistently, knock-down of p130Cas causes proliferative arrest in breast cancer cell lines harbouring oncogenic mutations in K-Ras, B-Raf, PTEN and PIK3CA (Pylayeva *et al.*, 2009), underlying a role for p130Cas as a general regulator of breast cancer cell growth induced by different oncogenes.

2.5 Role of p130Cas in TGF-beta signalling in breast cancer cells

Transforming growth factor-beta (TGF-beta) is a powerful suppressor of mammary tumorigenesis because of its ability to repress mammary epithelial cell proliferation, as well as through its creation of cell microenvironments that inhibit mammary epithelial cells (MECs) motility, invasion, and metastasis. Yet, paradoxically, cancer cells elicit mechanisms that subvert the tumour suppressing functions of TGF-beta, and in doing so, confer oncogenic and metastatic activities upon this multifunctional cytokine (Massague, 2008). In epithelial cells, integrin beta1 suppresses apoptosis and growth inhibition induced by TGF-beta (Zhang *et al.*, 2003). In this context p130Cas has been shown to be a crucial player by binding to Smad3, and preventing its phosphorylation by TGF-beta receptor. As a consequence, the transcription of the cyclin-dependent kinase inhibitors p15 and p21 is inhibited, resulting in cell cycle progression (Kim *et al.*, 2008). Recently, it has been reported that p130Cas over-expression in MECs shifts TGF-beta signalling from Smad2/SMAD3 phosphorylation to p38 MAPK activation, rendering MECs resistant to TGF-beta -induced growth arrest and enhancing their metastatic potential (Wendt *et al.*, 2009). Overall, p130Cas can act as a molecular rheostat that switches the tumour suppressor function of TGF-beta to a pro-metastatic role during breast cancer progression.

3. The ErbB2 oncogene in breast cancer

The ErbB2 oncogene is a member of the Epidermal Growth Factor Receptor (EGFR) family of receptor tyrosine kinases (RTKs). This family comprises four related members: EGFR, ErbB2 (also known as Neu, HER-2), ErbB3 (HER-3), and ErbB4 (HER-4) (Holbro *et al.*, 2003). Over-expressed and mutated ErbB2 has been found in human tumors and cancer cell lines (Mukohara; Yarden *et al.*, 2004). In addition, several studies have shown a strong correlation of ErbB2 over-expression with a negative clinical prognosis in breast cancer (Choi *et al.*, 2009; Mukohara). Significantly, ErbB-2 may be useful not only as a prognostic marker but also as a predictive marker, given that its elevated expression predicts tamoxifen resistance of the primary tumor and the response to anti-HER2 targeted therapy such as the monoclonal antibody Herceptin.

Further understanding of the mechanisms by which ErbB2 leads to tumorigenesis in the mammary gland comes from studies of ErbB2 mouse models. Expression of Neu mutation that promotes spontaneous receptor dimerization (NeuT), under the MMTV promoter, or more recently under the ErbB2 endogenous promoter (ErbB2/KI model), leads to the formation of mammary adenocarcinomas (Andrechek et al., 2000; Muller et al., 1998). Interestingly, the expression of the ErbB2 protooncogene in a MMTV-transgenic mice show late tumor latency with a low penetrance of lung metastasis, suggesting that gene amplification of the wild type receptor may be the main mechanism implicated in ErbB2-mediated tumorigenesis. Indeed, elevated protein and mRNA ErbB2 levels in the ErbB2/KI model also correlated with selective genomic amplification of the activated ErbB2 allele (Andrechek and Muller, 2000; Hodgson et al., 2005; Montagna et al., 2002). One of the most significant effects associated with ErbB2 activation is enhanced and sustained signal transduction cascades leading to the regulation a variety of cellular processes, including proliferation, apoptosis, cell polarity, migration and invasion (Feigin and Muthuswamy, 2009). Activation of specific ErbB homo- or heterodimer pairs leads to initiation of the mitogen activated protein kinase (MAPK) cascade, activation of phospholipase C gamma (PLCγ) and phosphatidylinositol 3 kinase (PI3K), as well as induction of the small GTPases Rho, Rac and Cdc42, among many other effectors   (Hynes and MacDonald, 2009; Kurebayashi, 2001). Several reports have demonstrated a role for these pathways in ErbB-induced cell migration.

3.1 p130Cas in ErbB2 dependent transformation

In the context of ErbB2 positive breast cancer, previous studies generated by our group placed p130Cas as an important regulator of ErbB2-dependent tumorigenesis. To investigate the mechanisms through which p130Cas is linked to tumorigenesis, we generated mouse mammary tumor virus (MMTV)-p130Cas mice overexpressing p130Cas in the mammary gland. MMTVp130Cas transgenic mice are characterized by extensive mammary epithelial hyperplasia during development and pregnancy and by delayed involution at the end of lactation. These phenotypes are associated with activation of Src kinase, Erk1/2 MAPK, and Akt pathways, leading to an increased rate of proliferation and a decreased apoptosis. A double-transgenic line derived from crossing MMTV-p130Cas with MMTV-HER2-Neu mice expressing the activated form of the HER2-Neu oncogene develops multifocal mammary tumors with a significantly shorter latency than the HER2-Neu parental strain alone (Figure 3). MECs isolated from tumors of double-transgenic mice display increased tyrosine phosphorylation, c-Src, and Akt activation compared with cells derived from HER2-Neu tumors. In addition, p130Cas down-regulation by RNA interference increases apoptosis in HER2-Neu-expressing cells, indicating that p130Cas regulates cell survival. These findings provide evidences for a role of p130Cas as a positive regulator of both proliferation and survival in normal and transformed mammary epithelial cells. Its overexpression contributes to HER2-Neu-induced breast tumorigenesis, thus identifying this protein as a putative target for clinical therapy (Cabodi et al., 2006).

More recent studies further assessed the functional role of p130Cas in ErbB2-dependent breast tumorigenesis by its silencing in breast cancer cells derived from mouse mammary tumours over-expressing ErbB2 (N202-1A cells), and by its re-expression in ErbB2-

transformed p130Cas-null mouse embryonic fibroblasts. We demonstrate that p130Cas is necessary for ErbB2-dependent foci formation, anchorage-independent growth and *in vivo* growth of orthotopic N202-1A tumours. Moreover intra-nipple injection of p130Cas-stabilized siRNAs in the mammary gland of MMTV-HER2-Neu mice decreases the growth of spontaneous tumours (Figure 4) (Cabodi *et al.*, 2010c).

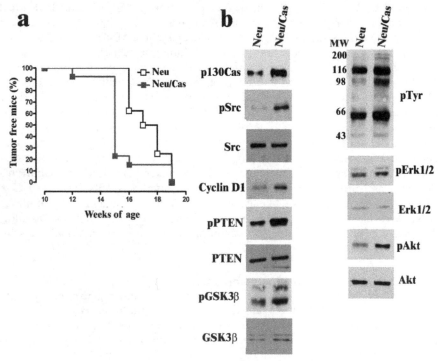

Fig. 3. Kinetics of tumor occurrence in p130Cas/HER2-Neu and HER2-Neu mice.
A) Tumor formation in p130Cas/HER2-Neu (gray line and black circles) and HER2-Neu (black line and empty squares) mice. Twenty mice were analyzed for each group. The difference of occurrence between the two groups is statistically significant, P < 0.001.
B) Independent epithelial cell culture were derived from four distinct tumors excised from p130Cas/HER2-Neu and HER2-Neu mice. Western blot analysis of protein extracts was done with the indicated antibodies and representative results are shown. MW, molecular weight markers. The figure is modified from Cabodi *et al.*, 2006.

To precisely underline the mechanism implicated in p130Cas/ErbB2-mediated transformation, cultures of MECs grown on three dimensional matrix, that share several properties with breast epithelial acini were evaluated. These in vitro three-dimensional acini-like structures provide a developmental context and serve as an important tool to study the biological effects of oncogenic signals. Most oncogenic signals that promote proliferative signals have the ability disrupt acini organization with oncogene-specific features. For instance, activation of ErbB2 induces formation of abnormal non invasive structures consisting of individual units (Muthuswamy *et al.*, 2001). Interestingly, in human mammary cells MCF10A.B2, the concomitant activation of ErbB2 and p130Cas over-expression provides invasive properties (Figure 5). Consistently, p130Cas drives N202-1A cells *in vivo* lung metastases formation. These results demonstrate that p130Cas is an essential transducer in ErbB2 transformation and highlight its potential use as a novel therapeutic target in ErbB2 positive human breast cancers (Cabodi *et al.*, 2010c).

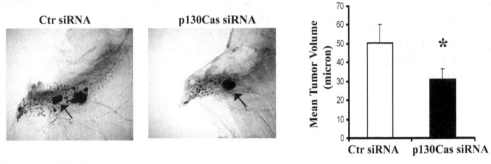

Fig. 4. p130Cas is required for *in vivo* ErbB2 tumorigenesis. Intra-nipple injection was performed in BalbC-NeuT female mice. Control (Ctr siRNA) or p130Cas stabilised siRNA (p130Cas siRNA) were injected once a week for 5 weeks starting from week 12. Left: Whole mount analyses of fixed mammary gland at week 18. The gland is composed of a tree-like structure of branching ducts. Small lesions that have histologic aspects of a solid carcinoma are visible. Black arrows indicate the lymph node. Ctr siRNA picture shows larger lesions on the right of the lymph node. Right: The histogram shows the mean tumour volume measured from two independent experiments with 8 mice per group. *p<0.0329 (two-tailed P value). The figure is modified from Cabodi *et al.*, 2010c.

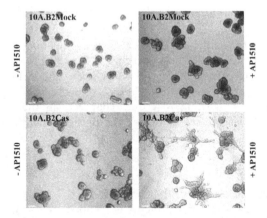

Fig. 5. p130Cas triggers acina invasion of ErbB2 transformed MCF10 cells. p130Cas over-expressing or Mock ErbB2 transformed MCF10 cells were plated on a Matrigel/collagen 1:1 matrix and left un-stimulated or activated for ErbB2 by treating with the small molecule AP1510. 3D invasive protrusions are present only in p130Cas over-expressing and ErbB2 activated acinar structures. The figure is modified from Tornillo *et al.*, 2010.

We further analysed the molecular mechanisms through which p130Cas controls ErbB2-dependent invasion in three-dimensional cultures of mammary epithelial cells. Concomitant p130Cas over-expression and ErbB2 activation enhance PI3K/Akt and Erk1/2 MAPK signalling pathways and promote invasion of mammary acini. By using pharmacological inhibitors, we demonstrate that both signaling cascades are required for the invasive behaviour of p130Cas over-expressing and ErbB2 activated acini. Erk1/2 MAPK and PI3K/Akt signaling triggers invasion involving mTOR/p70S6K and Rac1 activation, respectively (Figure 6). Moreover, in silico analyses indicate that p130Cas expression in ErbB2 positive human breast cancers significantly correlates with higher risk to develop distant metastasis, thus underlying the value of the p130Cas/ErbB2 synergism in regulating breast cancer invasion. In conclusion, high levels of p130Cas favour progression of ErbB2-transformed cells towards an invasive phenotype (Tornillo *et al.*, 2010).

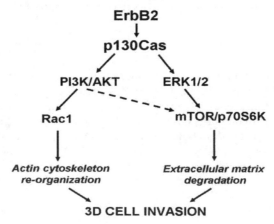

Fig. 6. Scheme illustrating the signaling pathways leading to 3D invasion of ErbB2 transformed MCF10 over-expressing p130Cas.

Both PI3K/Akt and Erk1/2 pathways are activated during invasion triggered by ErbB2 transformation of p130Cas over-expressing MEC. ErbB2/p130Cas/Erk1/2 MAPK signalling pathway preferentially targets mTOR/p70S6K, whereas the ErbB2/p130Cas/PI3K/Akt cascade triggers Rac1 activation. Both signaling pathways are required for mammary epithelia invasion in 3D suggesting that they cooperate in the regulation of different processes that ultimately lead to cell invasion. The figure is modified from Tornillo *et al.*, 2010.

4. p140Cap adaptor protein

4.1 p140Cap structure and phosphorylation
The human p140Cap (Cas associated protein) is codified by the gene Srcin1, previously known as SNIP, P140 or p140Cap. The Srcin1 gene is conserved in human, mouse, rat, dog, cow, and zebrafish and in human is localized on Chromosome 17 q21.1.
The p140Cap protein was originally identified in rat brain as SNIP, a Synaptosome-associated protein SNAP-25b-interacting protein implicated in regulated exocytosis (Chin *et al.*, 2000). The name p140Cap derives from its identification as a protein associated to

p130Cas by affinity cromatography and MALDI-Mass spectrometry in epithelial cells (Di Stefano, 2004). p140Cap is a multisite docking protein, composed by a putative N-terminal mirystilation site, a tyrosine-rich domain, two prolin-rich regions, a coil-coiled domain, two regions rich in charged amino acids and a putative actin binding site (Figure 1)(Chin *et al.*, 2000; Di Stefano *et al.*, 2004).

p140Cap is mainly expressed in brain, testis and epithelial rich tissues such as mammary gland, lung, colon and kidney (Chin *et al.*, 2000; Di Stefano *et al.*, 2004; Ito *et al.*, 2008). The protein is present at least in two N-terminal alternative and two C-terminal different isoforms. The presence of many conserved sequence motifs that could undergo extensive post-translational modification, mostly tyrosine and serine phosphorylation, led to predict that p140Cap could promotes protein–protein interactions, leading to the formation of multiprotein complexes. Indeed p140Cap is tyrosine phosphorylated in epithelial cells upon integrin-mediated adhesion and EGF receptor activation (Di Stefano *et al.*, 2004). In addition, global phospho-proteomic analysis of human brain extracts revealed that p140Cap is phosphorylated on serine 859 in the context of the sequence 857RGS*DELTVPR866 (DeGiorgis *et al.*, 2005). The same sequence has also been found phosphorylated in mouse brain (Collins *et al.*, 2005).

4.2 p140Cap interacting proteins

Since its discovery, many proteins have been shown to bind directly or to associate in molecular complexes with p140Cap. In normal epithelial cells, p140Cap was found associated to the adaptor protein p130Cas. Although *in vitro* binding studies indicate that p140Cap and p130Cas are not directly linked, their association is mediated by the last 217 amino acids of the p140Cap C-terminal region and the p130Cas region encompassing amino acids 544-678. Through the same C-terminal region, p140Cap binds directly to the SH3 domain of the Src kinase. Moreover in MCF7 cells p140Cap has been shown by Far Western Blotting to bind directly the kinase C-terminal Src kinase (Csk), a potent negative regulator of Src (Di Stefano *et al.*, 2007). The physiological significance of p140Cap interaction with Src and Csk relates to p140Cap ability to regulate Src activation and downstream signaling (see below).

By two hybrid screen in human brain, the C-terminal motif of p140Cap has also been found to associate with the SH3 domain of Vinexin (Ito *et al.*, 2008), belonging to a family composed of vinexin, c-Cbl associated protein/ponsin, and Arg-binding protein 2 (Kioka *et al.*, 2002; Matsuyama *et al.*, 2005). In non-neuronal cells, Vinexin is localized at focal adhesions and shown to be involved in growth factor- and integrin-mediated signal transduction, actin cytoskeletal organization, cell spreading, motility, and growth (Kioka *et al.*, 2002). Always in brain, p140Cap directly associates with all the members of the microtubule plus-end tracking protein EB family through a short 92 amino acid C-terminal region, likely through a positively charged S/P-rich region (Jaworski *et al.*, 2009). The p140Cap interaction with Vinexin and EB family proteins in tumour cells remains to be established.

Finally, in breast cancer cells, p140Cap has also been shown to bind with Cortactin (Damiano *et al.*, 2011). Cortactin is a major substrate of Src kinase and localizes to cortical actin structures where it regulates early cell migration and invasion by controlling actin assembly (Weed *et al.*, 2000; Wu and Parsons, 1993; Wu *et al.*, 1991). p140Cap/Cortactin association requires the second proline-rich domain of p140Cap and the Cortactin SH3 domain, suggesting a direct interaction between the two proteins. p140Cap binding to Cortactin controls invasion properties of breast cancer cells (Damiano *et al.*, 2011).

In conclusion, p140Cap is involved in direct interactions with several proteins (Figure 1). The p140Cap binding partners are mainly implicated in membrane fusion and actin cytoskeleton remodelling. p140Cap association to p130Cas, Src, Cortactin and the presence of a putative actin binding domain in the p140Cap sequence, suggest that p140Cap could be an actin binding protein. Indeed, p140Cap has been described to co-localize with actin stress fibers and cortical actin both in epithelial and in neuroectodermal cells (Chin *et al.*, 2000; Di Stefano *et al.*, 2004; Jaworski *et al.*, 2009).

4.3 140Cap in human breast cancer
So far, few data are available on p140Cap in human tumors. Immunohistochemistry analysis of normal mammary tissue show that p140Cap expression is confined to the luminal cells of alveoli, suggesting that in normal conditions p140Cap might play a role in mammary cell differentiation. In contrast, in human breast tumours p140Cap is not expressed in 70% of tumour specimens, showing an inverse correlation with the state of malignancy.

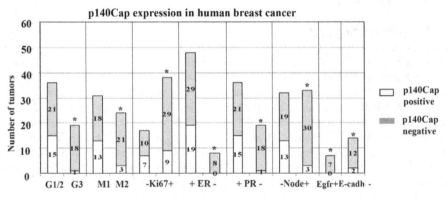

Fig. 7. p140Cap expression is lost in aggressive human breast cancers. In the histogram we reported the number of tumours positive (white) or negative (grey) for p140Cap expression according to tumour grade (low grade G1/G2, high grade G3), number of mitosis 10/10 HPS (M1 Mitosis < 10, M2 Mitosis>10), Ki67 proliferation index (Ki67+>24% , Ki67- <24%), Estrogen Receptor staining (ER-, ER+), Progesterone Receptor staining (PR-, PR+), infiltration in lymph nodes (Node+, Node-), EGFR staining (EGFR+), E-Cadherin staining (E-Cad-). The figure is modified from Damiano *et al.*, 2010.

Interestingly, 94.8% of aggressive G3 tumours, 87% of the Node +, 86.5% of tumours with a mitosis major number of 10/10HPF, and 76% of highly proliferative tumours (revealed by Ki67 staining), lose p140Cap expression. Moreover, none of the E-cadherin negative and EGFR positive tumours express p140Cap, suggesting mutually exclusive correlation between EGFR and p140Cap expression (Figure 7) (Damiano *et al.*, 2010). Therefore, although limited, these data point out that only low grade breast tumors express p140Cap. Further analysis is required to draw a general picture of the relevance of p140Cap in human breast cancers, and to delineate a potential use of p140Cap as a diagnostic and prognostic factor.

4.4 p140Cap modulates Src activity and EGFR signalling in breast cancer cells

The major function of the p140Cap adaptor is its ability to regulate Src kinase activation. In particular, in breast cancer cells, upon cell-matrix adhesion or EGF stimulation, p140Cap activates the Csk kinase, that phosphorylates the negative regulatory tyrosine 530 on the C-terminal domain of Src (Latour and Veillette, 2001) , resulting in inhibition of Src kinase. Consistently p140Cap silencing increases Src activation, leading to a fine tuning of integrin and growth factor receptor signalling (Figure 2) (Damiano *et al.*, 2010; Di Stefano *et al.*, 2007)

As a consequence, in breast cancer cells expressing high levels of p140Cap, upon integrin-mediated adhesion, the association between Src and Fak is impaired as well as integrin-dependent p130Cas phosphorylation (Figure 2). As described above p130Cas phosphorylation leads to the assembly of a p130Cas-Crk signalling complex that drives for cell migration and invasion through activation of Rac. Therefore elevated levels of p140Cap severely impair integrin-dependent Rac activity, while its down-regulation induces a sustained Rac activation (Di Stefano *et al.*, 2007).

In MCF7 breast cancer cells, p140Cap functionally interacts with E-cadherin and EGFR at the cell membrane, behaving as a new player in E-cadherin-dependent down-regulation of EGFR signalling. Indeed p140Cap-dependent inhibition of Src kinase activity results in E-cadherin immobilization at the cell membrane (Damiano *et al.*, 2010). E-cadherin is known to inhibit EGFR, either by interaction through the extracellular domains or by a beta catenin-dependent mechanism (Perrais *et al.*, 2007; Qian *et al.*, 2004; Takahashi and Suzuki, 1996). Consistently, EGFR activation, association and phosphorylation of Grb2 and Shc and Ras/Erk1/2 MAPK activities are profoundly impaired by p140Cap over-expression and enhanced by its silencing (Damiano *et al.*, 2010). Interestingly, rescue of Src activity and of E-cadherin mobility is sufficient to recover EGFR phosphorylation, but not Ras and Erk1/2 activation, that require an active RasV12, suggesting that p140Cap might regulate the Ras pathway through an additional mechanism. Therefore, in MCF7 cancer cells, p140Cap regulates EGFR signalling with dual mechanisms, involving both an E-cadherin-dependent inactivation of EGFR and a Ras-dependent inhibition of Erk1/2 activity (Damiano *et al.*, 2010).

Moreover, p140Cap expression also inhibits EGFR, Src and Erk phosphorylation in the highly aggressive MTLn3-EGFR breast cancer cells. Interestingly, in these cells, p140Cap affects also Cortactin phosphorylation in response to EGF (Damiano *et al.*, 2011).

4.5 p140Cap affects cell proliferation and in vivo tumour growth of breast cancer cells

The ability of p140Cap to regulate Src and Ras pathways profoundly affects cell proliferation. Elevated expression of p140Cap in both breast and colon cancer cells inhibits in vitro proliferation, but does not affect cell survival (Damiano *et al.*; Di Stefano *et al.*, 2007). Interestingly, p140Cap over-expression impairs colony formation in soft agar, while its silencing leads to a significantly increased number of colonies, demonstrating that p140Cap, likely through the regulation of integrin signalling, controls anchorage-independent growth (Di Stefano *et al.*, 2007). *In vivo* xenografts of breast and colon cancer cells show that cells expressing high levels of p140Cap are impaired in tumour formation. Consistently, p140Cap silencing in carcinoma cells dramatically increases *in vivo* tumour formation. Strikingly, p140Cap knock-down is sufficient for *in vivo* growth of MCF7 cells even in the absence of estrogen pellets, a condition in which control cells are unable to grow. These last findings also rise the possibility that p140Cap may regulate estrogen receptor signalling, contributing to breast cancer resistance to hormonal therapies. Thus these data provide evidence that p140Cap behaves mechanistically as a tumour suppressor molecule in breast and colon cancer cells, with a broad effect on cell proliferation and tumorigenesis.

4.6 p140Cap affects in vitro motility and invasion of breast cancer cells

As expected for the major role of Src in actin cytoskeleton dynamics and cell migration, high levels of p140Cap impair spreading and extension of lamellipodia and filopodia on extracellular matrix proteins of breast cancer cells. In addition, p140Cap over-expression also inhibits migration on fibronectin-coated transwells and invasion in Matrigel. Consistently, p140Cap silencing induces an increase in cell spreading in the early phases of cell adhesion, a fibroblastic-like shape and increased motility and invasion. Cells expressing a truncated form of p140Cap, lacking the Src-binding domain, restores integrin-dependent Src and Rac activation and are capable of migrating and invading properly (Di Stefano et al., 2007).

In addition, p140Cap specifically interferes with invasive and migratory properties of cancer cells blocking E-cadherin/EGFR cross-talk in both breast and colon cancer cells. The ability of p140Cap to immobilize E-cadherin at the cell surface strengthenes cell-cell adhesion and inhibition of cell scatter in response to EGF. Rescue of Src activity by the expression of a kinase-defective Csk mutant or by Csk silencing, recover E-cadherin mobility at the cell surface and the ability to scatter in response to EGF (Damiano et al., 2010)

Moreover, we recently identified p140Cap as a critical regulator of in vitro cell motility and invasion and in vivo metastasis formation of highly metastatic MTLn3-EGFR breast cancer cells. Our data show that increasing p140Cap expression in the highly aggressive MTLn3-EGFR cells results in an 80% decrease in in vivo lung metastasis formation (Figure 8).

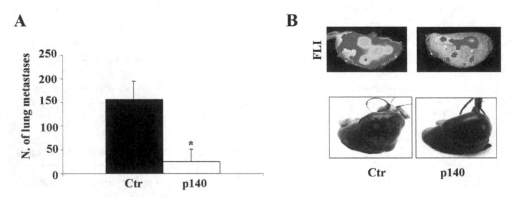

The figure is modified from Damiano et al., 2011.

Fig. 8. p140Cap over-expression inhibits spontaneous lung metastasis formation.
A) 5x10⁵ Ctr and p140 cells were injected subcutaneously in Rag2$^{-/-}$ γc$^{-/-}$ mice. Right panels: after sacrificing the mice, lungs were coloured with ink, metastasis were counted and the number of metastasis reported in the y axis of the histogram. Statistical significances were evaluated by Student's t-test: Ctr EGF vs p140 EGF (*p<0.05).
B) Upper panels: two representative pictures of lung metastases visualized with the FLI (GFP detection) after spontaneous metastasis assay with the MTLn3-EGFR Ctr and p140 cells. Lower panels: two representative pictures of the lungs coloured with ink are shown.

Consistently, p140Cap over-expressing MTLn3-EGFR cells show also reduced anchorage-independent cell growth, which is an *in vitro* characteristic that predicts the *in vivo* metastatic potential of many tumour cells. Furthermore, detailed *in vitro* analysis of cell migratory and invasive abilities showed that p140Cap over-expressing cells have an impaired capacity to migrate in response to EGF. Remarkably, p140Cap over-expressing cells display an increased number and area of focal adhesions, which correlate with the presence of actin stress fibers consistent with a less dynamic turnover of adhesive structures. Cortactin tyrosine phosphorylation has been shown to regulate MTLn3 cells invadopodia assembly and maturation (Oser *et al.*, 2009). Our results show that in p140Cap over-expressing cells cortactin phosphorylation in response to EGF is decreased. Indeed, the expression of the phosphomimetic cortactin mutant is sufficient to completely rescue the defects in migration and invasion of MTLn3-EGFR p140Cap over-expressing cells. Taken together, these data demonstrate that p140Cap suppresses the invasive properties of highly metastatic breast carcinoma cells by inhibiting cortactin-dependent cell motility (Damiano *et al.*, 2011).

5. Conclusions

As outlined in this chapter p130Cas and p140Cap adaptor proteins represent key elements in the control of cell migration and invasion in breast cancer cells. Interestingly, in breast cancers, p130Cas results frequently over-expressed, while p140Cap is not expressed in the more aggressive human breast cancers. Interestingly, Src kinase is a common target of these two proteins. However, even though both p130Cas and p140Cap have been described to bind to Src, they exert opposite roles on Src activity. Indeed p130Cas enhances and sustains Src activity, while p140Cap is a negative regulator of Src kinase. Therefore, it is likely that Src activity is finely tuned by p130Cas and p140Cap relative expression in cells in which they are co-expressed. As a consequence in breast tumors their reciprocal levels of expression might profoundly influence the ability of cancer cells to acquire invasive properties. Although still limited, the analysis of human breast tumors suggests that an overbalance towards p130Cas over-expression might represent a negative prognostic marker in human breast cancer specimens, indicating progression to a more aggressive phenotype.

6. Acknowledgement

This work was supported by EU FP7 Metafight project, AIRC, MUR (PRIN), Regione Piemonte – Progetti Sanità, Oncoprot, PiSTEM, Druidi and CIPE, Compagnia San Paolo, Torino. S. Cabodi and P. Defilippi are co-last authors.

7. References

Andrechek ER, Hardy WR, Siegel PM, Rudnicki MA, Cardiff RD, Muller WJ (2000). Amplification of the neu/erbB-2 oncogene in a mouse model of mammary tumorigenesis. *Proc Natl Acad Sci U S A* 97: 3444-9.

Andrechek ER, Muller WJ (2000). Tyrosine kinase signalling in breast cancer: tyrosine kinase-mediated signal transduction in transgenic mouse models of human breast cancer. *Breast Cancer Res* 2: 211-6.

Berx G, Raspe E, Christofori G, Thiery JP, Sleeman JP (2007). Pre-EMTing metastasis? Recapitulation of morphogenetic processes in cancer. *Clin Exp Metastasis* 24: 587-97.

Berx G, Van Roy F (2001). The E-cadherin/catenin complex: an important gatekeeper in breast cancer tumorigenesis and malignant progression. *Breast Cancer Res* 3: 289-93.

Bouton AH, Riggins RB, Bruce-Staskal PJ (2001). Functions of the adapter protein Cas: signal convergence and the determination of cellular responses. *Oncogene* 20: 6448-58.

Brabek J, Constancio SS, Shin NY, Pozzi A, Weaver AM, Hanks SK (2004). CAS promotes invasiveness of Src-transformed cells. *Oncogene* 23: 7406-15.

Buettner R, Mesa T, Vultur A, Lee F, Jove R (2008). Inhibition of Src family kinases with dasatinib blocks migration and invasion of human melanoma cells. *Mol Cancer Res* 6: 1766-74.

Burnham MR, Harte MT, Richardson A, Parsons JT, Bouton AH (1996). The identification of p130cas-binding proteins and their role in cellular transformation. *Oncogene* 12: 2467-72.

Cabodi S, del Pilar Camacho-Leal M, Di Stefano P, Defilippi P (2010a) Integrin signalling adaptors: not only figurants in the cancer story. *Nat Rev Cancer* 10: 858-70.

Cabodi S, Di Stefano P, Leal Mdel P, Tinnirello A, Bisaro B, Morello V *et al* (2010b) Integrins and signal transduction. *Adv Exp Med Biol* 674: 43-54.

Cabodi S, Morello V, Masi A, Cicchi R, Broggio C, Distefano P *et al* (2008). Convergence of integrins and EGF receptor signaling via PI3K/Akt/FoxO pathway in early gene Egr-1 expression. *J Cell Physiol*.

Cabodi S, Moro L, Baj G, Smeriglio M, Di Stefano P, Gippone S *et al* (2004). p130Cas interacts with estrogen receptor alpha and modulates non-genomic estrogen signaling in breast cancer cells. *J Cell Sci* 117: 1603-11.

Cabodi S, Tinnirello A, Bisaro B, Tornillo G, del Pilar Camacho-Leal M, Forni G *et al* (2010c) p130Cas is an essential transducer element in ErbB2 transformation. *FASEB J* 24: 3796-808.

Cabodi S, Tinnirello A, Di Stefano P, Bisaro B, Ambrosino E, Castellano I *et al* (2006). p130Cas as a new regulator of mammary epithelial cell proliferation, survival, and HER2-neu oncogene-dependent breast tumorigenesis. *Cancer Res* 66: 4672-80.

Cavallaro U, Christofori G (2004). Cell adhesion and signalling by cadherins and Ig-CAMs in cancer. *Nat Rev Cancer* 4: 118-32.

Chin LS, Nugent RD, Raynor MC, Vavalle JP, Li L (2000). SNIP, a novel SNAP-25-interacting protein implicated in regulated exocytosis. *J Biol Chem* 275: 1191-200.

Choi YH, Ahn JH, Kim SB, Jung KH, Gong GY, Kim MJ *et al* (2009). Tissue microarray-based study of patients with lymph node-negative breast cancer shows that HER2/neu overexpression is an important predictive marker of poor prognosis. *Ann Oncol* 20: 1337-43.

Collins MO, Yu L, Coba MP, Husi H, Campuzano I, Blackstock WP *et al* (2005). Proteomic analysis of in vivo phosphorylated synaptic proteins. *J Biol Chem* 280: 5972-82.

Damiano L, Di Stefano P, Camacho Leal MP, Barba M, Mainiero F, Cabodi S *et al* (2010) p140Cap dual regulation of E-cadherin/EGFR cross-talk and Ras signalling in tumour cell scatter and proliferation. *Oncogene* 29: 3677-90.

Damiano L, Le Devedec S, Di Stefano P, Repetto D, Lalai R, Truong L *et al* (2011). p140Cap suppresses the invasive properties of highly metastatic MTLn3-EGFR cells via impaired cortactin phosphorylation. *Oncogene*. In Press

DeGiorgis JA, Jaffe H, Moreira JE, Carlotti CG, Jr., Leite JP, Pant HC *et al* (2005). Phosphoproteomic analysis of synaptosomes from human cerebral cortex. *J Proteome Res* 4: 306-15.

Desgrosellier JS, Barnes LA, Shields DJ, Huang M, Lau SK, Prevost N *et al* (2009). An integrin alpha(v)beta(3)-c-Src oncogenic unit promotes anchorage-independence and tumor progression. *Nat Med* 15: 1163-9.

Di Stefano P, Cabodi S, Boeri Erba E, Margaria V, Bergatto E, Giuffrida MG *et al* (2004). P130Cas-associated protein (p140Cap) as a new tyrosine-phosphorylated protein involved in cell spreading. *Mol Biol Cell* 15: 787-800.

Di Stefano P, Damiano L, Cabodi S, Aramu S, Tordella L, Praduroux A *et al* (2007). p140Cap protein suppresses tumour cell properties, regulating Csk and Src kinase activity. *EMBO J* 26: 2843-55.

Dorssers LC, Van der Flier S, Brinkman A, van Agthoven T, Veldscholte J, Berns EM *et al* (2001). Tamoxifen resistance in breast cancer: elucidating mechanisms. *Drugs* 61: 1721-33.

Eliceiri BP, Puente XS, Hood JD, Stupack DG, Schlaepfer DD, Huang XZ *et al* (2002). Src-mediated coupling of focal adhesion kinase to integrin alpha(v)beta5 in vascular endothelial growth factor signaling. *J Cell Biol* 157: 149-60.

Feigin ME, Muthuswamy SK (2009). Polarity proteins regulate mammalian cell-cell junctions and cancer pathogenesis. *Curr Opin Cell Biol* 21: 694-700.

Giancotti FG (2003). A structural view of integrin activation and signaling. *Dev Cell* 4: 149-51.

Guo W, Giancotti FG (2004). Integrin signalling during tumour progression. *Nat Rev Mol Cell Biol* 5: 816-26.

Gutkind JS (2000). Regulation of mitogen-activated protein kinase signaling networks by G protein-coupled receptors. *Sci STKE* 2000: RE1.

Heasman SJ, Ridley AJ (2008). Mammalian Rho GTPases: new insights into their functions from in vivo studies. *Nat Rev Mol Cell Biol* 9: 690-701.

Hodgson JG, Malek T, Bornstein S, Hariono S, Ginzinger DG, Muller WJ *et al* (2005). Copy number aberrations in mouse breast tumors reveal loci and genes important in tumorigenic receptor tyrosine kinase signaling. *Cancer Res* 65: 9695-704.

Holbro T, Civenni G, Hynes NE (2003). The ErbB receptors and their role in cancer progression. *Exp Cell Res* 284: 99-110.

Holcomb M, Rufini A, Barila D, Klemke RL (2006). Deregulation of proteasome function induces Abl-mediated cell death by uncoupling p130CAS and c-CrkII. *J Biol Chem* 281: 2430-40.

Honda H, Oda H, Nakamoto T, Honda Z, Sakai R, Suzuki T *et al* (1998). Cardiovascular anomaly, impaired actin bundling and resistance to Src-induced transformation in mice lacking p130Cas. *Nat Genet* 19: 361-5.

Hsia DA, Mitra SK, Hauck CR, Streblow DN, Nelson JA, Ilic D *et al* (2003). Differential regulation of cell motility and invasion by FAK. *J Cell Biol* 160: 753-67.

Hynes NE, MacDonald G (2009). ErbB receptors and signaling pathways in cancer. *Curr Opin Cell Biol* 21: 177-84.

Hynes RO (2004). The emergence of integrins: a personal and historical perspective. *Matrix Biol* 23: 333-40.

Ito H, Atsuzawa K, Sudo K, Di Stefano P, Iwamoto I, Morishita R et al (2008). Characterization of a multidomain adaptor protein, p140Cap, as part of a pre-synaptic complex. *J Neurochem* 107: 61-72.

Janssen H, Marynen P (2006). Interaction partners for human ZNF384/CIZ/NMP4--zyxin as a mediator for p130CAS signaling? *Exp Cell Res* 312: 1194-204.

Jaworski J, Kapitein LC, Gouveia SM, Dortland BR, Wulf PS, Grigoriev I et al (2009). Dynamic microtubules regulate dendritic spine morphology and synaptic plasticity. *Neuron* 61: 85-100.

Kim W, Seok Kang Y, Soo Kim J, Shin NY, Hanks SK, Song WK (2008). The integrin-coupled signaling adaptor p130Cas suppresses Smad3 function in transforming growth factor-beta signaling. *Mol Biol Cell* 19: 2135-46.

Kioka N, Ueda K, Amachi T (2002). Vinexin, CAP/ponsin, ArgBP2: a novel adaptor protein family regulating cytoskeletal organization and signal transduction. *Cell Struct Funct* 27: 1-7.

Kiyokawa E, Hashimoto Y, Kobayashi S, Sugimura H, Kurata T, Matsuda M (1998). Activation of Rac1 by a Crk SH3-binding protein, DOCK180. *Genes Dev* 12: 3331-6.

Klemke RL, Leng J, Molander R, Brooks PC, Vuori K, Cheresh DA (1998). CAS/Crk coupling serves as a "molecular switch" for induction of cell migration. *J Cell Biol* 140: 961-72.

Kobashigawa Y, Sakai M, Naito M, Yokochi M, Kumeta H, Makino Y et al (2007). Structural basis for the transforming activity of human cancer-related signaling adaptor protein CRK. *Nat Struct Mol Biol* 14: 503-10.

Kostic A, Sheetz MP (2006). Fibronectin rigidity response through Fyn and p130Cas recruitment to the leading edge. *Mol Biol Cell* 17: 2684-95.

Kurebayashi J (2001). Biological and clinical significance of HER2 overexpression in breast cancer. *Breast Cancer* 8: 45-51.

Latour S, Veillette A (2001). Proximal protein tyrosine kinases in immunoreceptor signaling. *Curr Opin Immunol* 13: 299-306.

Massague J (2008). TGFbeta in Cancer. *Cell* 134: 215-30.

Matsuyama M, Mizusaki H, Shimono A, Mukai T, Okumura K, Abe K et al (2005). A novel isoform of Vinexin, Vinexin gamma, regulates Sox9 gene expression through activation of MAPK cascade in mouse fetal gonad. *Genes Cells* 10: 421-34.

Mitra SK, Hanson DA, Schlaepfer DD (2005). Focal adhesion kinase: in command and control of cell motility. *Nat Rev Mol Cell Biol* 6: 56-68.

Montagna C, Andrechek ER, Padilla-Nash H, Muller WJ, Ried T (2002). Centrosome abnormalities, recurring deletions of chromosome 4, and genomic amplification of HER2/neu define mouse mammary gland adenocarcinomas induced by mutant HER2/neu. *Oncogene* 21: 890-8.

Morello V, Cabodi S, Sigismund S, Camacho-Leal MP, Repetto D, Volante M et al (2011) beta1 integrin controls EGFR signaling and tumorigenic properties of lung cancer cells. *Oncogene*.

Moro L, Venturino M, Bozzo C, Silengo L, Altruda F, Beguinot L et al (1998). Integrins induce activation of EGF receptor: role in MAP kinase induction and adhesion-dependent cell survival. *Embo J* 17: 6622-32.

Mukohara T (2004) Mechanisms of resistance to anti-human epidermal growth factor receptor 2 agents in breast cancer. *Cancer Sci* 102: 1-8.

Muller WJ, Ho J, Siegel PM (1998). Oncogenic activation of Neu/ErbB-2 in a transgenic mouse model for breast cancer. *Biochem Soc Symp* 63: 149-57.

Muthuswamy SK, Li D, Lelievre S, Bissell MJ, Brugge JS (2001). ErbB2, but not ErbB1, reinitiates proliferation and induces luminal repopulation in epithelial acini. *Nat Cell Biol* 3: 785-92.

O'Neill GM, Fashena SJ, Golemis EA (2000). Integrin signalling: a new Cas(t) of characters enters the stage. *Trends Cell Biol* 10: 111-9.

Oser M, Yamaguchi H, Mader CC, Bravo-Cordero JJ, Arias M, Chen X et al (2009). Cortactin regulates cofilin and N-WASp activities to control the stages of invadopodium assembly and maturation. *J Cell Biol* 186: 571-87.

Peinado H, Olmeda D, Cano A (2007). Snail, Zeb and bHLH factors in tumour progression: an alliance against the epithelial phenotype? *Nat Rev Cancer* 7: 415-28.

Perrais M, Chen X, Perez-Moreno M, Gumbiner BM (2007). E-cadherin homophilic ligation inhibits cell growth and epidermal growth factor receptor signaling independently of other cell interactions. *Mol Biol Cell* 18: 2013-25.

Pylayeva Y, Gillen KM, Gerald W, Beggs HE, Reichardt LF, Giancotti FG (2009). Ras- and PI3K-dependent breast tumorigenesis in mice and humans requires focal adhesion kinase signaling. *J Clin Invest* 119: 252-66.

Qian X, Karpova T, Sheppard AM, McNally J, Lowy DR (2004). E-cadherin-mediated adhesion inhibits ligand-dependent activation of diverse receptor tyrosine kinases. *Embo J* 23: 1739-48.

Reynolds AB, Carnahan RH (2004). Regulation of cadherin stability and turnover by p120ctn: implications in disease and cancer. *Semin Cell Dev Biol* 15: 657-63.

Ridley AJ, Schwartz MA, Burridge K, Firtel RA, Ginsberg MH, Borisy G et al (2003). Cell migration: integrating signals from front to back. *Science* 302: 1704-9.

Riggins RB, Quilliam LA, Bouton AH (2003). Synergistic promotion of c-Src activation and cell migration by Cas and AND-34/BCAR3. *J Biol Chem* 278: 28264-73.

Sakai R, Iwamatsu A, Hirano N, Ogawa S, Tanaka T, Mano H et al (1994). A novel signaling molecule, p130, forms stable complexes in vivo with v- Crk and v-Src in a tyrosine phosphorylation-dependent manner. *Embo J* 13: 3748-56.

Salgia R, Avraham S, Pisick E, Li JL, Raja S, Greenfield EA et al (1996). The related adhesion focal tyrosine kinase forms a complex with paxillin in hematopoietic cells. *J Biol Chem* 271: 31222-6.

Sawada Y, Tamada M, Dubin-Thaler BJ, Cherniavskaya O, Sakai R, Tanaka S et al (2006). Force sensing by mechanical extension of the Src family kinase substrate p130Cas. *Cell* 127: 1015-26.

Streuli CH (2009). Integrins and cell-fate determination. *J Cell Sci* 122: 171-7.

Takahashi K, Suzuki K (1996). Density-dependent inhibition of growth involves prevention of EGF receptor activation by E-cadherin-mediated cell-cell adhesion. *Exp Cell Res* 226: 214-22.

Tikhmyanova N, Little JL, Golemis EA (2010) CAS proteins in normal and pathological cell growth control. *Cell Mol Life Sci* 67: 1025-48.

Tornillo G, Bisaro B, Camacho-Leal MD, Galie M, Provero P, Di Stefano P et al (2010) p130Cas promotes invasiveness of three-dimensional ErbB2-transformed mammary acinar structures by enhanced activation of mTOR/p70S6K and Rac1. *Eur J Cell Biol.*

Uberti B, Dentelli P, Rosso A, Defilippi P, Brizzi MF (2010) Inhibition of beta1 integrin and IL-3Rbeta common subunit interaction hinders tumour angiogenesis. *Oncogene* 29: 6581-90.

van der Flier S, van der Kwast TH, Claassen CJ, Timmermans M, Brinkman A, Henzen-Logmans SC *et al* (2001). Immunohistochemical study of the BCAR1/p130Cas protein in non-malignant and malignant human breast tissue. *Int J Biol Markers* 16: 172-8.

Weed SA, Karginov AV, Schafer DA, Weaver AM, Kinley AW, Cooper JA *et al* (2000). Cortactin localization to sites of actin assembly in lamellipodia requires interactions with F-actin and the Arp2/3 complex. *J Cell Biol* 151: 29-40.

Wendt MK, Smith JA, Schiemann WP (2009). p130Cas is required for mammary tumor growth and transforming growth factor-beta-mediated metastasis through regulation of Smad2/3 activity. *J Biol Chem* 284: 34145-56.

Wu H, Parsons JT (1993). Cortactin, an 80/85-kilodalton pp60src substrate, is a filamentous actin-binding protein enriched in the cell cortex. *J Cell Biol* 120: 1417-26.

Wu H, Reynolds AB, Kanner SB, Vines RR, Parsons JT (1991). Identification and characterization of a novel cytoskeleton-associated pp60src substrate. *Mol Cell Biol* 11: 5113-24.

Yarden Y, Baselga J, Miles D (2004). Molecular approach to breast cancer treatment. *Semin Oncol* 31: 6-13.

Zhang XA, He B, Zhou B, Liu L (2003). Requirement of the p130CAS-Crk coupling for metastasis suppressor KAI1/CD82-mediated inhibition of cell migration. *J Biol Chem* 278: 27319-28.

9

Endocrine Resistance and Epithelial Mesenchymal Transition in Breast Cancer

Sanaa Al Saleh and Yunus A. Luqmani
Faculty of Pharmacy, Kuwait University
Kuwait

1. Introduction

Estrogen plays a major part in the regulation of cell proliferation and survival, controlling female physiology, reproduction and behaviour (Musgrove and Sutherland, 2009). It however assumes a more malevolent role in its association with breast cancer pathogenesis. Consequently, therapies have been designed to block the actions of estrogen mediated through its receptors (ERα and ERβ), or to simply reduce its levels in the body (Zilli et al., 2009). Since Beatson (1896) first introduced ovariectomy over a century ago as the first therapeutic modality to reduce the adverse effects of estrogen, endocrine therapy has developed into the cornerstone of breast cancer treatment for those 60-70% of patients whose tumours over-express ER and/or progesterone receptor (PR) (Massarweh and Schiff, 2007; Zilli et al., 2009). For three decades, selective estrogen receptor modulators (SERMS), predominantly tamoxifen, have proved to be effective agents for the suppression of breast cancer growth in both early and advanced disease (Normanno et al., 2005). Tamoxifen has significantly improved the quality of life and survival of many patients with metastatic disease, as well as displaying prophylactic benefit, particularly in women with ductal carcinoma-*in situ* (Fisher et al., 1999).

However, about half of ER+ patients with advanced disease and nearly all patients with metastatic disease fail to respond to first-line tamoxifen therapy. About 40% of patients receiving tamoxifen as adjuvant therapy experience tumour relapse and die from their disease, and a third of women treated with tamoxifen for 5 years develop recurrent disease within 15 years (Normanno et al., 2005). The introduction of pure estrogen antagonists such as fulvestrant, to overcome the apparent disadvantage of tamoxifen with its partial agonist properties, did not resolve the resistance problem (Osborne and Schiff, 2011). Second line therapy with other endocrine agents designed to inhibit peripheral extra-gonadal synthesis of estrogen in postmenopausal women produces some beneficial effects but for the most part serves merely to delay onset of endocrine resistance (Massarweh and Schiff, 2007). This refractiveness to continued administration of anti-estrogens and aromatase inhibitors poses a significant therapeutic problem that has been addressed by a large number of studies. Several theories have been proposed to explain this phenomenon, based on observations made with a variety of *in vitro* cellular models (Normanno et al., 2005). The consensus opinion seems to be that whereas *de novo* resistance is most likely due to low levels of ER expression, *acquired* resistance is predominantly the consequence of an attenuated response to other peptide growth factors that normally play a subsidiary role in cell proliferation.

These molecules exert their action through a variety of trans-membrane receptors that possess intrinsic tyrosine kinase activity. Fig 1 depicts the various potential influences that govern the behaviour of breast cancer cells.

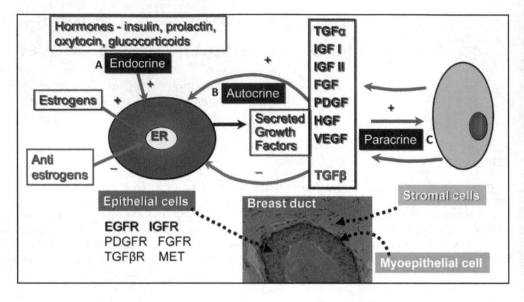

Fig. 1. Factors affecting growth and proliferation of breast cancer cells. Breast epithelial cells are subject to various influences that can either promote or inhibit cellular activity. (A) Endocrine stimulation by a variety of hormones, most significantly estrogen, promotes long term effects. (B) Autocrine stimulation involves, under various conditions, the production and secretion of a number of peptides that act back on the producer cell to modify its activity through membrane bound receptors that frequently possess intrinsic tyrosine kinase activity which initiates a signalling cascade that terminates in the action of transcriptional regulators to modify gene expression. (C) Paracrine stimulation is effected by the action of mediators which include the listed peptide growth factors as well as others originating from myoepithelia (in the normal breast) and stromal elements that include fibroblasts and macrophages in tumours. All of these pathways have been found to operate both *in vitro* (in tumour-derived cell lines) and *in vivo*, but their relative contributions vary considerably in both cases and may be influenced not only by biological heterogeneity but also by therapeutic interventions.

It is also a general experience that endocrine resistance is associated with increased aggressiveness and frequent metastasis (Hiscox et al., 2007), characteristics that more often typify ER-ve tumours. Identification of ligands, receptors and downstream signaling molecules with increased activity in the resistant phenotype, both in cell culture and in tumour biopsies, has highlighted a bewildering collection of molecules that may play a direct causative role, be a consequence or simply innocent bystanders in the progressive cellular change towards endocrine independence. For the purposes of therapeutic discrimination, attempts have been made to reduce this plethora, generated principally by microarray analyses (eg Charafe-Jauffret et al., 2006 ; Luqmani et al., 2009; Al Saleh, 2010) to a manageable number, and given the designation of 'gene signature' by virtue of selectively circumscribing a particular sub-group of patients.

In a separate scenario, new insights have been gained into our understanding of cell differentiation from studies that have demonstrated that epithelial cells have the potential to trans-differentiate into mesenchymal cells (epithelial to mesenchymal transition: EMT) and vice versa (mesenchymal to epithelial transition: MET). Many recent reports have indicated that this process, which was previously observed during transition between developmental stages, is synonymous with the process of tumour metastasis. Both processes share similar pathways of activation. Our recent data (Luqmani et al., 2009; Al Saleh, 2010; Al Saleh et al., 2011a) suggests that there may also be causal links between the development of endocrine resistance and the onset of EMT. In this report we summarise the molecular pathways of ER activity, the mechanisms proposed to account for resistance and finally review the evidence for the above hypothesis.

2. Mechanisms of estrogen receptor induced cell proliferation

ERα and ERβ are transcribed from distinct genes located on separate chromosomes (6 and 14, respectively) (Green et al., 1986; Kuiper et al., 1996). These receptors differ in their tissue distribution, with ERα being highly expressed in the pituitary gland, ovaries (thecal and interstitial cells), uterus, liver, kidneys, adrenals and the mammary glands while ERβ is found mainly in the prostate, bone, ovaries (granulosa cells), lungs and in various parts of the central and peripheral nervous system (Emmen et al., 2005; Kuiper et al., 1997). Nevertheless, ERα and ERβ do overlap in their expression in some tissues (Zilli et al., 2009). More importantly, the two receptors have different roles in breast development. Only ERα appears to be essential for ductal growth although both receptors are present in the breast. ERα-knockout mice show very little growth of mammary ducts, while ERβ-knockout mice develop a normal mammary gland with regular ductal branching (Förster et al., 2002; Lubahn et al., 1993). This suggests that ERβ might be exerting pro-differentiative and anti-proliferative functions. In addition, increased ERα/ERβ ratio in breast cancer as compared with benign tumours and normal tissues suggest that ERα is most closely associated with breast cancer pathogenesis, while ERβ can protect against the mitogenic activity of estrogens in pre-malignant lesions (Roger et al., 2001; Shaw et al., 2002). It has even been suggested that the estrogen-induced proliferation of ER+ breast cancer cells can be inhibited by ERβ over-expression (Ström et al., 2004; Williams et al., 2008). Thus ERα remains the main focus of attention in studies on breast cancer. Unless otherwise specified, 'ER' in this review will refer to ERα.

In what is now referred to as the nuclear or genomic action of ER, binding of estrogen induces activation of the receptor by initiating its dissociation from cognate heat shock proteins, and leads to conformational changes, dimerisation and autophosphorylation (Osborne & Schiff, 2005). The activated ER binds to estrogen response elements (EREs) located in the promoter regions upstream of estrogen-regulated genes. Frasor et al., (2003) observed from microarray analysis of gene expression in MCF-7 cells that about 70% of such estrogen-regulated genes were actually down-regulated following treatment with estradiol. Many of these genes are transcriptional repressors, or genes with anti-proliferative or pro-apoptotic function. On the other hand, there is increased expression of genes inducing cell proliferation and survival. Up-regulation of gene expression is mediated through two domains; activating function-1 (AF-1) and activating function-2 (AF-2). AF-1 is a hormone independent domain located at the N-terminus of the receptor with its function regulated by phosphorylation. AF-2 is the site where ligand-binding actually occurs and is therefore hormone dependant. Almost all gene promoters are activated through both AF-1 and AF-2, though some are activated independently by AF-1 or AF-2 (Gronemeyer 1991; Osborne et al., 2001). Subsequent to formation of the ER-ligand complex, binding of co-regulatory molecules such as nuclear-receptor co-activator 1 (NCOA1 or SRC1), NCOA2 (TIF2) and NCOA3 (AIB1, TRAM1, RAC3 or ACTR) (Leo & Chen 2000; McKenna et al., 1999) enhance the transcriptional activity of ER accompanied by increased activity of histone-acetyltransferase (HAT) at the promoter site. Other co-regulatory molecules can also partly suppress the transcriptional activity of ER by recruitment of histone-deacetylase complexes such as nuclear-receptor co-repressor 1 (NCOR1) and NCOR2 that influence ER-induced transcription (Chen & Evans, 1995; Horlein et al., 1995). Several of these groups of molecules have been reported to have prominent roles in cancer. AIB1 (SRC-3) is over-expressed in almost two thirds of all breast cancers and associated with a shorter disease-free survival in patients receiving tamoxifen as adjuvant treatment (Osborne et al., 2003). In untreated patients, high levels of AIB1 were associated with improved outcome, consistent with studies that suggest the possibility of an association between an enhanced agonistic effect of tamoxifen and the high levels of co-activators. However, ER can also co-operate with FOS/JUN and bind with other transcription factors such as AP-1 (activator protein-1) and SP-1 (specificity protein-1) at their specific sites on DNA (Kushner et al., 2000; Ray et al., 1997; Safe 2001) commonly designated as serum response elements (SRE).

In addition to its classical mode of action through a nuclear-located receptor, estrogen has also been reported to interact with membrane associated receptors, leading to a more rapid reaction than would be expected from a transcriptionally mediated response, such as initiation of cAMP production (Rosner et al., 1999; Zivadinovic et al., 2005) and activation of intrinsic kinases present in other plasma membrane receptors such as insulin-like growth factor-1 receptor (IGF-1R), epidermal growth factor receptor (EGFR) and ERBB2 (Bunone et al., 1996; Campbell et al., 2001; Font de Mora & Brown 2000) as well as receptors for fibroblast growth factor (FGF), platelet-derived growth factor (PDGF), vascular endothelial growth factor (VEGF) and hepatocyte growth factor (HGF). It has been suggested that interaction of SERMs including tamoxifen with such membrane associated receptors may be responsible for their agonist behaviour. There is however much controversy over this issue, with other studies discounting the involvement of such postulated receptors as G protein-coupled receptor as targets of estrogen action (Otto et al., 2008). However this may be, any non-genomic interactions of estrogen would depend on the levels of the above-mentioned kinases, and they will likely be modest in ER+ breast cancer cells that express low levels of tyrosine kinase receptors such as EGFR and ERBB2 (Normanno et al., 2005).

Ligand independent activation of ER can occur via the downstream signaling cascades transmitted through membrane receptor tyrosine kinases such as EGFR, ERBB2, and IGF1R In particular. MAPK/ERK, PI3K/AKT, p90RSK and p38 MAPK pathways can specifically activate ER at key positions (serine 118 and 167 and threonine 311) in the AF-1 domain and in other domains (Bunone et al., 1996; Campbell et al., 2001; Joel et al., 1998; Kato et al., 1995). Expression of ligands and receptors such as transforming growth factor-α (TGFα), IGF1 and IGF1R can be increased by estrogen and those can then initiate signalling while expression of other receptors such as EGFR and ERBB2 is decreased by estrogen signaling (Kushner et al., 2000; Massarweh et al., 2008; Umayahara et al., 1994; Vyhlidal et al., 2000; Yarden et al., 2001). In addition, activation of the PI3K/AKT and the p42/44 MAPK pathways by these receptors down-regulates the expression of ER and PR causing reduction in estrogen dependency while activating the transcriptional function of ER, which suggests a contribution of this cross talk to the relative resistance to endocrine therapies in tumours with amplified ERBB2 expression (Bayliss et al., 2007; Brinkman and El-Ashry, 2009; Creighton et al., 2010; Lopez-Tarruella and Schiff, 2007).

The two types of ER actions, genomic and non-genomic, are not mutually exclusive and do overlap. For example, ER induces the expression of transcripts for both TGFα and amphiregulin (Normanno et al., 1993; Saeki et al., 1991) which can both bind and activate EGFR resulting in activation of MAPK and AKT signaling which are also activated by direct interaction with ER (Salomon et al., 1995). ER binding to membrane caveolin-1 leads to the activation of specific G proteins resulting in the activation of SRC and in turn of matrix metalloproteinases that cleave transmembrane precursors of the EGFR ligand, heparin binding-EGF (HB-EGF) (Levin, 2003; Razandi et al., 2003). Fig 2 illustrates the major identified downstream events involving ER activation.

3. Mechanisms of endocrine resistance

It should be noted that most tumours are heterogeneously composed and a biphasic response to treatment could reflect the survival and eventual clonal outgrowth of an intrinsically resistant minor sub-population.

3.1 Alterations in ER expression or function

Since all endocrine therapies target ER, the expression of the latter is the main predictor of the outcome of such therapies. The *de novo* resistance is clearly caused by the lack of ER expression which can be due to histone deacetylation (Parl, 2003) or associated with aberrant methylation of ER CpG islands that deactivates chromatin (Ottaviano et al., 1994; Weigel & deConinck, 1993). Interestingly, ER expression can be restored in ER-ve breast cancer following co-treatment with DNMT1 and HDAC inhibitors (Robertson et al., 2000; Rountree et al., 2000; Yang et al., 2001).

It was initially thought that acquired resistance might be due to missing or non-functional variants of ER. However, only 17–28% of patients with acquired endocrine resistance lack ER expression (Gutierrez et al., 2005; Johnston et al., 1995). Furthermore, approximately 20% of tamoxifen-resistant patients will eventually respond to second-line treatment with aromatase inhibitors or fulvestrant (Howell et al., 2005; Osborne et al., 2002). Although a number of exon-deleted receptor isoforms have been described, their frequency is insufficient to account for resistance.

Furthermore, these mutations have been detected in ER-ve tumours (Herynk & Fuqua 2004). A mutation that results in a hypersensitive receptor that shows enhanced binding of co-activators in the presence of low estrogen levels (a single amino acid substitution changing lysine 303 to arginine) was found in 20 of 59 hyperplastic breast lesions (Fuqua et al., 2000). However, the role and frequency of such mutations in primary breast carcinomas and their relation to endocrine resistance needs to be explored in a larger number of patients.

Patients carrying inactive alleles of cytochrome P450 2D6 (CYP2D6) (approximately 8% of Caucasian women) fail to convert tamoxifen to its active metabolite, endoxifen (4-hydroxy-N-desmethyl-tamoxifen), and are consequently less responsive to tamoxifen, which is considered to be a significant factor in resistance to therapy (Hoskins et al, 2009). The baseline levels of endoxifen are elevated in patients carrying the wild-type CYP2D6 and who

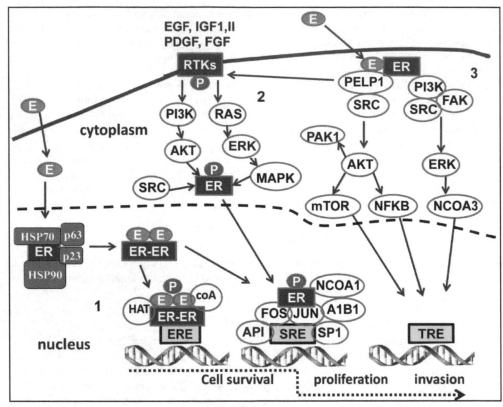

Fig. 2. Proposed cellular mechanisms mediated through the estrogen receptor. 1. Classical genomic mode of action, in which estrogen binds to an inactive ER complex, causing dissociation from heat shock and other cognate proteins, receptor dimerisation and phosphorylation (P). This can then interact directly with estrogen response elements (ERE) on target genes in concert with histone acetyl transferase (HAT) and several other co-activators (coA) or by association with the ubiquitous transcriptional factors FOS/JUN and with NCOA1 and AIB1 co-activators at API/SPI sites termed serum response element (SRE). 2. Cytoplasmically located ER can be phosphorylated by the action of AKT, SRC and ERK/MAPK serine/threonine kinases, downstream of signalling events initiated by various growth factors' interaction with their respective tyrosine kinase containing receptors and mediated through RAS or PI3K. This ligand- independent activated receptor can initiate transcription through the SRE. 3. Binding of estrogen to membrane–associated ER may induce assembly of complexes with either PI3K/FAK/SRC leading to activation through ERK of the transcriptional activator NCOA3 or with PELP1/SRC resulting in up-regulation of mTOR and NFKB through AKT. These mediate an action through other transcriptional response elements (TRE) on a variety of target genes without involving direct interaction of ER with chromatin. The latter mechanisms are referred to as the non-genomic pathways, that are postulated to explain those observed effects of estrogen which are too rapid to be accounted for by mechanism 1. Further 'crosstalk' between ER and RTKs may involve participation of PELP1.

had low levels of the metabolite when co-treated with paroxetine, a selective serotonin re-uptake inhibitor (prescribed to alleviate tamoxifen-associated hot flashes) that can inhibit CYP enzymes. Heterozygous patients showed a better outcome when treated with tamoxifen, as compared with untreated patients suggesting a role for cytochrome P450 enzyme variants in regulating the response to tamoxifen (Wegman et al., 2005).

The presence of ER variants was also hypothesized to have a role in endocrine resistance. A reduced response to endocrine therapy has been associated with the presence of a new truncated variant of ER, ER36, in addition to the full-length receptor (Shi et al., 2009).

3.2 Estrogen receptor β

It has been reported that ERß transcript levels were about 2-fold higher than those of ERα in tamoxifen-resistant as compared with tamoxifen-sensitive patients (Speirs et al., 1999) and that ERß bound to tamoxifen, raloxifen or the anti-estrogen ICI 164 384, increased transcription of AP-1-dependent genes (Paech et al., 1997). Other studies show that ERβ has a negative effect on ERα-promoted transcription (Hall & McDonnell 1999; Pettersson et al., 2000) or no correlation with response or resistance to endocrine treatment (Cappelletti et al., 2004). Development of antibodies distinguishing between the ER types and their variants has led to identification of responses in ERβ+ve but ERα-ve cancers and a potential role for the carboxy-terminally truncated variants of ERβ (ERβ2 and ERβ5) in tamoxifen responsiveness (Honma et al., 2008; Murphy and Watson, 2006). In addition to ERβ, the oestrogen-related receptor ERRγ was found to be over-expressed and mediated tamoxifen resistance in lobular invasive breast cancer models (Riggins et al., 2008).

3.3 Adaptation to estrogen withdrawal

Breast cancer cells can acquire a state of hypersensitivity to estrogen that renders them resistant to endocrine therapy. MCF7 cells cultured in estrogen-free medium to produce long-term estrogen deprived cells (LTED) mimics the effects of ablative endocrine therapy (Santen et al., 2003) and produces cells that are highly sensitised to substantially lower concentrations of estrogen as compared with wild-type MCF-7 cells (Masamura et al., 1995). Growth factor signalling and ER expression was significantly higher in these cells. Treatment with estrogen resulted in rapid association of ER and phosphorylation of SHC, an adaptor protein involved in tyrosine kinase receptor signalling, and increased activation of both SRC and the RAS/RAF/MEK/MAPK signalling pathways (Song et al., 2002a,b; Song et al., 2004). Exposure of these cells to fulvestrant blocked MAPK activation indicating that this pathway may be a downstream effector of the ER non-genomic pathway (Santen et al., 2003; Song et al., 2002a,). However, a high AKT and MAPK level in LTED cells was associated with increased resistance to endocrine therapy and a worse outcome.

In another version of MCF7 LTED cells, enhanced transcriptional activity of ER was associated with increased activation of growth factor pathways that in turn trans-activate ER (Johnston & Dowsett, 2003). After prolonged culture in the absence of estradiol, the ER in these cells functions independently from exogenous estradiol, which was suggested to be due to a super-sensitivity of LTED to residual estrogen present in the medium (Chan et al., 2002; Martin et al., 2003). These cells also showed increased levels of phosphorylation of ER at serine 118, a known target for several intracellular kinases. Furthermore, IGF-1R and ERBB2 signalling was significantly increased in these cells concurrently with increased MAPK activation. Interestingly, the phosphorylation of ER at serine 118 was blocked by

MAPK or EGFR/ERBB2 blockade but not by blocking MEK/MAPK or PI3K/AKT signalling, indicating that additional kinases might be involved in this hypersensitive state. Nicholson et al., (2004) also developed an MCF7 cell line (MCF-7X cells) that is resistant to estrogen withdrawal but not hypersensitive to it. These cells could be growth inhibited by fulvestrant, implying that the ER pathway is still involved in their proliferation. However, the PI3K/AKT pathway was demonstrated to be the main factor promoting their growth without the involvement of EGFR/ERBB2 or IGF-1R signalling, suggesting that the adaptation to estrogen withdrawal can occur in the absence of increased sensitivity to estrogen and does not require activation of classical growth factor receptors.

3.4 Estrogen receptor and co-regulators

Since ER action is mainly controlled through transcriptional factors and co-regulator molecules, it seems likely some of these may be implicated in endocrine resistance. For example, increased AP1 and NFKB transcriptional activity has been associated with endocrine resistance (Johnston et al., 1999; Zhou et al., 2007). And similarly when ER co-activators are over-expressed or phosphorylated. For example, NCOA3 (A1B1 or SRC3) over-expression leads to constitutive ER-mediated transcription, which confers resistance both *in vitro* and in xenograft models and is associated with reduced responsiveness to tamoxifen in patients (Ali & Coombes, 2002; Osborne et al., 2003; Ring & Dowsett, 2004). Another ER co-activator associated with resistance is PELP1 (Fig 2) which is a cytoplasmic scaffold protein that modulates ER interaction with SRC, leading to activation of SRC and the ERK family kinases and also promotes oestrogen activation of PI3K (Gururaj et al., 2006). Interestingly, ER cytoplasmic complex composed of ERα, PI3K, SRC and focal adhesion kinase (FAK; also known as pTK2) is formed as a result of the transient methylation of ER at R260 by protein arginine N-methyltransferase 1 (pRMT1). This complex activates AKT and could confer resistance to endocrine therapy but this methylation event which is frequent in breast cancer has yet to be linked to resistance (Le Romancer et al., 2008).

3.5 Growth factor receptor pathways

Perhaps the most important factors that affect the response to endocrine therapy are those that can modulate alternative proliferation and survival in the tumours in which the ER signalling pathway is effectively inhibited. These alternative growth pathways can do so by the establishment of a bidirectional cross talk with ER signalling. These pathways will act as ER-independent drivers of cancer proliferation and survival and are involved in both *de novo* and *acquired* resistance (Normanno et al., 2005). Increased expression of EGFR, ERBB2 and IGF1R along with their downstream components such as ERK and PI3K can modulate tamoxifen resistance (Faridi et al., 2003; Hutcheson et al., 2003; McClelland et al., 2001). ERBB2 has been reported to be over-expressed in association with down regulation of the X-linked tumour suppressor forkhead box p3 (FOXP3) and the zinc finger transcription factor GATA4 (Hua et al., 2009; Zuo et al., 2007). Other factors that might affect ERBB2 expression are the presence of the paired-domain transcription factor PAX2 and the ER co-activator NCOA3 which compete for binding and regulating ERBB2 transcription and, in turn, responsiveness to endocrine therapy. However, like GATA4 and FOXP3, PAX2 was also shown to be down-regulated in tamoxifen resistant breast cancers in the presence of NCOA3 and an over-expressed ERBB2 (Hurtado et al., 2008). The SRC substrates BCAR1 and BCAR3 have both been reported to elicit endocrine resistance *in vitro* (Dorssers et al., 1993). BCAR1 binds and activates SRC leading to phosphorylation of EGFR and the signal transducer and activator of transcription 5B (STAT5B) (Riggins et al., 2007). On the other hand, BCAR3 is believed to activate RAC and p21-activated kinase 1 (pAK1), which is a mediator of endocrine resistance itself through ER phosphorylation, and through the activation of SRC in association with BCAR1 (Cai et al., 2003; Rayala et al., 2006; Riggins et al., 2003; van Agthoven et al., 1998).

The de-regulation of several growth pathways including EGFR, ERBB2 and IGF1R are implicated in endocrine resistance (Faridi. et al., 2003; Miller et al., 2009). Many events might trigger this de-regulation such as activating mutations in PIK3CA and loss of heterozygosity or methylation of PTEN, activation of AKT, over-expression of ERBB2 and activation of IGF1R and ERBB3 following the loss of PTEN (Arpino et al., 2008; Miller et al., 2009; Riggins et al., 2007). However, following de-regulation of these pathways acquisition of endocrine resistance might be effected by a number of possible activities as summarised by Musgrove & Sutherland, (2009): "decreased ER expression mediated by ERK activation; loss of ER-mediated repression of EGFR and ERBB2 and consequent activation of mitogenic signalling cascades; ligand-independent activation of ER or its co-activators through phosphorylation; up-regulation of key cell cycle regulators, for example MYC and the D and E-type cyclins, through constitutive activation of mitogenic signalling pathways; and the inhibition of apoptosis through constitutive activation of survival signalling".

3.6 Cell cycle signalling molecules

In order for cancer cells to bypass the inhibition of cell proliferation elicited by endocrine agents, one would expect down-regulation of effector molecules involved in the induction of apoptosis while those involved in proliferation, especially during G1 phase, are up regulated. Over-expressed cell cycle regulators include MYC, cyclin E1, cyclin D1, cyclin D1b, as well as p21 and p27, and a de-activated RB gene (Prall et al., 1998; Wang et al., 2008). Over-expression of MYC and cyclin D1 leads to an abundance of CDK complexes that are directly associated with increased cellular proliferation and/or relief of the inhibitory effects of the negative cell cycle regulators p21 and p27, a phenomenon that is also achieved through activation of ERBB2, AKT and SRC (Caldon et al., 2009; Chu et al., 2008; Hui et al., 2002; Perez-Tenorio et al., 2006). Cyclin D1 can also interact with several transcription factors including ER and STAT3 (Coqueret et al., 2002). Tamoxifen actually enhances the binding of cyclin D1 to ER at the expense of STAT3, hence activating both transcription factors and consequently establishing endocrine resistance (Ishii et al., 2008). Other important molecules are those involved in apoptosis. In particular, the pro-apoptotic molecules such as BIK (BCL2-interacting killer) and caspase 9 are down regulated in endocrine resistant cancers while those which are considered as anti-apoptotic molecules such as BCL-XL and its second messenger ceramide, are up regulated (Mandlekar et al., 2001; Riggins et al., 2005) . The expression of these molecules is also affected by signalling through PI3K/AKT, TNF, IFN and NFKB.

4. Epithelial mesenchymal transition

The phenomenon of epithelial cells undergoing a transition towards a mesenchymal phenotype was first identified as programmed events occurring during embryonic developmental processes (Greenberg & Hay, 1982). Since then EMT has since been described in various pathological conditions. During the process of cancer metastasis, a minority of epithelial cells lose their apico-basal polarity, detach from adjacent cells, scatter and acquire increased motility and are able to invade into the extracellular matrix with subsequent penetration into the vasculature. This process is facilitated by a morphological transformation into a fibroblastoid structure that has all the hallmark features of EMT, Both processes share remarkable similarities, with characteristic phenotypic changes. These include the loss of cell-cell adhesion as a result of reduced E-cadherin in adherens junctions, occludins (OCLN) and claudins (CLDN) in tight junctions and desmoplakin (DSP) in desmosomes and down regulation of epithelial cytokeratins (KRT8, KRT18, and KRT19) and up-regulation of mesenchymal proteins most notably vimentin (VIM) and fibronectin and sometimes alpha smooth muscle actin (ACTA2) along with many other changes.

Fig 3 depicts the changes occurring during EMT. Multiple molecular mechanisms underlie EMT initiation and its reversal process, MET, which cancer cells are thought to undergo at sites where they form metastases, in order to re-establish cohesive colonies and initiate neo-vascularisation.

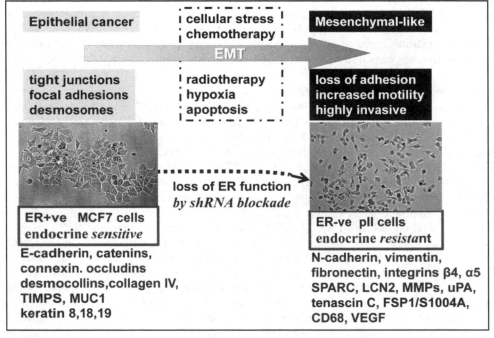

Fig. 3. Epithelial to mesenchymal transition. Loss of epithelial characteristics and breakdown of tissue architecture through dissolution of cell-cell junctions and loss of apico-basal polarity by detachment from the basement membrane can be initiated through a variety of diverse cellular insults which lead to transformation into a cell type that displays mesenchymal–like features. At a molecular level there is a certain uniformity of changes. Cells that have lost ER function and consequently acquired endocrine independence, in this case by shRNA- induced down-regulation (Al Saleh, 2010), show both the morphological appearance as well as the phenotypic changes that are characteristic of cells undergoing EMT. Several differences are indicated between MCF7 and pII cells that parallel those seen during EMT.

The transformation of epithelial cells into a mesenchymal-like form requires the participation of a complex network of both extra- and intra-cellular signals., Amongst the many identified are TGFβ, HGF, FGF, EGFR family members, IGF1 and 2, and PDGF (Thiery et al., 2002). An array of embryonic transcription factors such as the homeobox protein GOOSECOID (GSC), TCF3 (E47), the zinc-finger proteins SNAIL1 and SNAIL2 (previously SLUG), the basic helix-loop-helix protein TWIST1, the forkhead box proteins FOXC1 and FOXC2 , and the zinc-finger E-box-binding proteins ZEB1 and ZEB2 (SIP1) , are generated by the activity of these growth factor pathways, each of which is capable, on its own, of inducing an EMT.

There is increasing evidence of extensive crosstalk between these molecules, permitting the formation of an extensive signalling network responsible for establishing and maintaining a mesenchymal phenotype. (Moreno-Bueno et al., 2008; Peinado et al., 2007). In addition, some of these transcriptional activators such as TWIST are pivotal factors in overcoming cellular senescence (Ansieau et al., 2008) and in generating tumourigenic cancer stem cells (Mani et al., 2008). Interestingly, EMT-inducing transcription factors also confer stem cell characteristics on epithelial cells. For example, the receptor KIT which is an important factor for maintaining the stem cell state in the haematopoietic system has been shown to induce SNAIL2 expression in both mice (Perez-Losada et al., 2002) and humans (Sanchez-Martin et al., 2002). Many of these transcription factors exert repressive functions by binding to conserved E-box sequences in the promoter regions of such critical genes as CDHI (Gilles et al., 2003; Pieper et al., 1992).

4.1 Transforming Growth Factor β

TGFβ can independently promote an EMT phenotype in mouse mammary epithelial cells (Thuault et al., 2006; Waerner et al., 2006). This cytokine induces EMT by both SMAD-dependent and independent signalling events (Berx et al., 2007; Das et al, 2009; Santisteban et al., 2009). In advanced disease, TGF-β can stimulate invasion and metastasis of tumours that have become TGF-β insensitive which can be inhibited by ectopic expression of dominant negative TGF-β receptors (Ozdamar et al., 2005). TGF-β1 ligand activates a heteromeric receptor of two transmembrane serine/threonine kinases, type I and II receptors (TβRI and TβRII). TβRII transphosphorylates TβRI, activating its kinase function to exert its signalling effects. Activated TβRI phosphorylates the intracellular proteins SMAD 2 and 3 which then associate with SMAD 4, translocating to the nucleus where the complex interacts with other transcriptional co-activators and co-repressors to regulate expression of several genes (Onder et al., 2008). This type of signalling that depends on SMAD, up-regulates the expression of many transcription factors such as SNAIL1, SNAIL2, TWIST, and members of the ZFH family, ZEB1 and ZEB2 (Sarrio et al., 2008; Vandewalle et al., 2005; Yang et al., 2004) that are considered to be primary transcriptional inducers of EMT. TGFβ can also phosphorylate certain cytoplasmic proteins regulating cell polarity and tight junction formation. These include RAS/MAPK (Xue et al., 2003), integrin β-1 (Blanco et al., 2002), integrin-linked kinase (Hartwell et al., 2006), p38 MAPK (Mani et al., 2007), RHOA kinase (ROCK) (Moody et al., 2005), PI3K (Martin et al., 2003), JAGGED1/NOTCH (Come et al., 2006), SARA (Laffin et al., 2008), NFKB (Lester et al., 2007), PAR6 (Berx et al., 2001; Storci et al., 2008), pAR66A and ERK (Wu et al., 2009). Furthermore, EMT induced by the oncogenic stimulation by RAS and/or RAF activation in mammary, kidney and skin epithelial tissue was found to depend almost completely on TGF-β signaling (Moustakas and Heldin, 2009). TGFβ can also induce the activation of other signalling pathways that might participate in initiation of EMT such as the WNT and NOTCH pathways (Polyak and Weinberg, 2009). Figure 4 illustrates the major events that are thought to be critical in the trans-differentiation of epithelial cells.

4.2 AXL

As mentioned earlier, receptor tyrosine kinase activity is altered in breast cancer and is considered to be an important factor in endocrine resistance. These molecules are also implicated in EMT since they already play a pivotal role in embryogenesis. One interesting member of the TAM (Tyro-AXL-MER) receptor tyrosine kinases is AXL which exerts diverse effects in regulating cellular responses that include cell proliferation, cell survival, migration, autophagy, angiogenesis, natural killer cell differentiation and platelet aggregation (Linger et al., 2008). AXL was reported to be associated with EMT since it is activated in many signal transduction pathways including AKT, MAPK, NFKB, and STAT. (Hafizi et al., 2006). Furthermore, AXL expression alone is considered as a predictive marker for poor overall patient survival. It has also been reported that elevated AXL levels are needed for maintaining breast cancer invasiveness, growth in foreign microenvironments and metastatic potential. Endocrine-resistant breast cancer cells show highly elevated expression of AXL (Al Saleh et al., 2010).

4.3 E-cadherin and its transcriptional repressors

E-cadherin is a critical switch in EMT during early embryonic development. Its down-regulation in epithelial cells triggers acquisition of a fibroblastic phenotype, dissociation from the epithelium sheets and migration, vital steps in gastrulation, neural crest formation and organ development (Thiery, 2003). E-cadherin expression is often lost in aggressive breast cancers acquiring EMT which would result in the disassembly of inter-cellular adhesion complexes, loosening contacts between neighbouring epithelial cells and thus disrupting the overall tissue architecture. E-cadherin loss also causes the liberation of β-catenin to the nucleus and its subsequent activation of WNT signalling of other EMT inducers as described above. Furthermore, E-cadherin loss mediates EMT through the induction of its own transcriptional repressors, SNAIL, TWIST and ZEB1 (EF1), in a feed-forward loop that sustains E-cadherin repression and potentiates EMT (Onder et al., 2008).

An interesting connection between endocrine resistance and EMT is established through the connection between SNAIL, E-cadherin and metastasis-associated protein 3 (MTA3). MTA3, which is directly activated by ER, is a repressor of SNAIL, thereby also repressing EMT (Al Saleh et al., 2011). We have recently shown that down-regulation of ER in MCF7 cells leads to a reduction in both MTA1 and MTA3 and a concurrent rise in SNAIL2 (Al Saleh et al., 2011a).

Reduction of E-cadherin expression correlates with poor differentiation, invasiveness, aggressive metastatic behaviour, and an unfavourable prognosis (Berx et al., 2001; Wheelock et al., 2003); experimental knockdown of E-cadherin is sufficient to establish metastasis but not fully reverse EMT by itself. Interestingly, the down regulated expression of E-cadherin during EMT is a reversible process that arises through hypermethylation of the E-cadherin promoter or transcriptional repression although many lobular breast cancers appear to have lost the expression of E-cadherin through inactivating mutations and loss of heterozygosity (Berx et al, 2001).

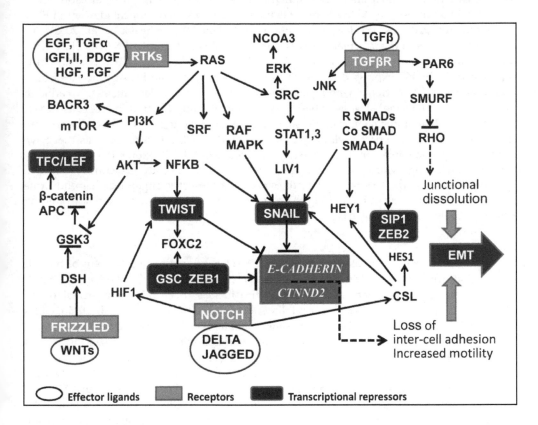

Fig. 4. Transduction pathways and effectors contributing to processes leading to EMT. A variety of growth factors (EGF, TGFα, IGFI, II, PDGF, HGF, FGF) binding to receptor tyrosine kinases (RTK) activate the central RAS pathway to promote transcription of SNAIL through the RAF/MAPK, the PI3K/AKT/NFKB or the SRC/LIV pathways. AKT, as well as WNTs acting through the FRIZZLED receptor, promote inhibition of GSK3 through DSH to promote re-localisation of β-catenin and generate TCF/LEF that also increases SNAIL. DELTA/JAGGED signalling through NOTCH also increases SNAIL via CSL as well as TWIST through HIF1. TGFβ signals through its receptor to increase SMAD family members that co-operatively promote both SNAIL as well as SIP1/ZEB2. It also acts through PAR6 to up-regulate the ubiquitin ligase SMURF that degrades RHO which is a key promoter of tight junctions, The transcriptional repressors SNAIL, TWIST, GSC, ZEB1,2 and TFC/LEF effectively down-regulate E-cadherin and associated molecules, which leads to loss of cell adhesion, permitting cell scattering, cellular motility and invasion through the action of up-regulated proteases. Not shown here, for clarity, is HEDGEHOG signalling which through GLI integrates with the RTK and WNT pathways to up-regulate SNAIL family members Evidence for the interactions illustrated is summarised in excellent reviews by Huber et al., 2005; Moustakes & Heldin, 2007 and Sabbah et al., 2008 and references therein.

The appearance of another mesenchymal marker, N-cadherin (CDH12) and/or cadherin-11 (CDH11), in a process termed 'cadherin switching', is also a well documented event in EMT (Gjerdrum et al., 2010; Sarrio et al., 2008; Sphyris and Mani, 2009; Wheelock et al., 2008). The expression of these mesenchymal markers during EMT is induced by SNAIL, ZEB2/SIP1 and SNAIL2 (Cano et al., 2000; Sarrio et al., 2008; Vandewalle et al., 2005). N-cadherin is reported to be highly expressed in invasive and metastatic human breast cancer cell lines and tumours and to correlate with aggressive clinical behaviour. Nevertheless, N-cadherin expression can be triggered in E-cadherin expressing cells and it could in fact cause EMT, impacting on their epithelial phenotype, suggesting a dominating role for this cadherin over the other, possibly in synergy with FGF2 (Hazan et al., 2000, 2004). MCF7 cells that have acquired endocrine independence through induced loss of ER expression also display cadherin switching which is accompanied by increased motility, F-actin cytoskeletal rearrangement and the loss of cellular adhesion molecules. It is suggested that endocrine resistance is a major event influencing the cells to move and invade into the surrounding tissues (Al Saleh, 2010; Al Saleh et al., 2011a).

4.4 Vimentin

A marker that is commonly used to characterise EMT is vimentin, a component of type III intermediate filaments and the archetypal mesenchymal marker (Trimboli et al., 2008). Elevated vimentin expression correlates well with increased cell migration, invasion and EMT induction in several breast cancer cell lines (Al Saleh, 2010; Al Saleh et al., 2011a; Gilles et al., 2003) in co-ordination with other mesenchymal markers such as tenascin C (Dandachi et al., 2001; Polette et al., 2007), which has been associated with over-expressed ERBB2 and down-regulated ER. The molecular events triggering vimentin expression during EMT are less well delineated in comparision to the mechanisms inducing E-cadherin down-regulation. The expression of vimentin is considered to be a late occurrence in EMT in a temporal sequence of genetic events starting from loss of epithelial markers followed by appearance of mesenchymal markers (Polette et al., 2007). Direct activation of vimentin expression in human breast tumour cells (Gilles et al., 2003) by β-catenin/T-cell factor/lymphocyte enhancer factor-1 is consistent with the activation of β-catenin as a downstream event from consequential loss of E-cadherin. The indirect promotion of vimentin expression by ZEB2/SIP1 during EMT in a β-catenin-independent manner (Bindels et al., 2006) suggests the existence of some trans-activators driving EMT which are associated with vimentin expression.

4.5 Matrix metalloproteinases and lipocalin

In order for cancer cells to metastasise, they need to penetrate into and through the extracellular matrix (ECM). This process is facilitated by the activity of matrix metalloproteinases (MMPs). A family of more than 28 MMPs have been reported to be up-regulated in nearly every tumour type and are closely involved in cancer progression through cleavage and release of bioactive molecules that inhibit apoptosis and stimulate cancer invasion and metastasis. For example, treatment of cells with MMP-3 results in an increased expression of the activated splice variant RAC1b, elevating the levels of cellular reactive oxygen species which, in turn, lead to increased expression of SNAIL and EMT initiation (Orlichenko et al., 2008). An MMP-9 associated protein, Lipocalin2 (LCN2), was also found to play a major role in cell regulation, proliferation, differentiation and regulation of EMT. It's over-expression in human breast cancer cells can cause up-regulation of vimentin and fibronectin while E-cadherin is down regulated (Yang et al., 2009). Furthermore, LCN2 over-expression significantly increases cell motility and invasiveness in previously non-invasive MCF-7 cells. Interestingly, siRNA-mediated LCN2 silencing inhibited cell migration and development of the mesenchymal phenotype in aggressive breast cancer cells. It was also reported that reduced expression of ER and increased expression of SNAIL2 was correlated with LCN2 expression while over-expression of ER in LCN-2 expressing cells was able to reverse EMT and reduce SNAIL2 expression, suggesting that ER negatively regulates LCN2-induced EMT (Yang et al, 2009).

4.6 Hypoxia

An interesting physiological mechanism that can cause EMT is hypoxia. It has been reported that tumour progression and metastasis is promoted by the stabilisation of the hypoxia-inducible factor-1α (HIF-1α). This transcription factor was shown to be associated with TWIST in inducing both EMT and tumour metastasis by hypoxia or over-expression of the former. Furthermore, the expression of TWIST was found to be regulated by HIF-1 binding to the hypoxia-response element (HRE) in the TWIST proximal promoter and is associated with it in inducing EMT or metastasis (Yang et al, 2008). Interestingly, the HIF-1α null mice phenotype resembles TWIST deficient mice. In addition, patients with head and neck cancer whose tumours co-express TWIST and HIF-1 had very poor prognosis suggesting a major role for these two genes in regulating EMT.

4.7 HOX genes

Another important set of genes in regulating EMT is the homeobox (HOX) gene family, master players in regulating embryonic development and maintaining homeostasis through strictly regulated expression in various tissues and organs during adult life. Several studies have demonstrated the association of HOX genes in the pathogenesis of multiple cancers. For example, HOXA7 and HOXD13 have been associated with lung cancer (Lechner et al., 2001), HOXC4 and HOXC8 in prostate cancer (Miller et al., 2003), HOXB7 in ovarian cancer (Naora et al, 2001) and HOXA10 in endometrial cancer (Yoshida et al., 2006). In one study 60% of their breast cancers had no HOXA5 expression (Raman et al., 2000) which causes p53-dependent apoptosis. HOXA5 was reported to cause cell death through the activation of the caspase pathways in HS578T cells expressing mutant p53 (Chen et al., 2004). HOXD10 was extensively reduced as malignancy increased in epithelial cells, and restoring its expression in MDA-MB-231 could significantly reduce the migration capacity of these highly aggressive cells (Carrio et al., 2005). HOXB13 over-expression was associated with increased MCF10A cell motility and invasion *in vitro*, while its ratio to interleukin-17β receptor was predictive of tumour recurrence during adjuvant tamoxifen monotherapy. HOXB7 is involved in tissue remodeling of the normal mammary gland (Ma et al., 2004) and is expressed at higher levels in metastatic breast tumours (Care et al., 1998, 2001). Furthermore, regulation of the expression of several growth and angiogenic factors, including basic FGF, VEGF, IL8, ANG1, ANG2, and MMP9 in SKBR3 breast cancer cells, depends on the over-expressed levels of HOXB7 which can result in the formation of vascularised tumours when grown as xenografts in nude mice. HOXB9 like HOXB7 can lead to increased cell motility and EMT (Hayashida et al., 2010).

4.8 NOTCH

DELTA/JAGGED acting through the NOTCH pathway are implicated in both cell fate in the normal human mammary gland (Raouf et al., 2008) and regulation of cancer stem cells (CSCs) in both ductal carcinoma *in situ* and in invasive carcinoma of the breast (Dontu et al., 2004; Stylianou et al., 2006). This pathway is known to be transcriptionally induced by TGFβ/SMAD signalling and contributes to EMT (Zavadil et al., 2004). This pathway is cell type specific and can be either oncogenic through activation of the NKFB pathway or it can be tumour suppressive. Wang et al., (2006) provided evidence demonstrating that NOTCH receptor signalling regulates SNAIL 1 and 2, ZEB1 and vimentin.

4.9 WNT

The WNT signalling pathway mediates several vital processes such as cell proliferation, migration, differentiation, adhesion and death (Vincan et al., 2008). In addition, this pathway can promote migration and EMT in breast cancer cells through the stabilisation or increased expression of SNAIL1 and 2 and TWIST (Onder et al., 2008; Vogelstein et al., 2004). SNAIL has been implicated in regulating WNT-1-induced EMT in MCF-7 cells. Furthermore, WNT signalling can also lead to the translocation of β-catenin to the nucleus where it can drive the expression of several EMT inducing transcription factors through the WNT induced inhibition of glycogen synthase kinase-3β (GSK3β)-mediated phosphorylation. However, β-catenin alone usually is not enough to induce EMT although in colorectal cancer WNT is indeed a silencer of its negative regulators SOX17 (Zhang et al., 2008), SFRPS18, 19 and DKK1 (Aguilera et al., 2006). Interestingly, both SFRP1 and DKK1 are frequently silenced by methylation in breast cancer.

4.10 miRNA

It is well established that non-protein coding micro (mi) RNAs play a significant role in regulation of gene expression and cellular protein levels. They are now also being increasingly recognised as major regulators of EMT and metastasis, specifically the miR-200 family (miR-200a, miR-200b, miR-200c, miR-141, miR-429 and miR-205 (Gregory et al, 2008; Park et al., 2008). Members from the miR-200 family and miR-205 are associated with increased expression of E-cadherin and decreased vimentin. In addition, these miRNAs also target the expression of ZEB1 and ZEB2, the E-cadherin transcriptional repressors. Expression levels of miR-205 and of some members of the miR-200 family were also found to vary inversely with vimentin expression in primary serous papillary carcinomas of the ovary (Park et al., 2008). In another study, EMT was induced through either TGFβ or the tyrosine phosphatase pEZ in Madin–Darby canine kidney (MDCK) cells. The levels of both miR-205 and miR-200 family members was down-regulated after EMT induction while their ectopic expression induced MET (Gregory et al., 2008).

One way that natural antisense transcripts can play a major role in EMT is by targeting the regulation of ZEB2 expression. This was documented when EMT was induced in a human colorectal cancer cell line by SNAIL. ZEB2 levels were found to be directly increased after EMT initiation which was explained as the result of the action of a natural antisense transcript that prevented the splicing of a large intron in the 5' untranslated region (UTR) that contains an internal ribosomal entry site which lowers ZEB2 levels in epithelial cells through the inhibition of ribosome scanning. During EMT activation, the antisense transcript levels are increased. They bind to the 5'UTR and inhibit splicing, preserving the internal ribosomal entry site sequence and thereby increasing the translational efficiency of ZEB2 which then directly inhibits E-cadherin expression, maintaining an EMT state (Beltran et al., 2008).

Although these RNA molecules are associated with the regulation of EMT and MET, other miRNAs such as miR-10b are reportedly associated with metastasis and invasion. It inhibits HOX10 translation while increasing RHOC when induced by TWIST (Ma et al., 2007). Another miRNA that seems to increase the metastatic potential of cancer cells is miR-29a; up-regulated in a mesenchymal metastatic RASXT mammary cell line compared to epithelial EpRas cells. In addition, over-expression of miR-29a suppresses expression of tristetraprolin, a regulator of epithelial polarity and metastasis, and leads to EMT and metastasis through RAS signalling. This correlates with data from breast cancer patients showing enhanced miR-29a and reduced tristetraprolin levels (Gebeshuber et al., 2009). In contrast to miR-10b, miR-335 was found to be a suppressor of invasion and metastasis through modulation of the expression of the 'six gene signature' set: COL1A1, MERTK, PLCB1, PTPRN2, TNC and SOX4 which are considered predictive markers of metastasis and invasion. miR-335 was also reported to suppress invasion and metastasis in MDAMB231, a highly metastatic and invasive ER-ve breast cancer cell line (Tavazoie et al., 2008).

4.11 Epithelial to mesenchymal transition and breast cancer stem cells

An interesting idea that has emerged recently suggests the possibility that cancer cells undergoing EMT acquire stem cell-like characteristics. The breast cancer stem cell (BCSCs) hypothesis contends that breast cancer is derived from a single tumour initiating cell with stem cell-like properties.

BCSCs are characterized as CD24$^{-/low}$ and CD44$^+$ cells which are associated with basal subtype breast cancer. It was first reported by Al-Hajj et al., (2003) when they showed that a CD44$^+$/CD24$^{-/low}$ sub-population of breast cancer cells could produce tumours in a xenograft model more effectively. These cells are regarded as the 'metastatic component' of the cancer, particularly in breast neoplasms as they are the only subset of cells with potential to initiate new tumour growth. This was further supported by analysis of genetic profiles of CD44$^+$ breast cancer cells which showed enrichment with stem-cell markers and displayed activated TGFβ signalling with lung metastasis and poor clinical outcomes (Sheridan et al., 2006; Shipitsin et al., 2007). Furthermore, it has been reported that metaplastic and claudin-low breast cancers are enriched with markers of EMT and display stem cell characteristics suggesting that cancer cells undergoing EMT exhibit stem cell-like characteristics (Prat et al., 2010). In addition to that, inducing EMT in immortalized human mammary epithelial cells with either TGFβ, SNAIL1 and TWIST confers stem cell characteristics with increased formation of mammospheres in three dimensional culture and ductal outgrowths in xenotransplants (Mani et al., 2008; Morel et al, 2008). Interestingly, BCSCs isolated from primary tumors and normal breast tissue showed an increased expression of the mesenchymal markers TWIST1 and 2, FOXC2, SNAIL1, ZEB2, vimentin and fibronectin while epithelial cells (which are CD44$^-$/CD24$^+$) isolated from differentiated carcinoma do not (Mani et al., 2008). Furthermore, hypoxia-induced SNAIL2 expression has also been associated with acquisition of a basal-like breast cancer phenotype with high levels of the stem cell regulatory genes CD133 and BMI1 (Storci et al., 2008). Inhibition of WNT signalling through LRP6 was found to reduce stem cell-like properties and cause EMT reversal, restoration of the epithelial phenotype, and suppression of SNAIL2 and TWIST expression (DiMeo et al., 2009) in a mouse model of breast cancer metastasis to the lung.

It has also been reported that a CD24$^{-/low}$/CD44$^+$ *in vivo* tumour out- growth which is enriched with EMT markers results from CD8 T-cell-mediated immune response to epithelial breast cancer which would develop characteristics of aggressive carcinomas including potent tumourigenicity, ability to re-establish an epithelial tumour, and enhanced resistance to drugs and radiation (Sheridan et al., 2006; Santisteban et al., 2009). Moreover, breast cancer cells disseminated into the circulation and bone marrow are enriched with CD44$^+$CD24$^-$ antigen phenotype (Balic et al., 2006)

EMT induction may be a contributory factor to the decreased efficacy of chemotherapy in breast (Cheng et al., 2007), colorectal (Yang et al., 2006) and ovarian cancer (Kajiyama et al., 2006) while introduction of TWIST into breast cancer cells has been shown to induce paclitaxel resistance. In addition, AKT2 expression, which was amplified in breast cancer has also been correlated with acquired paclitaxel resistance (Cheng et al., 2007). Interestingly, acquisition of enhanced EGFR/ERBB2 signalling in ER+ breast cancer with tamoxifen resistance has been suggested to result from the selection of a more stem cell-like phenotype. EGFR expression is seen in stem cells of the normal mammary gland in both mice and humans (Asselin-Labat et al., 2006; Hebbard et al., 2000) whilst ER is predominantly expressed in the more differentiated luminal cells (Hebbard et al., 2000; Shipitsin et al., 2007). Furthermore, the EGFR pathway is also activated in CSCs of DCIS of the breast and there is emerging evidence for a role of the ERBB2 pathway in the function of CSCs. Expression of ERBB2 and presence of ALDH1+ CSCs was positively correlated in one series of 491 breast cancer patients (Ginestier et al., 2007). The CSC populations of four ERBB2+ breast cancer cell lines have been shown to express more ERBB2 mRNA and protein in comparison to the non-CSC population. Furthermore, trastuzumab was also shown to reduce mammosphere-forming ability and tumourigenicity on serial xenotransplantation (Magnifico et al., 2009). Interestingly, ERBB2+ tumours that received treatment with lapatinib showed decreased EMT related genes in comparison to CD24$^{low/-}$/CD44$^+$ post treatment tissues from patients that received standard anthracycline-taxane chemotherapy. In addition, the γ secretase inhibitor DAPT or a NOTCH 4 neutralizing antibody significantly reduced mammosphere formation in DCIS. NOTCH pathway antagonism has been reported to enhance the reduction of mammosphere formation in ERBB2 over-expressing cell lines induced by trastuzumab (Magnifico et al, 2009).

Colorectal and lung tumours undergoing EMT display decreased sensitivity to EGFR kinase inhibitors, possibly by the activation of downstream targets PI3K and AKT (Barr et al., 2008). In breast cancer, CD44$^+$/CD24$^{-/low}$ CSCs acquire resistance against the chemotherapeutic agents docetaxel, doxorubicin and cyclophosphamide (Li et al., 2008). Furthermore, a proportion of CD44$^+$/CD24$^{-/low}$ cells increase in breast cancer patients following treatment with these anti-cancer drugs suggesting that breast cancer cells may acquire resistance to both conventional and targeted therapies upon conversion to a mesenchymal-like phenotype. This in turn would suggest that any EMT inducing factors such as TWIST and ERBB2 are crucial players in inducing cancer stem cells.

An analysis of a panel of breast cancer cell lines of luminal, intermediate and basal phenotypes showed a significant increase in the fraction of CSCs (CD44$^+$/CD24$^{low/-}$/ESA$^+$) in basal type breast cancers compared to hormone-sensitive luminal cancers (Fillmore & Kuperwasser, 2008). In addition, the number of CSCs and cell line tumourigenicity in *in vivo* models was correlated positively (Fillmore et al., 2008).

A functionally redundant ER in endocrine-resistant breast cancer might promote a more mesenchymal stem-cell-like phenotype based on the observation that ER negatively regulates the expression of the key EMT transcription factors including SNAIL1 and SNAIL2 (Dhasarathy et al., 2007; Ye et al., 2008). Furthermore, tamoxifen resistant MCF7 cells have been reported to show an enhanced mammosphere formation capacity in comparison to the tamoxifen sensitive cells which suggests an increased CSC fraction (Storci et al., 2008). EMT may facilitate the generation of CSCs with mesenchymal and self-renewal properties necessary for dissemination and initiation of metastasis. (Hollier et al., 2009; Mani et al, 2008). An immunohistochemical analysis of 479 invasive breast carcinomas showed a high expression of the EMT-induced markers vimentin, α-smooth muscle actin, N-cadherin, CDH1, SPARC, laminin and fascin, in comparison to the low expression of E-cadherin in these CD44+/CD24- basal-like breast tumours. These tumours have the ability to form distant metastases hence exhibiting a worse prognosis (Perou et al., 2000; Sorlie et al., 2001). In a study on 117 samples of primary invasive breast carcinomas, nuclear staining of the EMT inducing transcription factor FOXC2 showed a significant correlation with CD44+CD24- basal-like subtypes (Mani et al., 2007). Another study on 226 blood samples from 39 patients with metastatic breast cancer showed that the majority of the circulating tumour cells (CTCs) exhibited EMT and CSC characteristics (Aktas et al., 2009). CTCs were present in 69 of 226 (31%) blood samples taken from patients with metastatic breast cancer to investigate the expression of TWIST, AKT2, and PI3Kα and ALDH1 which is considered to be a stem cell marker. In the CTC-positive group, 62% were positive for the EMT markers and 69% for ALDH1, while in the CTC-negative group the proportions were 7 and 14%, respectively (Aktas et al., 2009). The CTCs have also been shown to have a reduced expression of epithelial-specific cytokeratins (Pantel et al., 2008). Interestingly, disseminated tumour cells (DTCs) over-expressed TWIST. Assessment of occurrence of bone marrow metastases indicated that TWIST+ cells were present prior to chemotherapy and this was significantly associated with relapse (Watson et al., 2007).

EMT undergoing CTCs have also been shown to resist apoptosis. One study reported that following the induction of EMT by TGFβ in the EpH-4 and nMuMG murine mammary epithelial cell lines, they tended to acquire resistance to ultraviolet light induced apoptosis (Robson et al., 2006). Likewise, down regulation of the expression of LET-7 miRNA in breast cancer cell lines increased their metastatic potential and the resistance to therapy, in association with the acquisition of stem cell characteristics and EMT-associated gene expression profiles (Yu et al., 2007). Furthermore, the factors that can induce a full EMT; TGFβ, WNT, HEDGEHOG, NOTCH, and RAS signaling pathways, are all considered to be involved in the induction and maintenance of stem cell niches (Fuxe et al., 2010). There is however some data showing that TGFβ stimulation of transformed human breast epithelial cells can result in the loss of stem cell-like properties including the ability to form mammospheres (Tang et al., 2007).

5. Endocrine resistance and EMT

It is becoming increasingly apparent that acquired endocrine resistance is a multi-factorial stepwise progression that can be triggered through a number of distinct pathways, that *in vitro*, can be manipulated. Whether it is the actual loss of ER due to transcriptional or translational down-regulation, or functional redundancy of ER (which seems to be the more frequent occurrence *in vivo*), either scenario would have the same end result in terms of independence from estrogen. It is therefore pertinent to ask what happens to a cell that experiences loss of ER. As described in preceding sections this issue has been addressed by various cell models that have been made endocrine resistant by exposure to antiestrogens or by deprivation of estradiol, but rarely by the direct prevention of ER synthesis.

We have explored this avenue by modifying MCF7 cells by transfection with shRNA generating plasmids targeting the ER mRNA (Al Azmi, 2006; Luqmani et al., 2009; Al Saleh et al., 2011a). As expected, stably transfected cell lines with constitutive reduction of ER (termed pII) exhibit a loss of response to either estradiol or tamoxifen/fulvestrant and hypersensitivity to EGF and IGF1 (Salloum, 2010). There is reduction in the classical ER-regulated markers such as pS2, cathepsin D, PR and PRLR. Like the tumour-derived naturally ER-ve MDAMB231 cell line, these (acquired) endocrine resistant cells show increased motility and ability to invade simulated components of the ECM mimicking the behaviour of aggressive ER-ve/EGFR+ve tumours. Both of these activities as well as cellular proliferation are reduced by various tyrosine kinase inhibitors that are known to block, in particular, EGFR and VEGFR phosphorylation (Al Saleh, 2010) supporting the data mentioned in preceding sections. However, the most striking features of pII cells was initially noted in their morphological appearance (see Fig 3), assuming a more elongated spindly shape and failure to form the compact colonies characteristic of MCF7 cells, with re-arrangement of the actin cytoskeleton giving rise to increased incidence of lamellipodia and microspikes, features closely associated with cellular motility (Parker et al., 2002).

Microarray analysis confirmed that pII cells had assumed a phenotype that is generally seen for mesenchymal cells, with transcriptional loss of genes normally associated with epithelial cells. Lack of colony formation can be explained by loss of E-cadherin and many other factors responsible for normal cell-cell adhesion including catenins, laminin, type IV collagen, desmogleins, desmocollins, occludins, connexion 2b claudins and MUC1. Likewise, archetypical epithelial components such as keratins 8, 18 and 19 and tissue inhibitors of metallo-proteinases are all reduced. On the other hand, we observed an increased expression of mesenchymal markers such as N cadherin, vimentin, fibronectin, integrins β4 and α5, tenascin, SPARC, PLAU, VEGF, CD68, FSP1/S100A4, LCN2 and various metalloproteinases In short, we are seeing all the hallmarks of cells undergoing EMT with acquisition of the phenotype characterising the group of basal-like 'claudin low' tumours such as the triple negative (ER-ve, PR-ve, ERBB2-ve) metaplastic tumours described by Hennessy et al., (2009). A similar conclusion was reached by Gadalla et al., (2005) who observed an EMT-like transition with loss of E-cadherin and reduction in CD24 induced by ER silencing. However, they did not observe the increase in CD44 that we and others have widely reported.

An interesting molecule whose expression was found to be substantially repressed in our pII cells (Al Saleh et al., 2011a) is GATA3, a zinc finger transcription factor that plays an important role as a regulator of mammary gland formation and development (Kouros-Mehr et al., 2008) and has been implicated in both EMT and breast cancer metastasis. GATA3 is a positive transcriptional regulator of ER expression whilst simultaneously itself being a target gene for the ER complex. Its expression has been linked to favourable outcome of endocrine therapy (Parikh et al., 2005). Several studies have shown association of GATA3 with ER+ tumours (eg, Mehra et al., 2005). Yan et al., (2010) recently demonstrated that not only was GATA3 expression abolished in ER-ve cell lines but also correlated with E-cadherin. siRNA-induced silencing of GATA3 resulted in fibroblastic-like transformation of MCF7 cells. On the other hand, restoration of GATA3 expression in ER-ve cells led to renewal of epithelial characteristics as typified by increased levels of E-cadherin and decrease of N-cadherin, vimentin and MMP9 with parallel reduction of tumour forming capacity of MDAMB231 cells injected into xenografted mice. These studies elegantly support the notion that ER regulated events is intimately involved in the same processes that lead to EMT and very crucially, that these events are reversible.

Another significant group of genes variously implicated in EMT that is elevated in pII cells is included in the '24 gene signature' of genes proposed as predictive of invasiveness (Zajchowski et al., 2001): integrin, TIMP-2 and TIMP-3, MT1-MMP, PAI-1, Osteonectin/SPARC, thrombospondin-1, collagen (VI) α1 and collagen (I) α2. pII also display the '9 gene signature' of down-regulated or low expressing genes (E-cadherin, CLDN7, CRB3, KRT8, TACSTD1, IRF6, SPINT2, MAL2 and MARVELD3) that was found by Katz et al., (2011) to be common between their C35 transfected cells and claudin-low tumours. Evidence that the latter represent EMT is now substantial and supported by *in vitro* observations (Prat et al., 2010; Taube et al., 2010).

Substantial reduction in ER expression has been observed in modified MCF7 sub-lines resistant to the mitotic inhibitors paclitaxel and docetaxel and the anthracycline doxorubicin (Iseri et al., 2011). Microarray analysis showed up-regulation of SNAIL2, CDH2, VIM, CLDN1, CLDN11, EGFR, FGFR1, SMAD3 and TGFBR2 and down-regulation of E-cadherin, OCLN, CLDN3, CLDN4, and CLDN7. This data bears remarkable resemblance to the profile for pII cells with the common denominator being loss of ER.

This brings us finally to the group of transcriptional repressors that have been coined as the 'mediators of EMT' and discussed above, so far a relatively smaller group that unify a much larger and diverse array of signalling molecules involved in their regulation. Of the key factors identified in cadherin switching, ZEB1, ZEB2/SIP1 and SNAIL2 (Onder et al, 2008) are all significantly elevated in our endocrine resistant pII cells. These observations lead us to conclude that there is a high degree of synonimity between endocrine resistance and EMT, both effected by functional loss of ER and both resulting in increased propensity for tumour dissemination through the actions of a common set of mediators. The repression of SNAIL by the ER dependent MTA3 (Fujita et al., 2003), a subunit of the Mi-2/NuRD histone deacetylase complex, which could well be regarded, among others, as a guardian of the epithelial phenotype (?) may be worthy of further attention. Interestingly, another family member, MTA1, is described as a potent inhibitor of nuclear ER function through cytoplasmic sequestration of the receptor and this may provide an explanation for resistance in ER+ cells as MTA1 would indirectly reduce the levels of MTA3 thereby relieving SNAIL repression.

There have also been intriguing suggestions regarding the origin of the mesenchymal-like cells, with the attractive view of these as a possibly slow growing pre-existing CSC sub-population within the tumour (Lim et al., 2010; May et al., 2011). In such a scenario there is no induced EMT as such, but a gradual emergence of a group of cells already bearing these properties, to become the dominant group. Similar ideas have often been suggested to explain the re-emergence of 'drug–regressed' tumours as an expansion of a pre-existing intrinsically resistant cell population once the sensitive cells have been eliminated. However, attractive as this may be, in the alternative scheme elaborated by May et al., (2011) there would be a reversion of such 'MaSCs' back to an epithelial phenotype at the site of metastatic growth in a reverse MET transition, which raises the question that If cells can undergo MET then why not EMT, and there is no necessity to postulate the existence of *a priori* mesenchymal cells. Moreover, the *in vitro* data demonstrates quite clearly that an actual EMT transition does take place as the initial population of cells is relatively homogeneous with respect to being epithelial in nature. Most if not all of the cells in culture can simultaneously undergo EMT whereas it is very likely that only a very small fraction of cells in a tumour acquire all of the characteristics enabling them to undergo a full transition, which may be why such mesenchymal-like cells have not been routinely reported by pathologists (Thompson et al., 2008).

6. Summary

The persistent problem of drug resistance and in particular the therapeutic failure of endocrine agents presents serious therapeutic issues especially in view of the success of this type of intervention in a significantly large proportion of women with breast cancer. Many studies have focused on elucidating the mechanisms responsible for *de novo* and *acquired* independence from estrogen. Consensus of opinion favours the view that signaling pathways mediated through a variety of peptide growth factors is largely responsible for the aggressive proliferation of tumours that have ceased to depend upon the ER, although no single unifying or even major factor has been identified. Somewhat in parallel, the last few years have witnessed an increasing number of reports describing the relatively recently recognized phenomenon of EMT, highlighting its similarity to the events leading to tumour invasion and vascular dissemination. Many of the key mediators of EMT particularly the transcriptional repression of E-cadherin by SNAIL appear to be critical steps in tumour progression. The association of mesenchymal-like features such as cadherin switching, loss of adhesion proteins and CD24, increased vimentin and fibronectin, with ER-ve tumours, have been sporadically, almost anecdotally reported in the literature over the last decade or more. We have now found evidence to show that the acquisition of endocrine independence, due to induced ER loss, by previously ER+ breast cancer cells, is accompanied by all the hallmark features of EMT. Although it is still far from clear whether the two processes are occurring side by side or whether either is causal of the other, it seems reasonable to conclude that loss of ER can directly trigger EMT. It remains to be seen whether restoration of ER in the trans-differentiated cells can reverse EMT and allow the cells to regain estrogen dependence.

7. Acknowledgements

We thank Kuwait University Research Administration for financial support in the form of Grant YM08/09.

8. References

Aguilera O, Fraga MF, Ballestar E, Paz MF, Herranz M, et al: Epigenetic inactivation of the Wnt antagonist DICKKOPF-1 (DKK-1) gene in human colorectal cancer. Oncogene 25: 4116–4121, 2006.

Aktas B, Tewes M, Fehm T, Hauch S, Kimmig R & Kasimir-Bauer S: Stem cell and epithelial-mesenchymal transition markers are frequently over-expressed in circulating tumor cells of metastatic breast cancer patients. Breast Cancer Res 11:R46, 2009.

Al Saleh S, Sharaf LH & Luqmani YA: Signalling pathways involved in endocrine resistance in breast cancer and associations with epithelial to mesenchymal transition. Int J Oncol 38(5):1197-217, 2011.

Al Saleh S, Al Mulla F & Luqmani YA: Estrogen receptor silencing induces epithelial to mesenchymal transition in human breast cancer cells. PLoS One 6(6):e20610. 2011a. 2011a.

Al Saleh S: Association of functional loss of estrogen receptor with an epithelial to mesenchymal transition in human breast cancer. MSc thesis, Kuwait University, 2010.

Al-Hajj M, Wicha MS, Benito-Hernandez A, Morrison SJ & Clarke MF: Prospective identification of tumorigenic breast cancer cells. Proc Natl Acad Sci USA 100:3983-3988, 2003.

Ali S & Coombes RC: Endocrine-responsive breast cancer and strategies for combating resistance. Nature Rev. Cancer 2: 101–112, 2002.

Ansieau S, Bastid J, Doreau A, Morel AP, Bouchet BP, et al: Induction of EMT by twist proteins as a collateral effect of tumor-promoting inactivation of premature senescence. Cancer Cell 14:79–89, 2008.

Arpino G, Wiechmann L, Osborne CK & Schiff R: Crosstalk between the estrogen receptor and the HER tyrosine kinase receptor family: molecular mechanism and clinical implications for endocrine therapy resistance. Endocr Rev 29: 217-233, 2008.

Asselin-Labat ML, Shackleton M, Stingl J, Vaillant F, Forrest NC, et al: Steroid Hormone Receptor Status of Mouse Mammary Stem Cells. J Natl Cancer Inst 98(14): 1011-1014, 2006.

Balic M, Lin H and Young L, et al: Most early disseminated cancer cells detected in bone marrow of breast cancer patients have a putative breast cancer stem cell phenotype. Clin Cancer Res 12: 5615–21, 2006.

Barr S, Thomson S, Buck E, Russo S, Petti F, et al. Bypassing cellular EGF receptor dependence through epithelial-to-mesenchymal-like transitions. Clin Exp Metastasis 25: 685–693, 2008.

Bayliss J, Hilger A, Vishnu P, et al: Reversal of the estrogen receptor negative phenotype in breast cancer and restoration of antiestrogen response. Clin Cancer Res 13:7029–36, 2007

Beatson GT: on the treatment of inoperable cases of carcinoma of the mamma: suggestions for a new method of treatment with illustrative cases. Lancet 2: 104-107, 1896.

Beltran M, Puig I, Peña C, García JM, Alvarez AB et al: A natural antisense transcript regulates Zeb2/Sip1 gene expression during Snail1- induced epithelial-mesenchymal transition. Genes Dev 22: 756-769, 2008.

Berx G & van Roy F: The E-cadherin/catenin complex: an important gatekeeper in breast cancer tumorigenesis and malignant progression. Breast Cancer Res 3: 289-293, 2001.

Berx G, Raspe E, Christofori G, Thiery JP & Sleeman JP: Pre-EMTing metastasis: recapitulation of morphogenetic processes in cancer. Clin Exp Metastasis 24: 587-597, 2007.

Bindels S, Mestdagt M, Vandewalle C, et al: Regulation of vimentin by SIP1 in human epithelial breast tumor cells. Oncogene 25: 4975-4985, 2006.

Blanco MJ, Moreno-Bueno G, Sarrio D, Locascio A, Cano A, Palacios J & Nieto MA: Correlation of Snail expression with histological grade and lymph node status in breast carcinomas. Oncogene 21: 3241-3246, 2002

Brinkman JA & El-Ashry D: ER re-expression and resensitization to endocrine therapies in ERnegative breast cancers. J. Mammary Gland Biol. Neoplasia 14:67–78, 2009.

Bunone G, Briand PA, Miksicek RJ & Picard D: Activation of the unliganded estrogen receptor by EGF involves the MAP kinase pathway and direct phosphorylation. EMBO J 15: 2174-2183, 1996.

Cai D, Iyer A, Felekkis KN, Near RI, Luo Z, et al: AND-34/BCAR3, a GDP exchange factor whose over-expression confers antiestrogen resistance, activates Rac, PAK1, and the cyclin D1 promoter. Cancer Res 63: 6802-6808, 2003.

Caldon CE, Sergio CM, Schütte J, Boersma MN, Sutherland RL, et al: Estrogen regulation of cyclin E2 requires cyclin D1, but not c-Myc. Mol Cell Biol 29:4623–4639, 2009.

Campbell RA, Bhat-Nakshatri P, Patel NM, Constantinidou D, Ali S and Nakshatri H: Phosphatidylinositol 3-kinase/akt- mediated activation of estrogen receptor α: a new model for anti-estrogen resistance. J Biol Chem 276: 9817-9824, 2001

Cano A, Perez-Moreno MA, Rodrigo I, Locascio A, Blanco MJ, et al: The transcription factor Snail controls epithelial-mesenchymal transitions by repressing E-cadherin expression. Nat Cell Biol 2: 76-83, 2000.

Cappelletti V, Celio L, Bajetta E, Allevi A, Longarini R, et al: Prospective evaluation of estrogen receptor-beta in predicting response to neoadjuvant antiestrogen therapy in elderly breast cancer patients. Endocr-Relat Cancer 11:761–770, 2004.

Care A, Felicetti F, Meccia E, et al: HOXB7: a key factor for tumor-associated angiogenic switch. Cancer Res 61: 6532-6539, 2001.

Care A, Silvani A, Meccia E, Mattia G, Peschle C & Colombo MP: Transduction of the SkBr3 breast carcinoma cell line with the HOXB7 gene induces bFGF expression, increases cell proliferation and reduces growth factor dependence. Oncogene 16: 3285-3289, 1998.

Carrio M, Arderiu G, Myers C & Boudreau NJ: Homeobox D10 induces phenotypic reversion of breast tumor cells in a three-dimensional culture model. Cancer Res 65: 7177-7185, 2005.

Chaffer CL, Thompson EW & Williams ED. Mesenchymal to epithelial transition in development and disease. Cells Tissues Organs 185: 7–19, 2007.

Chan CM, Martin LA, Johnston SR, Ali S & Dowsett M: Molecular changes associated with the acquisition of estrogen hypersensitivity in MCF-7 breast cancer cells on long-term estrogen deprivation. J Steroid Biochem Mol Biol 81: 333–341, 2002.

Charafe-Jauffret E, Ginestier C, Monville F, Finetti P, Adélaïde J, et al: Gene expression profiling of breast cell lines identifies potential new basal markers. Oncogene 25(15):2273-84, 2006.

Chen H, Chung S & Sukumar S: HOXA5-induced apoptosis in breast cancer cells is mediated by caspases 2 and 8. Mol Cell Biol 24: 924-935, 2004.

Chen JD &Evans RM: A transcriptional co-repressor that inter-acts with nuclear hormone receptors. Nature 377: 454-457, 1995.

Cheng GZ, Chan J, Wang Q, Zhang W, Sun CD & Wang LH: Twist transcriptionally up-regulates AKT2 in breast cancer cells leading to increased migration, invasion, and resistance to paclitaxel. Cancer Res 67(5): 1979–1987, 2007.

Chu IM, Hengst L & Slingerland JM: The Cdk inhibitor p27 in human cancer: prognostic potential and relevance to anticancer therapy. Nature Rev Cancer 8: 253–267, 2008.

Come C, Magnino F, Bibeau F, et al: SNAIL and SNAIL2 play distinct roles during breast carcinoma progression. Clin Cancer Res 12: 5395-5402, 2006.

Coqueret O: Linking cyclins to transcriptional control. Gene 299: 35–55, 2002.

Creighton CJ, Fu X, Hennessy BT, et al: Proteomic and transcriptomic profiling reveals a link between the PI3K pathway and lower estrogen-receptor (ER) levels and activity in ER+ breast cancer. Breast Cancer Res 12(3):R40, 2010.

Dandachi N, Hauser-Kronberger C, More E, et al: Co-expression of tenascin-C and vimentin in human breast cancer cells indicates phenotypic transdifferentiation during tumour progression: correlation with histopathological parameters, hormone receptors, and onco-proteins. J Pathol 193: 181-189, 2001.

Das S, Becker B, Hoffmann FM & Mertz JE: Complete reversal of epithelial to mesenchymal transition requires inhibition of both ZEB expression and the Rho pathway. BMC Cell Biol 10: 94-112, 2009.

Dhasarathy A, Kajita M & Wade PA: The transcription factor snail mediates epithelial to mesenchymal transitions by repression of estrogen receptor-alpha. Mol Endocrinol 21: 2907 2918, 2007.

DiMeo TA, Anderson K, Phadke P, et al: A novel lung metastasis signature links wnt signalling with cancer cell self-renewal and epithelial-mesenchymal transition in basal-like breast cancer. Cancer Res 69: 5364-5373, 2009.

Dontu G, Jackson KW, McNicholas E, Kawamura MJ, Abdallah WM, Wicha MS, et al: Role of Notch signaling in cell-fate determination of human mammary stem/progenitor cells. Breast Cancer Res 6: R605-R615, 2004.

Dorssers LC, van Agthoven T, Dekker A, van Agthoven TL & Kok EM: Induction of antiestrogen resistance in human breast cancer cells by random insertional mutagenesis using defective retroviruses: identification of bcar-1, a common integration site. Mol. Endocrinol 7: 870-878, 1993.

Emmen JM, Couse JF, Elmore SA, Yates MM, Kissling GE & Korach KS: In vitro growth and ovulation of follicles from ovaries of estrogen receptor (ER){alpha} and ER{beta} null mice indicate a role for ER{beta} in follicular maturation. Endocrinology 146: 2817-2826, 2005.

Faridi J, Wang L, Endemann G & Roth RA: Expression of constitutively active Akt-3 in MCF-7 breast cancer cells reverses the estrogen and tamoxifen responsivity of these cells in vivo. Clin Cancer Res 9: 2933–2939, 2003.

Fillmore CM & Kuperwasser C: Human breast cancer cell lines contain stem like cells that self-renew, give rise to phenotypically diverse progeny & survive chemotherapy. Breast cancer res 10(2) : R25, 2008.

Fillmore CM & Kuperwasser C: Human breast cancer cell lines contain stem-like cells that self-renew, give rise to pheno-typically diverse progeny and survive chemotherapy. Breast Cancer Res 10: R25, 2008.

Fisher B, Dignam J, Wolmark N, Wickerham, DL, Fisher ER, et al: Tamoxifen in treatment of intraductal breast cancer. National Surgical Adjuvant Breast and Bowel Project B-24 randomised controlled trial. Lancet 12; 353(9169):1993-2000.

Font de Mora J & Brown M: AIB1 is a conduit for kinase-mediated growth factor signaling to the estrogen receptor. Mol Cell Biol 20: 5041-5047, 2000.

Forster C, Makela S, Warri A, Kietz S, Becker D, Hultenby K, Warner M & Gustafsson JA: Involvement of estrogen receptor beta in terminal differentiation of mammary gland epithelium. Proc Natl Acad Sci USA 99:15578-15583, 2002.

Frasor J, Danes JM, Komm B, Chang KC, Lyttle CR & Katzenellenbogen BS: Profiling of estrogen up- and down-regulated gene expression in human breast cancer cells: insights into gene networks and pathways underlying estrogenic control of proliferation and cell phenotype. Endocrinology 144: 4562–4574, 2003.

Fujita N, Jaye DL, Kajita M. Geigerman C, Moreno CS, et al: MTA3, a Mi-2/NuRD Complex Subunit, Regulates an Invasive Growth Pathway in Breast Cancer. Cell 113: 207–219, 2003.

Fuqua SA, Wiltschke C, Zhang QZ, Borg A, Castles CG, et al: A hypersensitive estrogen receptor-alpha mutation in premalignant breast lesions. Cancer Res 60:4026–4029, 2000.

Fuxe J, Vincent T, & de Herreros AJ: Transcriptional crosstalk between TGFβ and stem cell pathways in tumor cell invasion: role of EMT promoting Smad complexes. Cell Cycle 9 (12): 2363–2374, 2010.

Gadalla SE, Alexandraki A, Lindström MS, Nistér, M & Ericsson C: Uncoupling of the ERα regulated morphological phenotype from the cancer stem cell phenotype in human breast cancer cell lines. BBRC 405 (4): 581-587 , 2005.

Gebeshuber CA, Zatloukal K & Martinez J: miR-29a suppresses tristetraprolin, which is a regulator of epithelial polarity and metastasis, EMBO Rep 10(4):400-5, 2009.

Gilles C, Polette M, Mestdagt M, et al: Transactivation of vimentin by beta-catenin in human breast cancer cells. Cancer Res 63: 2658-2664, 2003.

Ginestier C, Hur MH, Charafe-Jauffret E, Monville F, Dutcher J, et al: ALDH1 is a marker of normal and malignant human mammary stem cells and a predictor of poor clinical outcome. Cell Stem Cell 1: 555-567, 2007.

Gjerdrum C, Tiron C, Høiby T, Stefansson I, Haugen H, et al: Axl is an essential epithelial-to-mesenchymal transition-induced regulator of breast cancer metastasis and patient survival. Proc Natl Acad Sci USA 107: 1124-1129, 2010.

Green S, Walter P, Kumar V, Krust A, Bornert JM, Argos P & Chambon P: Human oestrogen receptor cDNA: Sequence, expression and homology with v-erb. Nature (Lond.) 320:134–139, 1986.

Greenberg G & Hay ED: Epithelia suspended in collagen gels can lose polarity and express characteristics of migrating mesenchymal cells. J Cell Biol 95: 333-339, 1982.

Gregory PA, Bracken CP, Bert AG & Goodall GJ: MicroRNAs as regulators of epithelial-mesenchymal transition. Cell Cycle 7: 3112–3118, 2008.

Gronemeyer H: Transcription activation by estrogen and proges-terone receptors. Ann Rev Genet 25: 89-123, 1991.

Gururaj AE, Rayala SK, Vadlamudi RK & Kumar R: Novel mechanisms of resistance to endocrine therapy: genomic and nongenomic considerations. Clin Cancer Res 12: 1001s–1007s, 2006.

Gutierrez MC, Detre S, Johnston S, Mohsin SK, Shou J, et al: Molecular changes in tamoxifen-resistant breast cancer: relation-ship between estrogen receptor, HER-2, and p38 mitogen-activated protein kinase. J Clin Oncol 23: 2469-2476, 2005.

Hafizi S & Dahlbäck B: Signaling and functional diversity within the Axl subfamily of receptor tyrosine kinases. Cytok Growth Factor Rev 17: 295-304, 2006.

Hall JM & McDonnell DP: The estrogen receptor beta-isoform (ERbeta) of the human estrogen receptor modulates ERalpha transcriptional activity and is a key regulator of the cellular response to estrogens and antiestrogens. Endocrinology 140: 5566–5578, 1999.

Hartwell KA, Muir B, Reinhardt F, et al: The Spemann organizer gene, Goosecoid, promotes tumor metastasis. Proc Natl Acad Sci USA 103: 18969-18974, 2006.

Hay ED. An overview of epithelio-mesenchymal transformation. Acta Anat (Basel) 154:8–20, 1995.

Hazan RB, Phillips GR, Qiao RF, Norton L & Aaronson SA: Exogenous expression of N-cadherin in breast cancer cells induces cell migration, invasion, and metastasis. J Cell Biol 148: 779-790, 2000.

Hazan RB, Qiao R, Keren R, Badano I, & Suyama K: Cadherin switch in tumour progression. Ann NY Acad Sci 1014: 155-163, 2004.

Hebbard L, Steffen A, Zawadzki V, Fieber C, Howells N, et al: CD44 expression and regulation during mammary gland development and function, J Cell Sci 113(14):2619-2630, 2000.

Hennessy BT, et al: Characterization of a naturally occurring breast cancer subset enriched in epithelial-to-mesenchymal transition and stem cell characteristics. Cancer Res 69:4116-4124, 2009.

Herynk, MH & Fuqua SA: Estrogen receptor mutations in human disease. Endocr Rev 25: 869-898, 2004.

Hiscox S, Borley A, Nicholson RI & Barett-Lee P: Epithelial-mesenchymal transition (EMT) and its involvement in acquired endocrine resistance in breast cancer.Chapter 5. In: Cancer Drug Resistance Research perspectives. Torres LS (ed.) Nova Science Publishers, New York, pp81-95, 2007.

Hollier BG, Evans K & Mani SA: The epithelial-to-mesen-chymal transition and cancer stem cells: a coalition against cancer therapies. J Mamm Gland Biol Neoplasia 14: 29-43, 2009.

Honma N, Horii R, Iwase T, Saji S, Younes M, et al. Clinical importance of estrogen receptor-β evaluation in breast cancer patients treated with adjuvant tamoxifen therapy. J Clin Oncol 26: 3727-3734, 2008.

Horlein AJ, Naar AM, Heinzel T, Torchia J, Gloss B, et al: Ligand-independent repression by the thyroid hormone receptor mediated by a nuclear receptor co-repressor. Nature 377: 397-404, 1995.

Hoskins JM, Carey LA & McLeod HL. CYP2D6 and tamoxifen: DNA matters in breast cancer. Nature Rev Cancer 9:576-586, 2009.

Howell A, Pippen J, Elledge RM, Mauriac L, Vergote I, Jones SE, et al: Fulvestrant vs anastrozole for the treatment of advanced breast carcinoma: a prospectively planned combined survival analysis of two multicenter trials. Cancer 104: 236-239, 2005.

Hua G, Zhu B, Rosa F, Deblon N, Adélaïde J, et al: A negative feedback regulatory loop associates the tyrosine kinase receptor ERBB2 and the transcription factor GATA4 in breast cancer cells. Mol Cancer Res 7: 402-414, 2009.

Huber MA, Kraut N & Beug H: Molecular requirements for epithelial–mesenchymal transi tion during tumor progression. Curr Opin Cell Biol 17: 548-558, 2005.

Huber MA, Azoitei N, Baumann B, Grünert S, Sommer A, et al: NF-kappaB is essential for epithelial-mesenchymal transition and metastasis in a model of breast cancer progression. J Clin Invest Hui R, Finney GL, Carroll JS, Lee CS, Musgrove EA & Sutherland RL.: Constitutive overexpression of cyclin D1 but not cyclin E confers acute resistance to antiestrogens in T-47D breast cancer cells. Cancer Res 62: 6916-6923, 2002.

Hui R, Finney GL, Carroll JS, Lee CS, Musgrove EA & Sutherland RL: Constitutive overexpression of cyclin D1 but not cyclin E confers acute resistance to antiestrogens in T-47D breast cancer cells. Cancer Res 62:6916-6923, 2002.

Hurtado A, Holmes KA, Geistlinger TR, Hutcheson IR, Nicholson RI, et al: Regulation of ERBB2 by oestrogen receptor-PAX2 determines response to tamoxifen. Nature 456: 663–666, 2008.

Hutcheson IR, Knowlden JM, Madden TA, Barrow D, Gee JM, et al.: Oestrogen receptor-mediated modulation of the EGFR/MAPK pathway in tamoxifenresistant MCF-7 cells. Breast Cancer Res Treat 81: 81–93, 2003.

Iseri OD, Kars DM, Arpaci F, Atalay C, Pak I & Gunduz U: Drug resistant MCF-7 cells exhibit epithelial-mesenchymal transition gene expression pattern. Biomed Pharmacother: 65(1):40-45, 2011.

Ishii Y, Waxman S & Germain D: Tamoxifen stimulates the growth of cyclin D1-overexpressing breast cancer cells by promoting the activation of signal transducer and activator of transcription. Cancer Res 68: 852–860, 2008.

Joel PB, Smith J, Sturgill TW, Fisher TL, Blenis J & Lannigan DA: pp90rsk1 regulates estrogen receptor mediated transcription through phosphorylation of Ser-167. Mol Cell Biol 18: 1978-1984, 1998.

Johnston SR, Saccani-Jotti G, Smith IE, Salter J, Newby J, et al: Changes in estrogen receptor, progesterone receptor, and pS2 expression in tamoxifen resistant human breast cancer, Cancer Res 55: 3331–3338, 1995.

Johnston SR, Lu B, Scott GK, Kushner PJ, Smith IE, et al: Increased activator protein-1 DNA binding and c-jun NH2-terminal kinase activity in human breast tumors with acquired tamoxifen resistance. Clin Cancer Res 5: 251-256, 1999.

Johnston SR & Dowsett M: Aromatase inhibitors for breast cancer: lessons from the laboratory. Nature Reviews Cancer 3:821–831, 2003.

Kalluri R & Weinberg RA. The basics of epithelial–mesenchymal transition. J Clin Invest Jun 119(6): 1420–8, 2009.

Kato S, Endoh H, Masuhiro Y, Kitamoto T, Uchiyama S, et al: Activation of the estrogen receptor through phosphorylation by mitogenactivated protein kinase. Science 270: 1491-1494, 1995.

Kajiyama H, Hosono S, Terauchi M, Shibata K, Ino K, Yamamoto E, et al: Twist expression predicts poor clinical outcome of patients with clear cell carcinoma of the ovary. Oncology 71:394–401, 2006.

Kouros-Mehr H, Kim JW, Bechis SK, & Werb Z: GATA-3 and the regulation of the mammary luminal cell fate. Curr Opin Cell Biol 20: 164–170, 2008.

Kuiper GG, Enmark E, Pelto-Huikko M, Nilsson S & Gustafsson JA: Cloning of a novel receptor expressed in rat prostate and ovary. Proc Natl Acad Sci USA 93: 5925–5930, 1996.

Kuiper GG, Carlsson B, Grandien K, Enmark E, Häggblad J, et al: Comparison of the ligand binding specificity and transcript tissue distribution of estrogen receptors α and β. Endocrinology 138: 863–870, 1997.

Kushner PJ, Agard DA, Greene GL, Scanlan TS, Shiau AK, et al: Estrogen receptor pathways to AP-1. J Steroid Biochem Mol Biol 74: 311-317, 2000.

Laffin B, Wellberg E, Kwak HI, et al: Loss of singleminded-2s in the mouse mammary gland induces an epithelial-mesenchymal transition associated with up-regulation of slug and matrix metalloprotease 2. Mol Cell Biol 28: 1936-1946, 2008.

Le Romancer M, Treilleux I, Leconte N, Robin-Lespinasse N, et al: Regulation of estrogen rapid signaling through arginine methylation by PRMT1. Mol Cell 31: 212-221, 2008.

Lechner JF, Fugaro JM, Wong Y, Pass HI, Harris CC & Belinsky SA: Perspective: cell differentiation theory may advance early detection of and therapy for lung cancer. Radiat Res 155: 235-238, 2001

Leo C & Chen JD: The srcfamily of nuclear receptor co- activators. Gene 245: 1-11, 2000.

Lester RD, Jo M, Montel V, et al: uPAR induces epithelial mesenchymal transition in hypoxic breast cancer cells. J Cell Biol 178: 425-436, 2007.

Levin ER: Bidirectional signaling between the estrogen receptor and the epidermal growth factor receptor. Mol Endocrinol 17: 309-317, 2003.

Li X, Lewis MT, Huang J, Gutierrez C, Osborne CK, et al. Intrinsic resistance of tumorigenic breast cancer cells to chemotherapy. J Natl Cancer Inst 100: 672–679, 2008.

Lim E, Wu D, Pal B, Bouras T, Asselin-Labat ML, et al: Transcriptome analyses of mouse and human mammary cell subpopulations reveal multiple conserved genes and pathways. Breast Cancer Res 12:R21, 2010.

Linger RM, Keating AK, Earp HS & Graham DK: TAM receptor tyrosine kinases: biologic functions, signalling, and potential therapeutic targeting in human cancer. Adv Cancer Res 100: 35-83, 2008

Lopez-Tarruella S & Schiff R: The dynamics of estrogen receptor status in breast cancer: reshaping the paradigm. Clin. Cancer Res. 13:6921–25, 2007.

Lubahn DB, Moyer JS, Golding TS, Couse JF, Korach KS & Smithies O: Alteration of reproductive function but not prenatal sexual development after insertional disruption of the mouse estrogen receptor gene. Proc Natl Acad Sci USA 90: 11162–11166, 1993.

Luqmani YA, Al Azmi A, Al Bader M, Abraham G & El Zawahri M: Modification of gene expression induced by siRNA targeting of estrogen receptor in MCF7 human breast cancer cells. Int J Oncol 34: 231-242, 2009

Ma L, Teruya-Feldstein J & Weinberg RA: Tumour invasion and metastasis initiated by microRNA-10b in breast cancer. Nature 449: 682–688, 2007.

Ma XJ, Wang Z, Ryan PD, et al: A two-gene expression ratio predicts clinical outcome in breast cancer patients treated with tamoxifen. Cancer Cell 5: 607-616, 2004.

Magnifico A, Albano L, Campaner S, Delia D, Castiglioni F, et al: Tumor-initiating cells of HER2-positive carcinoma cell lines express the highest oncoprotein levels and are Trastuzumab sensitive. Clin Cancer Res 15: 2010-2021, 2009.

Mandlekar S & Kong AN: Mechanisms of tamoxifen induced apoptosis. Apoptosis 6: 469–477, 2001.

Mani SA, Yang J, Brooks M, et al: Mesenchyme Forkhead 1 (FOXC2) plays a key role in metastasis and is associated with aggressive basal-like breast cancers. Proc Natl Acad Sci USA 104: 10069-10074, 2007.

Mani SA, Guo W, Liao MJ, Eaton EN, Ayyanan A, et al: The epithelial-mesenchymal transition generates cells with properties of stem cells. Cell 133: 704-715, 2008.

Martin LA, Farmer I, Johnston SR, Ali S, Marshall C & Dowsett M: Enhanced estrogen receptor (ER) alpha, ERBB2, and MAPK signal transduction pathways operate during the adaptation of MCF-7 cells to long term estrogen deprivation, J. Biol. Chem. 278:30458–30468, 2003.

Masamura S, Santner SJ, Heitjan DF & Santen RJ: Estrogen deprivation causes estradiol hypersensitivity in human breast cancer cells. J Clin Endocrinol Metab 80:2918–2925, 1995.

Massarweh S & Schiff R: Unraveling the mechanisms of endocrine resistance in breast cancer: new therapeutic opportunities. Clin Cancer Res 13(7):1950-4, 2007.

Massarweh S, Osborne CK, Creighton CJ, Qin L, Tsimelzon A, et al: Tamoxifen resistance in breast tumors is driven by growth factor receptor signaling with repression of classic estrogen receptor genomic function. Cancer research 68(3):826-33, 2008.

May CD, Sphyris N, Evans KW, Werden SJ, Guo W, & Mani SA: Epithelial mesenchymal transition and cancer stem cells: a dangerously dynamic duo in breast cancer progression. Breast Cancer Res 13(1):202-211, 2011.

McClelland RA, Barrow D, Madden TA, Dutkowski CM, Pamment J, et al: Enhanced epidermal growth factor receptor signaling in MCF7 breast cancer cells after long-term culture in the presence of the pure antiestrogen ICI 182,780 (Faslodex). Endocrinology 142: 2776-2788, 2001.

McKenna NJ, Lanz Rb & O'Malley BW: Nuclear receptor co-regulators: cellular and molecular biology. Endocr Rev 20: 321-344, 1999.

Mehra R, Varambally S, Ding L, Shen R, Sabel MS, et al: Identification of GATA3 as a breast cancer prognostic marker by global gene expression meta-analysis. Cancer Res 65: 11259-11264, 2005.

Miller GJ, Miller HL, van Bokhoven A, et al: Aberrant HOXC expression accompanies the malignant phenotype in human prostate. Cancer Res 63: 5879-5888, 2003.

Moody SE, Perez D, Pan TC, Sarkisian CJ, Portocarrero CP, et al: The transcriptional repressor Snail promotes mammary tumour recurrence. Cancer Cell 8: 197-209, 2005.

Morel AP, Lievre M, Thomas C, et al: Generation of breast cancer stem cells through epithelial-mesenchymal transition. PLoS One 3: e2888, 2008.

Moreno-Bueno G, Portillo F & Cano A: Transcriptional regulation of cell polarity in EMT and cancer. Oncogene 27: 6958-6969, 2008.

Moustakas A & Heldin CH: Signaling networks guiding epithelial-mesenchymal transitions during embryogenesis and cancer progression. Cancer Sci 98:1512-1520, 2007.

Moustakas A & Heldin CH: The regulation of TGFβ signal transduction. Development 136: 3699-3714, 2009.

Murphy LC & Watson PH: Is oestrogen receptor-β a predictor of endocrine therapy responsiveness in human breast cancer? Endocr Relat Cancer 13: 327-334, 2006.

Musgrove EA & Sutherland RL: Biological determinants of endocrine resistance in breast cancer. Nat Rev 9: 631-643, 2009.

Naora H, Yang YQ, Montz FJ, Seidman JD, Kurman RJ & Roden Rb: A serologically identified tumor antigen encoded by a homeobox gene promotes growth of ovarian epithelial cells. Proc Natl Acad Sci USA 98: 4060-4065, 2001.

Nicholson RI, Staka C, Boyns F, Hutcheson IR & Gee JM: Growth factor-driven mechanisms associated with resistance to estrogen deprivation in breast cancer: new opportunities for therapy. Endocr Relat Cancer 11: 623-641, 2004.

Normanno N, Qi CF, Gullick WJ, Persico G, Yarden Y, et al: Expression of amphiregulin, cripto-1 and heregulin-a in human breast cancer cell lines. Int J Oncol 2: 903-911, 1993.

Normanno N, Di Maio M, De Maio E, De Luca A, De Matteis A, et al: Mechanisms of endocrine resistance and novel therapeutic strategies in breast cancer. Endocr Relat Cancer 12: 721-747, 2005.

Onder TT, Gupta PB, Mani SA, Yang J, Lander ES & Weinberg RA: Loss of E-cadherin promotes metastasis via multiple downstream transcriptional pathways. Cancer Res 68: 3645-3653, 2008.

Orlichenko LS & Radisky DC: Matrix metalloproteinases stimulate epithelial-mesenchymal transition during tumour development. Clin Exp Metastasis 25: 593-600, 2008.

Osborne CK, Schiff R, Fuqua SA & Shou J: Estrogen receptor: current understanding of its activation and modulation. Clin. Cancer Res: 7 (Suppl 12): S4338–S4342, 2001.

Osborne CK, Pippen J, Jones SE, Parker LM, Ellis M, et al : Double-blind, randomized trial comparing the efficacy and tolerability of fulvestrant versus anastrozole in postmenopausal women with advanced breast cancer progressing on prior endocrine therapy: results of a North American trial. Int J Oncol 20: 3386–3395, 2002.

Osborne CK, Bardou V, Hopp TA, Chamness GC, Hilsenbeck SG, et al: Role of the estrogen receptor coactivator AIB1 (SRC-3) and HER-2/neu in tamoxifen resistance in breast cancer. J Natl Cancer Inst 95, 353–361, 2003.

Osborne CK & Schiff R: Estrogen-receptor biology: continuing progress and therapeutic implications. J Clin Oncol 23:1616–1622, 2005.

Osborne CK & Schiff R: Mechanisms of endocrine resistance in breast cancer. Ann Rev Med. 62:233-47, 2011.

Ottaviano YL, Issa JP, Parl FF, Smith HS, Baylin SB & Davidson NE: Methylation of the estrogen receptor gene CpG island marks loss of estrogen receptor expression in human breast cancer cells. Cancer Res 54: 2552–2555, 1994.

Otto C, Rohde-Schulz B, Schwarz G, Fuchs I, Klewer M, et al: G Protein-Coupled Receptor 30 Localizes to the Endoplasmic Reticulum and Is Not Activated by Estradiol. Endocrinology 149 (10): 4846-4856, 2008.

Ozdamar B, Bose R, Barrios-Rodiles M, Wang HR, Zhang Y & Wrana JL: Regulation of the polarity protein Par6 by TGFbeta receptors controls epithelial cell plasticity. Science 307: 1603-1609, 2005.

Parker KK, Lepre Brock A, Brangwynne C, Mannix RJ et al : Directional control of lamellipodia extension by constraining cell shape and orienting cell tractional forces. FASEB J 16: 1195-1204, 2002.

Paech K, Webb P, Kuiper GG, Nilsson S, Gustafsson J, et al: Differential Ligand activation of estrogen receptors ERalpha and ERbeta at AP-1 sites. Science 277:1508–1510, 1997.

Pantel K, Brakenhoff RH & Brandt B: Detection, clinical relevance and specific biological properties of disseminating tumour cells. Nat Rev Cancer 8:329-340, 2008.

Parikh P, Palazzo JP, Rose LJ, Daskalakis C, & Weigel RJ: J Am Coll Surg 200: 705–710, 2005.

Park SM, Gaur AB, Lengyel E & Peter ME: The miR-200 family determines the epithelial phenotype of cancer cells by targeting the E-cadherin repressors ZEB1 and ZEB2. Genes Dev 22: 894–907, 2008.

Parl FF: Multiple mechanisms of estrogen receptor gene repression contribute to ER-negative breast cancer. Pharmacogenomics J 3:251–253, 2003.

Peinado H, Olmeda D & Cano A: Snail, Zeb and bHLH factors in tumour progression: an alliance against the epithelial phenotype? Nature Rev Cancer 7: 415–428, 2007.

Perez-Losada J, Sanchez-Martin M, Rodriguez-Garcia A, Sanchez M, Orfao A, et al. Zinc-finger transcription factor Slug contributes to the function of the stem cell factor c-kit signaling pathway. Blood 100: 1274–1286, 2002.

Pérez-Tenorio G, Berglund F, Esguerra Merca A, Nordenskjöld B, Rutqvist LE, et al: Cytoplasmic p21WAF1/CIP1 correlates with Akt activation and poor response to tamoxifen in breast cancer. Int J Oncol 28: 1031–1042, 2006.

Perou CM, Sørlie T, Eisen MB, van de Rijn M, Jeffrey SS, et al: Molecular portraits of human breast tumours. Nature 406:747–752, 2000.

Pettersson K, Delaunay F & Gustafsson JA: Estrogen receptor β acts as a dominant regulator of estrogen signalling. Oncogene 19: 4970–4978, 2000

Pieper FR, Van de Klundert FA, Raats JM, et al: Regulation of vimentin expression in cultured epithelial cells. Eur J Biochem 210: 509-519, 1992

Pluijm G. Epithelial plasticity, cancer stem cells and bone metastasis formation. Bone 48: 37-43, 2011

Polette M, Mestdagt M, Bindels S, et al: Beta-catenin and ZO-1: shuttle molecules involved in tumor invasion-associated epithelial-mesenchymal transition processes. Cells Tiss Organs 185: 61-65, 2007.

Polyak K & Weinberg RA: Transitions between epithelial and mesenchymal states: acquisition of malignant and stem cell traits. Nat Rev Cancer 9: 265-273, 2009.

Prall OWJ, Rogan EM, Musgrove EA, Watts CKW & Sutherland RL: c-Myc or cyclin D1 mimics estrogen effects on cyclin E-Cdk2 activation and cell cycle reentry. Mol Cell Biol 18: 4499-4508, 1998.

Prat A, Parker JS, Karginova O, Fan C, Livasy C, Herschkowitz JI, et al: Phenotypic and molecular characterization of the claudin-low intrinsic subtype of breast cancer. Breast Cancer Res 12:R68, 2010.

Raman V, Martensen SA, Reisman D, et al: Compromised HOXA5 function can limit p53 expression in human breast tumours. Nature 405: 974-978, 2000.

Raouf A, Zhao Y, To K, Stingl J, Delaney A, Barbara M, Iscove N, et al: Transcriptome analysis of the normal human mammary cell commitment and differentiation process. Cell Stem Cell 3: 109-118, 2008.

Ray P, Ghosh SK, Zhang DH & Ray A: Repression of inter-leukin-6 gene expression by17 beta-estradiol: inhibition of the DNA-binding activity of the transcription factors NF-IL6 and NF-kappa B by the estrogen receptor. FEBS Lett 409: 79-85, 1997.

Rayala SK, Molli PR & Kumar R: Nuclear p21- activated kinase 1 in breast cancer packs off tamoxifen sensitivity. Cancer Res 66: 5985-5988, 2006.

Razandi M, Pedram A, Park ST & Levin ER: Proximal events in signaling by plasma membrane estrogen receptors. J Biol Chem 278: 2701-2712, 2003.

Riggins RB, Quilliam LA & Bouton AH: Synergistic promotion of c-Src activation and cell migration by Cas and AND-34/BCAR3. J Biol Chem 278: 28264-28273, 2003.

Riggins RB, Zwart A, Nehra R & Clarke R: The nuclear factor κB inhibitor parthenolide restores ICI 182,780 (Faslodex; fulvestrant)-induced apoptosis in antiestrogen-resistant breast cancer cells. Mol. Cancer Ther 4: 33-41, 2005.

Riggins RB, Schrecengost RS & Guerrero MS and Bouton AH: Pathways to tamoxifen resistance. Cancer Lett 256: 1-24, 2007.

Riggins RB, Lan PJ, Klimach U, Zwart A, Cavalli RL et al: ERRγ mediates tamoxifen resistance in novel models of invasive lobular breast cancer. Cancer Res. 68:8908-8917, 2008.

Ring A & Dowsett M: Mechanisms of tamoxifen resistance. Endocr Relat Cancer 11: 643-658, 2004.

Robertson KD, Ait-Si-Ali S, Yokochi T, Wade PA, Jones PL & Wolffe AP: DNMT1 forms a complex with Rb, E2F1 and HDAC1 and represses transcription from E2F-responsive promoters. Nature Genet 25:338-342, 2000.

Robertson JF, Osborne CK, Howell A, Jones SE, Mauriac L, et al: Fulvestrant vs anastrozole for the treatment of advanced breast carcinoma: a prospectively planned combined survival analysis of two multicenter trials. Cancer 104: 236-239, 2005.

Robson EJ, Khaled WT, Abell K & Watson CJ: Epithelial-to-mesenchymal transition confers resistance to apoptosis in three murine mammary epithelial cell lines. Differentiation 74: 254-264, 2006.

Roger P, Sahla ME, Mäkelä S, Gustafsson JA, Baldet P & Rochefort H: Decreased expression of estrogen receptor beta protein in proliferative preinvasive mammary tumors. Cancer Res 61:2537–2541, 2001.

Rosner W, Hryb DJ, Khan MS, Nakhla AM & Romas NA: Androgen and estrogen signaling at the cell membrane via G-proteins and cyclic adenosine monophosphate. Steroids 64: 100–106, 1999.

Rountree MR, Bachman KE & Baylin SB: DNMT1 binds HDAC2 and a new co-repressor, DMAP1, to form a complex at replication foci. Nature Genet 25:269–277, 2000.

Saeki T, Cristiano A, Lynch MJ, Brattain M, Kim N, et al: Regulation by estrogen through the 50-flanking region of the transforming growth factor alpha gene. Mol Endocrinol 5: 1955-1963, 1991.

Sabbah M, Emami S, Redeuilh G, Julien S, Prévost G, et al. (2008) Molecular signature and therapeutic perspective of the epithelial-to-mesenchymal transitions in epithelial cancers. Drug Resistance Updates 11: 123–151.

Safe S: Transcriptional activation of genes by 17 betaestradiol through estrogen receptor-Sp1 interactions. Vitam Horm 62: 231-252, 2001.

Salloum A (2010). Responsiveness to growth stimulators of MCF7 breast cancer cells transfected with estrogen receptor siRNA constructs. MSc Thesis Kuwait University.

Salomon DS, Brandt R, Ciardiello F & Normanno N: Epidermal growth factor-related peptides and their receptors in human malignancies. Crit Rev Oncol Hemat 19: 183-232, 1995.

Sánchez-Martín M, Rodríguez-García A, Pérez-Losada J, Sagrera A, Read AP, et al: SLUG (SNAI2) deletions in patients with Waardenburg disease. Hum. Mol. Genet 11: 3231–3236, 2002.

Santen RJ, Song RX, Zhang Z, Kumar R, Jeng MH, et al: Adaptive hypersensitivity to estrogen: mechanism for superiority of aromatase inhibitors over selective estrogen receptor modulators for breast cancer treatment and prevention. Endocr Relat Cancer 10:111–130, 2003.

Santisteban M, Reiman JM, Asiedu MK, et al: Immune-induced epithelial to mesenchymal transition in vivo generates breast cancer stem cells. Cancer Res 69: 2887-2895, 2009.

Sarrio D, Rodriguez-Pinilla SM, Hardisson D, Cano A, Moreno-Bueno G &Palacios J: Epithelial-mesenchymal transition in breast cancer relates to the basal-like phenotype. Cancer Res 68: 989-997, 2008.

Shaw JA, Udokang K, Mosquera JM, Chauhan H, Jones JL & Walker RA: Oestrogen receptors alpha and beta differ in normal human breast and breast carcinomas, J. Pathol. 198: 450–457, 2002.

Sheridan C, Kishimoto H, Fuchs RK, Mehrotra S, Bhat-Nakshatri P, et al: CD44+, CD24– breast cancer cells exhibit enhanced invasive properties: an early step necessary for metastasis. Breast Cancer Res 8: R59, 2006.

Shi L, Dong B, Li Z, Lu Y, Ouyang T, Li J, Wang T, et al. Expression of ER-α36, a novel variant of estrogen receptor α, and resistance to tamoxifen treatment in breast cancer. J Clin Oncol 27:3423–3429, 2009.

Shipitsin M, Campbell LL, Argani P, Weremowicz S, Bloushtain-Qimron N, et al: Molecular definition of breast tumor heterogeneity. Cancer Cell 11: 259-273, 2007.

Song RX, Santen RJ, Kumar R, Adam L, Jeng MH, Masamura S & Yue W: Adaptive mechanisms induced by long-term estrogen deprivation in breast cancer cells. Molecular and Cell Endocrinol 193:29–42, 2002a.

Song RX, McPherson RA, Adam L, Bao Y, Shupnik M, et al: Linkage of rapid estrogen action to MAPK activation by ERalpha-Shc association and Shc pathway activation. Mol Endocrinol 16:116–127, 2002b.

Song RX, Barnes CJ, Zhang Z, Bao Y, Kumar R & Santen RJ: The role of Shc and insulin-like growth factor 1 receptor in mediating the translocation of estrogen receptor alpha to the plasma membrane. Proc Natl Acad Sci USA 101:2076–2081, 2004.

Sorlie T, Tibshirani R, Parker J, Hastie T, Marron JS, et al: Repeated observation of breast tumor subtypes in independent gene expression data sets. Proc Natl Acad Sci USA 100: 8418-8423, 2003.

Speirs V, Parkes AT, Kerin MJ, Walton DS, Carleton PJ, Fox JN & Atkin SL: Co expression of estrogen receptor α and β: poor prognostic factors in human breast cancer? Cancer Res 59: 525-528, 1999.

Sphyris N & Mani SA: The importance of the epithelial-mesenchymal transition in breast cancer. Curr Breast Cancer Rep 1: 229-237, 2009.

Storci G, Sansone P, Trere D, et al: The basal-like breast carcinoma phenotype is regulated by Slug gene expression. J Pathol 214: 25-37, 2008.

Ström A, Hartman J, Foster JS, Kietz S, Wimalasena J &Gustafsson JA: Estrogen receptor beta inhibits 17beta-estradiol-stimulated proliferation of the breast cancer cell line T47D. Proc Natl Acad Sci USA 101:1566-1571, 2004.

Stylianou S, Clarke RB & Brennan K: Aberrant activation of notch signalling in human breast cancer. Cancer Res 66: 1517-1525, 2006.

Tang B, Yoo N, Vu M, et al: Transforming growth factor- β can suppress tumorigenesis through effects on the putative cancer stem or early progenitor cell and committed progeny in a breast cancer xenograft model. Cancer Res 67(18):8643–8652, 2007.

Taube JH, Herschkowitz JI, Komurov K, Zhou AY, Gupta S et al: Core epithelial-to-mesenchymal transition interactome gene-expression signature is associated with claudin-low and metaplastic breast cancer subtypes. Proc Natl Acad Sci USA 107:15449-15454, 2010.

Tavazoie SF, Alarcón C, Oskarsson T, Padua D, Wang Q, et al: Endogenous human microRNAs that suppress breast cancer metastasis. Nature 451:147–152, 2008.

Thiery JP: Epithelial-mesenchymal transitions in tumor progression. Nat Rev Cancer 2: 442–454, 2002.

Thiery JP: Epithelial-mesenchymal transitions in development and pathologies. Curr Opin Cell Biol 15: 740-746, 2003.

Thiery JP, Acloque H, Huang RY & Nieto MA. Epithelial–mesenchymal transitions in development and disease. Cell 139(5):871–90, 2009.

Thompson EW & Williams ED. EMT and MET in carcinoma- clinical observations, regulatory pathways and new models. Clin Exp Metastasis 25(6):591–2, 2008.

Thuault S, Valcourt U, Petersen M, Manfioletti G, Heldin C H & Moustakas A: Transforming growth factor-beta employs HMGA2 to elicit epithelial- mesenchymal transition. J Cell Biol 174: 175-83, 2006

Trimboli AJ, Fukino K, de Bruin A, Wei G, Shen L, Tanner SM, et al: Direct evidence for epithelial-mesenchymal transitions in breast cancer. Cancer Res 68: 937-945, 2008.

Umayahara Y, Kawamori R, Watada H, Imano E, Iwama N, et al: Estrogen regulation of the insulin-like growth factor I gene transcription involves an AP-1 enhancer. J Biol Chem 269:16433-16442, 1994.

van Agthoven T, van Agthoven TL, Dekker A, van der Spek PJ, Vreede L, et al: Identification of BCAR3 by a random search for genes involved in antiestrogen resistance of human breast cancer cells. EMBO J 17, 2799–2808, 1998.

Vandewalle C, Comijn J, De Craene B, Vermassen P, Bruyneel E, et al: SIP1/ZEB2 induces EMT by repressing genes of different epithelial cell-cell junctions. Nucl Acids Res 33: 6566-6578, 2005.

Vincan E & Barker N: The upstream components of the Wnt signalling pathway in the dynamic EMT and MET associated with colorectal cancer progression. Clin Exp Metastasis 25: 657–663, 2008.

Voduc D, Cheang M & Nielsen T: Cancer Epidemiol. Biomarkers Prev 17: 365–373, 2008.

Vyhlidal C, Samudio I, Kladde M & Safe S: Transcriptional activation of transforming growth factor by estradiol: requirement for both a GC-rich site and an estrogen response element half-site. Mol Endocrinol 24: 329–338, 2000.

Waerner T, Alacakaptan M, Tamir I, Oberauer R, Gal A, et al: a cytokine essential for EMT, tumor formation, and late events in metastasis in epithelial cells. Cancer Cell 10:227- 39, 2006.

Wang Y, Dean JL, Millar EKA, Tran TH, McNeil CH, et al: Cyclin D1b is aberrantly regulated in response to therapeutic challenge and promotes resistance to estrogen antagonists. Cancer Res. 68: 5628–5638, 2008.

Wang Z, Bannerji S, Li Y, Rahman KMW, Zhang Y & Sarkar FH: Down-regulation of notch-1 inhibits invasion by inactivation of nuclear factor-kappaB, vascular endothelial growth factor, and matrix metalloproteinase-9 in pancreatic cancer cells. Cancer Res. 66: 2778–2784, 2006.

Watson MA, Ylagan LR, Trinkaus KM, Gillanders WE, Naughton MJ, et al: Isolation and molecular profiling of bone marrow micrometastases identifies TWIST1 as a marker of early tumor relapse in breast cancer patients. Clin Cancer Res 13:5001-5009, 2007.

Wegman P, Vainikka L, Stal O, Nordenskjold B, Skoog L, et al: Genotype of metabolic enzymes and the benefit of tamoxifen in postmenopausal breast cancer patients. Breast Cancer Res 7:R284–290, 2005.

Wei Yan, Qing Jackie Cao, Richard B. Arenas, Brooke Bentley & Rong Shao: GATA3 Inhibits Breast Cancer Metastasis through the Reversal of Epithelial Mesenchymal Transition. J Biol Chem 285 (18): 14042–14051, 2010

Weigel RJ & deConinck EC: Transcriptional control of estrogen receptor in estrogen receptor-negative breast carcinoma. Cancer Res 53:3472-3474, 1993.

Weigel NL & Zhang Y: Ligand-independent activation of steroid hormone receptors. J Mol Med 76: 469–479, 1998.

Wheelock MJ & Johnson KR: Cadherins as modulators of cellular phenotype. Annu Rev Cell Dev Biol 19: 207-235, 2003.

Wheelock MJ, Shintani Y, Maeda M, Fukumoto Y & Johnson KR: Cadherin switching. J Cell Sci 121: 727-732, 2008.

Williams C, Edvardsson K, Lewandowski SA, Ström A & Gustafsson JA: A genome-wide study of the repressive effects of estrogen receptor beta on estrogen receptor alpha signaling in breast cancer cells. Oncogene 27:1019–1032, 2008

Wu Y, Deng J, Rychahou PG, et al: Stabilization of snail by NF-kappaB is required for inflammation-induced cell migration and invasion. Cancer Cell 15: 416-428, 2009.

Xue C, Plieth D, Venkov C, et al: The gatekeeper effect of epithelial-mesenchymal transition regulates the frequency of breast cancer metastasis. Cancer Res 63: 3386-3394, 2003.

Yang D, Fan F, Camp ER et al: Chronic oxaliplatin resistance induces epithelial-to-mesenchymal transition in colorectal cancer cell lines. Clinical Cancer Research 12(14): 4147–4153, 2006.

Yang J, Mani SA, Donaher JL, Ramaswamy S, Itzykson RA, et al: Twist, a master regulator of morphogenesis, plays an essential role in tumour metastasis. Cell 117: 927-939, 2004.

Yang J &Weinberg RA: Epithelial-mesenchymal transition: at the crossroads of development and tumor metastasis. Dev Cell 14:818-829, 2008.

Yang J, Bielenberg Diane R. Rodig SJ, Doiron R, et al: Lipocalin 2 promotes breast cancer progression. Proc Natl Acad Sci USA 106: 3913-3918, 2009.

Yang MH, Wu MZ, Chiou SH, Chen PM, Chang SY, et al: Direct regulation of Twist by HIF-1alpha promotes metastasis. Nat Cell Biol 10: 295-305, 2008.

Yang X, Phillips DL, Ferguson AT, Nelson WG, Herman JG & Davidson NE: Synergistic activation of functional estrogen receptor (ER)-alpha by DNA methyltransferase and histone deacetylase inhibition in human ER-alpha-negative breast cancer cells. Cancer Res 61: 7025–7029, 2001.

Yarden RI, Wilson MA & Chrysogelos SA: Estrogen suppression of EGFR expression in breast cancer cells: a possible mechanism to modulate growth. J Cell Biochem 81: 232–246, 2001.

Ye Y, Xiao Y, Wang W, Yearsley K, Gao JX & Barsky SH: ERalpha suppresses slug expression directly by transcriptional repression. Biochem J 416: 179-187, 2008.

Yoshida H, Broaddus R, Cheng W, Xie S & Naora H: Deregulation of the HOXA10 homeobox gene in endometrial carcinoma: role in epithelial-mesenchymal transition. Cancer Res 66: 889-897, 2006.

Yu F, Yao H, Zhu P, Zhang X, Pan Q, et al: let-7 regulates self renewal and tumorigenicity of breast cancer cells. Cell 131:1109- 1123, 2007.

Zavadil J, Cermak L, Soto-Nieves N & Bottinger EP: Integration of TGF- beta/Smad and Jagged1/Notch signalling in epithelial-to-mesenchymal transition. Embo J 23: 1155-65, 2004.

Zhang W, Glöckner SC, Guo M, Machida EO, Wang DH, et al: Epigenetic inactivation of the canonical Wnt antagonist SRY-box containing gene 17 in colorectal cancer. Cancer Res. 68:2764–2772, 2008.

Zhou Y, Yau C, Gray JW, Chew K, Dairkee SH, et al: Enhanced NFκB and AP-1 transcriptional activity associated with anti-estrogen resistant breast cancer. BMC Cancer 7: 59-64, 2007.

Zilli M, Grassadonia A, Tinari N, Giacobbe AD, Gildetti S, et al: Molecular mechanisms of endocrine resistance and their implication in the therapy of breast cancer. Biochim Biophys Acta 1795: 62-81, 2009.

Zivadinovic D, Gametchu B & Watson CS: Membrane estrogen receptor-α levels in MCF-7 breast cancer cells predict cAMP and proliferation response. Breast Cancer Res. 7(1): R101–R112, 2005.

Zuo T, Wang L, Morrison C, Chang X, Zhang H, et al: FOXP3 is an X-linked breast cancer suppressor gene and an important repressor of the HER-2/ErbB2 oncogene. Cell 129: 1275–1286, 2007.

Zajchowski DA, Bartholdi MF, Gong Y, Webster L, Liu HL, et al: Identification of gene expression profiles that predict the aggressive behaviour of breast cancer cells. Cancer Res 61: 5168-5178, 2001.

10

Breast Cancer Metastasis: Advances Through the Use of In Vitro Co-Culture Model Systems

Anthony Magliocco and Cay Egan
University of Calgary
Canada

1. Introduction

Worldwide, breast cancer is the most frequent cancer diagnosed in women and is the second-most leading cause of cancer related deaths in women (Jemal, Bray et al. 2011). Death from breast cancer is most often the result of the spread of the primary tumour to distant sites, where the cancer cells lodge and develop into metastases. Depending on the site of the metastasis, the patient may live for years with reduced quality of life and needing increased health care resources. There is clearly a need for a greater understanding of the molecular events involved in breast cancer metastasis in order to improve treatment options for breast cancer patients and develop therapies aimed at preventing breast cancer metastasis.

Here we will summarize what is known about the molecular basis of breast cancer metastasis and discuss the use of *in vivo* and primarily *in vitro* model systems to study it.

2. Current knowledge

2.1 Metastasis

As early as 1889, Stephen Paget observed that some cancers metastasized preferentially to specific organs, and developed his theory of "seed and soil"(Paget 1889). The essential tenet of this theory was that cancer cells (seeds) disseminate throughout the body from their point of origin but can only develop metastatic satellites in appropriate stromal environments (soils). The many advances in our understanding of the molecular and cellular bases of breast cancer metastasis has led to a somewhat more complex picture, and the processes involved are still not completely understood. Breast cancer can spread to any secondary site in the body but metastases appear preferentially in bone, lung and liver (Rabbani and Mazar 2007). Presumably these sites provide a microenvironment favourable for the growth and development of breast cancer cells (Nguyen, Bos et al. 2009).

There are two prevailing models of breast cancer metastasis; one suggesting a linear progression and the other a parallel progression. The linear progression model advances the idea that cells in the primary tumour accumulate progressive mutations in a stepwise manner in genes regulating some aspect of cell growth and division such as oncogenes and tumour suppressor genes. Some cells eventually become able to proliferate autonomously; they expand clonally and leave the primary site to travel through lymphatic or vascular systems to a distant organ where they develop into a secondary metastatic growth. This model implies that cells at the primary site must undergo a number of rounds of division before they become autonomous and so development of metastasis is linked to primary tumour size with metastases more likely to develop from larger primary tumours. In support of this model it has long been known that there is a close association between tumour size and the possibility of development of metastasis, and tumour size is used as part of histological classification (1983; Rakha, Reis-Filho et al. 2010). The model also suggests that cells being shed by the primary tumour are fully metastatic and that cells that have metastasized to a secondary site should also be able to leave that site to set up at a tertiary site (Klein 1998; Klein 2009). Mutations in genes such as BRCA1, BRCA2, p53 and RB and amplification of the HER-2 receptor at the site of the primary tumour have been identified as being predictive of poorer outcome for breast cancer patients, consistent with this model (Slamon, Clark et al. 1987; Ross and Fletcher 1999; Bordeleau, Lipa et al. 2007; Bosco and Knudsen 2007; Kumar, Walia et al. 2007; Baker, Quinlan et al. 2010).

The parallel progression model suggests that tumour cells may disseminate from the site of the primary tumour very early in its development and may be subsequently genetically modified in the metastatic niche where they later settle (Klein 2009). This model predicts that disseminated tumour cells in the blood or lymph should be detectable very early in development of the primary tumour and that cells at the site of metastasis could be genetically divergent from those at the site of the primary tumour. In support of this model it has been shown in a HER-2 mouse model and in women with ductal carcinoma *in situ*, that disseminated tumour cells in bone and micro metastases could be detected from the time of earliest epithelial alterations at the site of the primary tumour. The numbers of disseminated tumour cells in this study were found to be the same for small and large tumours (Husemann, Geigl et al. 2008), suggesting that shedding of cells from the tumour mass was independent of primary tumour size. In a qualitative and quantitative study of 12,423 women with breast cancer, J. Engel *et. al.* (Engel, Eckel et al. 2003) determined that systemic disease was already present at the time of diagnosis in women who went on to develop metastases, again suggesting cells left the primary tumour early during its development.

The advent of single-cell genomics has allowed comparison of the characteristics of disseminated tumour cells in the blood and lymph and cells at the site of the primary tumour and these have been found to be genetically divergent in some cases (Klein, Seidl et al. 2002; Klein 2003; Fuhrmann, Schmidt-Kittler et al. 2008; Klein 2009; Klein and Stoecklein 2009), indicating that early clonal divergence and parallel progression may occur in some breast cancers. Disseminated tumour cells may also differ genetically from cells that eventually develop into a metastasis in the same patient (Stoecklein and Klein 2010). This could reflect the requirement for the disseminated tumour cells to undergo whatever genetic changes are necessary for them to adapt and be able to successfully grow in the new microenvironment. If that is the case it follows that the genetic aberrations found in the primary tumour may not reflect those seen in the metastasis and this has been found to occur (Tortola, Steinert et al. 2001; Albanese, Scibetta et al. 2004; Gow, Chang et al. 2009; Stoecklein and Klein 2010). In colorectal cancer, mutations in B-raf, K-ras and p53 seen in the primary tumour may be absent or altered in the metastasis. In some cases mutations in the metastasis may be absent in the primary tumour (Tortola, Steinert et al. 2001; Albanese, Scibetta et al. 2004; Stoecklein and Klein 2010). In a study of non-small-cell lung cancer where EGFR mutation status is used as a determinant for treatment with tyrosine kinase inhibitors, 27% of paired primary/metastasis samples (n=67 patients) were found to be discordant with respect to EGFR mutation status (Gow, Chang et al. 2009). This is of concern in a time of more personalized treatment, where often it is the genetic signature of the primary tumour alone on which outcome predictions or treatment options are based.

2.2 Metastasis suppressor genes

Evidence suggests that less than 1% of breast cancer cells that enter the circulatory system are capable of generating metastatic foci (Fidler 1970; Fidler and Nicolson 1977). Often disseminated breast tumour cells that have settled in the microenvironment at the site of metastasis will lie dormant for years in patients with no evidence of disease before developing into a clinically significant metastatic focus, indicating they are capable of escaping early systemic therapies that target rapidly proliferating cells at the site of the primary tumour (Pantel, Schlimok et al. 1993; Klein, Seidl et al. 2002; Riethdorf, Wikman et al. 2008; Morgan, Lange et al. 2009). As they remain quiescent for some period of time this also suggests that they, or the cells in their microenvironment, or both undergo genetic changes which allow them to progress to a metastatic phenotype (Riethdorf, Wikman et al. 2008) (Riethdorf, Wikman et al. 2008; Klein 2009; Nguyen, Bos et al. 2009; Smith and Theodorescu 2009; Rose and Siegel 2010; Stoecklein and Klein 2010). A class of genes that has been implicated in the regulation of this process is metastasis suppressor genes (Smith and Theodorescu 2009). These are genes that inhibit metastasis but do not affect the ability of cells to produce a primary tumour, and they play key roles in invasion, dissemination, arrest, survival and colony formation. Their function must be lost or inhibited for a metastasis to develop and they represent fertile new ground for the development of anti-metastatic therapeutics.

A number of metastasis suppressor proteins have been reported to inhibit breast cancer metastasis. Reduced levels of nm23 family proteins in the primary tumour have been reported to correlate with more aggressive phenotype in breast cancer patients (Galani, Sgouros et al. 2002; Terasaki-Fukuzawa, Kijima et al. 2002; Steeg, Ouatas et al. 2003; Peihong and Perry 2007), although conflicting results have also been presented (Charpin, Garcia et al. 1998; Belev, Aleric et al. 2002; Sgouros, Galani et al. 2007). The results seen in mouse models are more straightforward, where breast cancer cells with low expression of nm23 are more metastatic than those with high levels (Leone, Flatow et al. 1993; Bhujwalla, Aboagye et al. 1999; Tseng, Vicent et al. 2001). In vitro models have revealed that nm23 acts by reducing breast cancer cell motility and invasiveness (MacDonald, Freije et al. 1996; Russell, Pedersen et al. 1998; Steeg, Ouatas et al. 2003; Horak, Lee et al. 2007).

For Breast Cancer Metastasis Suppressor-1 (BRMS1), the clinical data reporting it to be a metastasis suppressor protein in breast cancer tumour samples is also conflicting (Kelly, Buggy et al. 2005; Hicks, Yoder et al. 2006; Lombardi, Di Cristofano et al. 2007). Again, its role in mouse models is clearer, where higher expression in breast cancer xenografts clearly resulted in reduced metastasis (Hedley, Vaidya et al. 2008; Hurst, Xie et al. 2008; Phadke, Vaidya et al. 2008). The stage at which BRMS1 suppresses metastasis is less clear, as it appears to affect a number of steps in the process of metastasis (Stafford, Vaidya et al. 2008). At least two of its functions appear to be increasing anoikis of cells free in the vascular system and inhibition of colonization of disseminated cells (Phadke, Vaidya et al. 2008). KAI1 (CD82, Tetraspannin), has also been clearly verified as a breast cancer metastasis suppressor in clinical samples, where decreased expression correlates with poor outcome (Yang, Welch et al. 1997; Christgen, Christgen et al. 2009; Malik, Sanders et al. 2009). Similar to BRMS1, KAI1 appears to act in multiple ways to inhibit metastasis and reduce breast cancer cell adhesion, migration and invasion *in vitro* (Malik, Sanders et al. 2009) and metastasis in mouse models *in vivo* (Yang, Wei et al. 2001). Other metastasis suppressor genes implicated in inhibiting breast cancer metastasis include KISS1 (Harms, Welch et al. 2003), MTSS1 (Parr and Jiang 2009) and alpha2beta1 integrin (Ramirez, Zhang et al. 2011), although their roles, at least in breast cancer have been less well studied.

As can be seen, the determination of the role of metastasis suppressor genes in metastasis using clinical samples is often confusing. This seemingly conflicting data may be a result of the many different experimental approaches to examining clinical samples; whether the samples are frozen or paraffin embedded and formalin fixed, whether mRNA or protein levels are the final determinant of expression (and these do not always correlate well), the type of extraction procedures used, and the source of the antibodies and staining methods for immunohistochemistry. The other difficulty with clinical samples is that they are almost exclusively derived from the primary tumour site, as biopsies of metastases are rarely carried out. Metastasis suppressor genes by definition do not inhibit events at the site of the primary tumour but must be inhibited for metastasis to take place. This inhibition may allow invasion of the circulatory system from the site of the primary tumour, survival through the process of transportation to the site of metastasis and evasion of the immune system, arrest within the metastatic niche, extravasion from the circulatory system or growth in the new environment (Kaplan, Psaila et al. 2006; Rabbani and Mazar 2007). Inhibition of expression at any step following detachment from the primary tumour would not likely be detected in the primary tumour.

3. Model systems of metastasis

It is evident that disseminated tumour cells in the blood and lymph and cells at the site of metastasis may diverge in phenotype from cells at the site of the primary tumour and from each other. Metastasis suppressor genes represent some of the genes with altered expression and one possibility of targeting metastasis therapeutically is to induce their re-expression or reiterate their function at the site of metastasis (Steeg, Ouatas et al. 2003; Stafford, Vaidya et al. 2008; Smith and Theodorescu 2009). To effectively select therapeutic targets it will be important to better understand their functions in the microenvironment of the site of metastasis. It is also known that the stromal environment surrounding the tumour cell is an active collaborator in the development of the metastasis. It is imperative to examine interactions between tumour cells and the stromal cells in the metastatic niche to understand what changes the stromal cells induce in the tumour cells and what changes the tumour cells induce in the stromal cells. *In vivo* and *in vitro* model systems have long been used as pre-clinical models to study breast cancer metastasis and ways of treating or preventing it.

3.1 In vivo mouse models

The use of mouse models in studying human breast cancer metastasis has the very great advantage of being able to study the entire process of metastasis from development of the primary tumour to the final development of the metastasis. It is possible to label the tumour cells with a variety of probes including green fluorescent protein (GFP) or luciferase and there are many excellent imaging techniques such as magnetic resonance, computed tomography and ultrasound available for live animal imaging to follow the progress of the tumour cells in the mouse. Live imaging is an advantage as progress can be monitored in one mouse over a period of time rather than sacrificing a number of mice at different time points. One of the major disadvantages in using mouse models to study human cancer metastasis is that mice are not human, and there is no guarantee that the metastasis will develop in them in a way that recapitulates what happens in a human body. Mice do develop breast cancer as a heterogeneous disease, similar to humans (Andrechek and Nevins 2010), but there are significant differences between mice and humans in the capacity of the primary cells for transformation, the size of tumours, expression of hormone receptors and preferential sites of homing for breast cancer. For researching metastasis of human cells, immunodeficient mouse strains need to be used, taking the model a further step away from what happens in a human host. In addition human breast cancer cell lines may not accurately reflect the biological characteristics of in-vivo breast cancer such as natural evolution and tumor diversity. Given that caveat, mouse models are very important for testing pre-clinical data before moving on to clinical trials or human tumour tissue samples. There are many technical issues to take into account when considering the use of a mouse model to study breast cancer metastasis. Those are beyond the scope of this chapter but are very fully reviewed by Danny Welch (Welch 1997). Mouse models have been particularly useful in identifying molecules important for a number of steps in metastasis, such as epithelial to mesenchymal transition (EMT), invasion, extravasation and intravasation (Vernon, Bakewell et al. 2007). One approach to modeling metastasis is to use xenografts, where human tumour cells are injected subcutaneously or into the mammary fat pad of a mouse and allowed to develop a primary tumour that spontaneously metastasizes. A second approach is to inject tumor cells directly into the venous system, using tail vein injection or cardiac puncture. Tail vein injection results primarily in metastasis to the lung, but cardiac puncture results preferentially in bone metastasis. This approach obviates the need for development of the primary tumour but is not useful for studying some of the early steps of metastasis. The artificial injection of tumor cells directly into the venous system may produce pseudometastasis through a process of embolization rather than true physiological metastasis. A third approach is to utilize genetically engineered mice that have had a tumour suppressor gene deleted or an oncogene activated in an organ specific manner.

Xenograft models and venous injections most generally use breast cancer cell lines, many of which are maintained and sold by the American Type Culture Collection (ATCC). These cell lines have a variety of gene expression profiles that identify them as similar to luminal, basal A or basal B [subtypes initially defined in tumour samples in 2006 (Fridlyand, Snijders et al. 2006)] and they show a variety of receptor and p53 profiles (Neve, Chin et al. 2006). Gene expression in these cell lines can be modified by over expression or deletion and the effect of the altered gene on metastasis can be monitored following injection. Although the resulting tumours are considered to metastasize "spontaneously", the injected cell lines are an artificial starting material as they have been cultured for long periods of time *in vitro* and do not resemble a spontaneously arising tumour. One of the advantages of xenograft models is that the cells of the primary tumour must interact with the stromal cells surrounding the tumour and must also interact with the stromal cells at the site of the metastasis for a productive metastasis to develop. A great deal of information about the interactions of human tumour cells and stromal cells has been accumulated by injecting human tumour cells and human mesenchymal stem stromal cells together in xenograft models [reviewed in (El-Haibi and Karnoub 2010)]. By using the same cell lines and different routes of injection it is possible to determine whether a gene is necessary for early steps of metastasis or whether it is involved in later steps (Chabottaux, Ricaud et al. 2009).

Genetically engineered mice, whether transgenic or gene knockout animals, have an advantage over xenograft models in that they illustrate the metastasis of tumours that arise in the mouse mammary gland as a result of internal genetic changes and not exogenously injected cells. This is more representative of how tumours develop from the very beginning of the metastatic process. To limit expressed genes to the breast of the transgenic mouse a breast-specific promoter such as the Mouse Mammary Tumour Virus (MMTV) promoter or the Whey Acidic Protein promoter (WAP) is generally utilized (Kim and Baek 2010). As the tumour arises from mouse cells, immunocompetent mice can be used and the effects of an intact immune system on the process of metastasis can be determined. There are many strains of mice available with well defined genetic backgrounds, enabling researchers to study the effects of differing genetic backgrounds on the development of metastasis arising from gain or loss of the gene of interest (Husemann and Klein 2009). Mice carrying different transgenes or knockouts can be crossed with each other to determine if there is an additive or synergistic effect of the different genes on development of metastasis (Vernon, Bakewell et al. 2007). Gene expression or deletion can be temporally regulated, using an MMTV promoter either alone or directing expression of the Cre/loxP system for somatic deletion. The MMTV promoter becomes active only after puberty, preventing the oncogene or tumour suppressor gene of interest from causing embryonic lethality. One of the drawbacks to using a genetically engineered mouse model is in testing therapeutic compounds. These mice develop subtypes of breast cancer similar to, but not identical with the subtypes seen in human breast tumours. Also, most tumours arising in genetically engineered mice lack expression of the estrogen receptor and thus fail to recapitulate human tumours that are estrogen receptor positive. Cytogenetic and genetic backgrounds are different between mice and humans as well and this could lead to misinterpretation of the usefulness and safety of a therapeutic compound (Kim and Baek 2010).

3.2 In vitro co-culture systems
3.2.1 Three-dimensional co-culture
Normal breast epithelial cells grown in three dimensional cultures will spontaneously aggregate to form hollow, cyst-like acini. The cells develop apicobasal polarization and are tightly regulated with respect to growth and proliferation thus reiterating several important features of glandular epithelium *in vivo*. For this reason these models represent a physiologically relevant system that is a reasonable alternative to expensive *in vivo* experimental systems. Some breast cancer cell lines such as MDA-MB-435 also form acinar structures in three dimensions (Glinsky, Huflejt et al. 2000) but others (DU4475) form clusters and cords (Langlois, Holder et al. 1979).
For cells to grow as aggregates in three dimensions they need to be in an environment where the adhesive forces between the cells are greater than their affinity for the substrate they are plated on. Some of the commonly used techniques include embedding the cells completely in a reconstituted basement membrane substrate such as Matrigel or collagen I, or growing them on a thin layer of solidified reconstituted basement membrane in a dilute solution of basement membrane in medium (liquid overlay) (Hebner, Weaver et al. 2008). Three dimensional aggregates can also be obtained using spinner culture flasks, where they are maintained in suspension by constant rotation. Some of the recently developed methods include growing the cells on pre-fabricated scaffolds of extracellular matrix that recreate the natural structure of a living tissue, and a NASA developed Rotary Cell Culture System

where the cells are grown in simulated microgravity in liquid medium (Kim, Stein et al. 2004).

Monotypic three-dimensional cell cultures have been the primary model used in the study of human breast cancer. These studies have revealed a great deal about the functions of oncogenes, tumour suppressor genes, reversion of tumour phenotypes, how cells escape from proliferative arrest, invasive and migratory behaviour and epithelial to mesenchymal transition [reviewed in (Weaver, Fischer et al. 1996; Debnath and Brugge 2005)]. Fewer researchers have used heterotypic co-culture models in three dimensions. Some of the approaches are summarized here.

Some studies have concentrated on the relationship between breast tumour cells and stromal fibroblasts as it has long been known that alterations in the stroma can alter tumour cell behaviour and disease progression. A research group at the Lawrence Berkeley Laboratory in Berkeley, California used three dimensional co-cultures to determine the origin of myofibroblasts in breast cancer. These are interstitial cells frequently found in the stroma of breast neoplasias that were, at that time, of uncertain origin. They isolated fibroblasts, vascular smooth muscle cells and pericytes from normal stroma and grew them in collagen gels with MCF-7 or HMT-3909 S13 breast cancer cell lines in co-culture for fourteen days. They found that it was primarily the fibroblasts that were converted to myofibroblasts and that only five percent of the fibroblasts closest to the spherical colonies made by the tumour cells were converted, suggesting a concentration gradient of factors released by the tumour cells was responsible for the conversion (Ronnov-Jessen, Petersen et al. 1995). A second group in Regensburg, Germany grew tumour cell lines and normal, breast tumour derived or skin fibroblasts as separate spherical colonies in three dimensional liquid overlay co-cultures. Interestingly, only two of the breast cancer cell lines tested, MCF-7 and SK-BR-3 cells, could infiltrate either the breast or the skin fibroblast spheroids under these experimental conditions. MCF-7 cells are normally considered to have low metastatic potential and only occasionally invaded the fibroblast spheroids whereas SK-BR-3 cells are highly metastatic and extensively infiltrated the fibroblast spheroids. Induction of the myofibroblastic phenotype by the tumour cells was only induced in the normal or tumour-derived fibroblasts, and not the skin fibroblasts (Kunz-Schughart, Heyder et al. 2001).

Another research group at Universitat Halle in Halle, Germany investigated the properties of mesenchymal stem cells in three dimensional co-cultures with MCF-7 or MDA-MB-231 breast cancer cell lines. In their experiments they found that within two hours of plating mesenchymal stem cells with MCF-7 spheroids or MDA-MB-231 aggregates the mesenchymal stem cells could invade the cancer cell masses. Using a Transwell assay, with breast cancer cell lines grown in the bottom well, they were able to show that the breast cancer lines attracted the mesenchymal stem cells indicating they were secreting a chemoattractant (Dittmer, Hohlfeld et al. 2009).

Researchers at The Pennsylvania State University have developed a specialized bioreactor for long term (up to ten months) co-culture of MDA-MB-231 breast tumour cells with murine osteoblasts. They have determined that the osteoblast cultures develop over time in the same way as in natural bone including development of ossification and phenotypic transformation into osteocytes. They differentially labelled the bone cells and the breast cells with green fluorescent protein and Alexa Fluor 568 respectively and were able to follow the real-time cancer cell invasion and colonization of the osteoblast tissue. They observed that important pathologic events such as cancer cells infiltrating the bone cells in single file and microtumour formation that are seen clinically were reproduced their in vitro system. They also observed that breast cancer cell colonization of the bone cells depended strongly on the maturity of the osteoblastic culture (Dhurjati, Krishnan et al. 2008; Mastro and Vogler 2009; Krishnan, Shuman et al. 2010).

A novel approach to three dimensional co-culturing of cells was developed by researchers at the University of Wisconsin-Madison in Madison, Wisconsin. They used a ninety-six arrayed single channel microchannel plate for co-culturing cells in 2ul collagen matrices and compared their results to conventional co-culturing of cells in collagen in six-well tissue culture plates. T47D breast cancer cells were co-cultured with human mammary fibroblasts and growth properties and inhibition of growth by small molecule inhibitors were compared between the two systems and found to be the same. The microchannel model has a number of advantages over conventional three dimensional co-culture systems in that it requires fewer resources, uses fewer cells, creating the possibility of using patient samples, and it is amenable for using high throughput screening of potential therapeutics (Bauer, Su et al. 2010). It will be interesting to follow future developments in the use of three dimensional heterotypic co-cultures in breast cancer research as this model system appears to have great potential.

3.2.2 Two-dimensional co-culture

By far the most commonly used *in vitro* co-culture model in the study of breast cancer metastasis is two-dimensional. Cells of various origins are cultured directly with breast cancer cells or in separate layers, as in Transwell plates. The measured outcomes in two dimensional co-cultures relate to breast cell growth, proliferation, adhesion, colony formation, migration and invasion. Signalling between cell types can be modified using gene overexpression or knock-down assays, or by adding inhibitory or stimulatory antibodies or other soluble compounds or drugs to the assay system. Some of the many and varied approaches are outlined below.

Researchers in Munster and Witten, Germany were interested in the role played by the HER-2 receptor in extravasation from the primary tumour through the venular wall. They modeled the venular wall using human umbilical vein endothelial cells grown on porous membranes coated with basement membrane extracellular matrix. They co-cultured these calls with breast cancer cell lines and with disaggregated tumour cells from twenty-three patients. They found that cell lines or patient samples with higher levels of HER-2 expression were significantly more invasive than cells with lower HER-2 expression. Interestingly, they also noted that there were subpopulations within individual breast cancers that had high HER-2 expression, and presumably high metastatic potential (Roetger, Merschjann et al. 1998).

A study was carried out in Milan, Italy, to investigate the interactions between hormone-dependent MCF-7 and ZR75.1 cells and hormone-independent MDA-MB-231 or BT20 breast cancer cells. Using a modified Transwell plate and measuring cell growth in the bottom well under serum-free conditions, they determined that the hormone-independent cell lines were capable of inducing cell growth in the hormone-dependent cells, in the absence of estrogen. Growth of the hormone-dependent cell lines could be further stimulated by the addition of transforming growth factor alpha to the medium. Their results confirmed the importance of paracrine interactions between cells in heterogeneous tumours and suggested an important role for transforming growth factor alpha in these interactions (Cappelletti, Ruedl et al. 1993).

Two dimensional co-culture systems are amenable to the use of primary tumour cells. A research group in Manchester, UK used primary epithelial cells from tumorous, benign or normal breast tissue in co-culture with human bone marrow or mammary fibroblasts from normal or malignant breast tissue. They found that breast epithelial cells from tumour tissue adhered preferentially to bone stroma over breast fibroblasts. The epithelial cells from normal or benign breast showed no preference for any of the stromal substrates. Interestingly, although breast tumour epithelial cells adhered preferentially to bone cells, this stromal environment did not provide a preferential growth platform (Brooks, Bundred et al. 1997). A similar study was carried out in Marseilles, France to determine the effect of stromal and epithelial cells from normal and tumorous breast tissue on growth of breast cancer cell lines. Fibroblasts from normal breast tissue but not conditioned medium from normal breast tissue were able to inhibit the growth of MCF-7 cells suggesting complex paracrine interactions between the two cell types. Normal fibroblasts did not inhibit the growth of immortalized S2T2 cells. Normal breast epithelial cells or the conditioned medium from them could inhibit a number of breast cancer cell lines suggesting that both fibroblasts and epithelial cells could have growth regulatory roles in the breast.

Many researchers co-culture breast cancer cell lines with bone-derived mesenchymal stem cells (MSCs) as these have been shown to have a profound effect on breast cancer metastasis. These cells were first observed by Friedenstein in 1976 (Friedenstein, Gorskaja et al. 1976) and have come to be defined as non-hematopoietic cells derived from bone stroma that are spindle-shaped and can be separated from other bone stromal cells by their tendency to adhere to plastic tissue culture plates. They have the stem cell characteristics of being able to differentiate into multiple cell lineages such as osteoblasts, chondrocytes, adipocytes and myoblasts and they express a consistent set of marker proteins on their surface (Brooks, Bundred et al. 1997; Pittenger, Mackay et al. 1999). Mesenchymal stem cells have been used in a number of laboratories in co-culture experiments with breast cancer cell lines or primary tumour cells and have been found to influence breast cancer cell adhesion, morphology, gene expression, proliferative capacity and growth characteristics (Brooks, Bundred et al. 1997; Hombauer and Minguell 2000; Fierro, Sierralta et al. 2004; Oh, Moharita et al. 2004). They have been shown in vivo to be able to migrate to sites of tissue damage and to primary tumour sites, and to modify the ability of breast cancer tumours to metastasize to other organs, making them potentially interesting vehicles for cell-based anti-tumour agents (Ferrari, Cusella-De Angelis et al. 1998; Hall, Dembinski et al. 2007; Rhodes and Burow 2010). They have also been shown in one research study to stimulate epithelial to mesenchymal transition in breast cells which may make them less suitable for use in drug delivery (Martin, Dwyer et al. 2010).

We use MSCs in a two dimensional co-culture model designed to determine factors that affect breast cancer cell behaviour in a microenvironment resembling breast cancer metastasis to bone; one of the most common sites of breast cancer metastasis. Our source of bone cells is from reamings from hip and knee replacement surgeries that are carried out on a regular basis in local hospitals rather than the more commonly used bone marrow aspirates that are more difficult to obtain. We wanted to determine that bone marrow cells that we derived from bone reamings resembled bone cells that were normally biologically involved in breast cancer metastases to bone. Breast cancer bone metastases are frequently characterized by the presence of a desmoplastic response, where normal haematopoietic tissue is replaced by activated fibroblastic cells. Adherent fibroblastic cells were isolated from both hip and knee bone reaming samples with a successful recovery rate of approximately 62% (8/13 patients). Microscopically, recovered cells that grew as a monolayer were observed to be morphologically heterogeneous, spindle shaped and fibroblast-like in appearance (Figure 1A) similar in appearance to mesenchymal stem cells previously reported in the literature (Wagner and Ho 2007; Wagner, Roderburg et al. 2007).

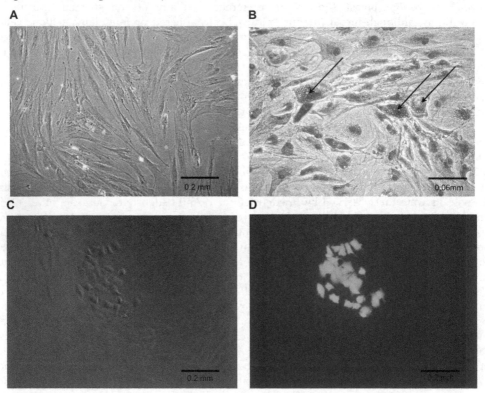

Fig. 1. Characterization of mesenchymal stem cells (MSCs) and breast cancer cell colonies plated on MSCs. MSCs growing as a monolayer are morphologically heterogeneous, spindle-shaped and fibroblast-like (A). MSCs can be induced to differentiate into adipocytes (B). Arrows indicate accumulations of lipid-rich vacuoles. Colonies of breast cancer cells growing on a lawn of MSCs can be visualized by light microscopy by their different refractive index (C) or, if they are stably transfected with GFP can be visualized using fluorescent microscopy (D).

To determine the multipotent potential of the bone cells adipogenic differentiation was induced in the isolated bone marrow derived cell cultures by treatment with Adipogenic Differentiation Medium (Fisher Scientific, SH3088602) according to the manufacturer's instructions. Induction was apparent by the accumulation of lipid-rich vacuoles within cells (Figure 1B). The content of the observed vacuoles was stained with Oil Red O dye and was localized to inside the cells where cell nucleus and membrane were counterstained with haematoxylin. This is consistent with our bone cell cultures having some of the multipotent characteristics of mesenchymal stem cells and we will refer to them as MSCs.

One of the usual characteristics to measure when breast cancer cells are grown on any stroma includes the ability of the breast cancer cells to form colonies on that stroma cell type. This can be determined using limiting dilution analysis. We used statistical analysis for limiting dilution assays adapted from the method described by Lefkovits and Waldmann (Lefkovits and Waldmann 1999). Limiting dilution analysis software developed by P. Rovenksy, J. Rubes, and T. Beran and included with the Lefkovits and Waldmann textbook was used for chi square and frequency calculations.

A modified limiting dilution analysis (LDA) method was used to evaluate the frequency of a given event in a population. We evaluated proliferation/survival of individual cancer cells, where binomial colony formation events were defined as 1) a *positive event* being the presence of colony ≥ 8 cells in size after the indicated time (days) period, and a 2) a *negative event* being the absence of any colonies or a colony <8 cells after the indicated time (days) period.

For co-cultures, 1000 cells/well of substratum cells were seeded in 96-well plates and allowed to attach and grow over 2 day period. After 2 days, the wells were washed twice using PBS and various dilutions of the breast cancer cell lines (1, 2, 4, 5, 7, 10 cells/well) were added in 100uL volume of serum-free Opti-MemI media per well (Gibco cat. #31985). The plates were incubated for an indicated time period at 37°C and 5% CO_2. Each well was analysed for the presence of colonies using an inverted microscope (100X magnification). Breast cancer cells were identified by morphology and a different refractive index when compared to the large flattened MSCs. An example is presented in Figure 1C and D.

Each well was scored as positive or negative based on the above established criteria. The data was tabulated and frequencies were determined using a Poisson distribution:

$$F_r = \frac{\mu^r}{r!} e^{-\mu}$$

Frequencies were calculated using the aforementioned LDA software package with a linear regression through the origin. Graphical representations of the distributions were also plotted on the μ vs. $-\ln F_0$ graphs. The accuracy of the fitted line was evaluated using a chi-squared test for goodness of fit

$$(X^2 = \frac{df \times V}{\sigma^2})$$

based on a 95% confidence interval of accepting the null hypothesis that the best line of fit accurately represents the observed data. The null hypothesis was accepted (line of best fit accurately represents the data that follows single-hit kinetics) when the p-value was greater than 0.05.

Inter-trial frequencies were compared based on the overlap of the 95% confidence limits of the slopes based upon evaluation of the reliability of the regression line estimates. Confidence limits of the slope (a) were calculated using the following equations,

$$a_{upper} = a + t_{\frac{\alpha}{2}, n-1} \sqrt{\frac{1}{(n-1)(\frac{\sum y_i^2}{\sum x_i^2} - a^2)}} \quad ,$$

$$a_{lower} = a - t_{\frac{\alpha}{2}, n-1} \sqrt{\frac{1}{(n-1)(\frac{\sum y_i^2}{\sum x_i^2} - a^2)}}$$

so that new slopes (a_{lower}, a_{upper}) define the boundaries of the fan. The values for the area α or $\alpha/2$ were obtained from the Student's t-test table. The overall frequency for each cell line was calculated using pooled data from experiments using the above described analysis.

Using limiting dilution analysis we determined, for example, that one MCF-7 cell in every fourteen could develop a productive colony on MSCs but only one MCF-7 cell in every thirty could develop a colony on HS68 fibroblasts, indicating that bone stroma was the preferential stroma to colonize (Figure 2).

Another characteristic very often measured in two dimensional co-cultures involves the ability of one cell type or conditioned medium from a cell type to influence the migratory capacities of another cell type. This is sometimes done with a wound healing assay where a confluent culture of one type of cells is disrupted by scratching cells off the tissue culture plate surface in a straight line and then measuring how long it takes the "wound" to fill in with new cells under conditions of differing types of conditioned media.

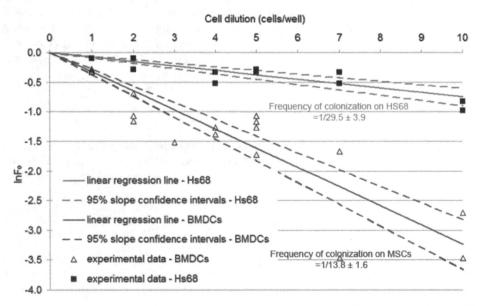

Fig. 2. Limiting Dilution Analysis (LDA) of MCF-7 Breast cancer cells grown on MSCs (blue) or HS68 fibroblast cells (red) indicates that the breast cancer cells can colonize wells having MSCs as a substrate at a significantly higher frequency than they can colonize wells in which HS68 cells have been plated as a substrate.

An alternative and more quantitative way to measure cell migration is in a Transwell or Boyden Chamber assay. Here, cells of interest are placed in the lower well of a Transwell plate and allowed to grow for some time to provide conditioned medium (Figure 3A). Cells to be tested for migratory capacity are placed on a porous membrane in the upper chamber and are allowed to migrate through the membrane for a given period of time. An example of MCF-7 breast cancer cells migrating through pores in response to MSCs or HS68 fibroblasts is given in Figure 3, where it can be seen that the breast cancer cells migrate preferentially in response to bone stromal cells.

A variation on the Transwell migration assay is an invasion assay where the cells must invade through a Matrigel layer before migrating through the pores. Usually an invasion assay and a migration assay are carried out at the same time under the same conditions and invasion is measured as a percentage of number of cells invading/migrating.

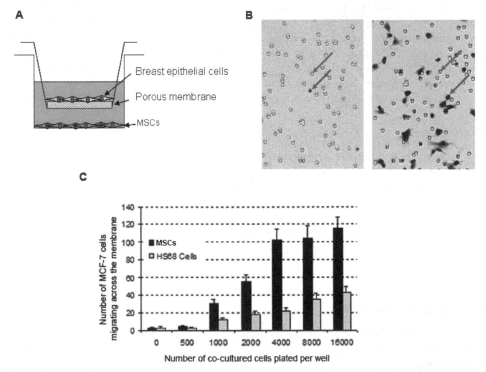

Fig. 3. Use of a Transwell Assay to determine the migration of MCF-7 breast cancer cells in response to MSCs or HS68 cells. A schematic diagram to illustrate the assay design (A). The Transwell membrane when stained and photographed from an inferior aspect has 8um pores (red arrows) and cells that have migrated through the pores can be visualized and counted (blue arrows). More cells migrate through the Transwell membrane in response to MSCs than in response to HS68 cells (C). Error bars indicate standard error of the mean.

One of the advantages of using a two dimensional co-culture system using Transwell plates is the ability to separate the cells after exposure to each other for analysis by western blot, PCR analysis or microarray analysis of differentially expressed genes. Another advantage is the ability to separate cells to determine which cell type is expressing a factor that regulates invasion or migration. For example, the bone remodeling protein Osteopontin is produced by bone cells and breast cancer cells. There are a number of reports in the literature suggesting Osteopontin produced by breast cancer cells regulates their migratory properties and contributes to the aggressiveness of the disease (Sharp, Sung et al. 1999; Chakraborty, Jain et al. 2008; Hedley, Welch et al. 2008; Patani, Jouhra et al. 2008; Ribeiro-Silva and Oliveira da Costa 2008). In our co-culture model we found, at least in the breast/bone microenvironment, that it was Osteopontin produced by the bone cells, not the breast cells that increased breast cancer cell migration (Koro, Parkin et al. 2010).

4. Future directions

It is becoming evident that gene expression at the site of breast cancer metastasis may not be the same as at the site of the primary tumour and we need better ways to treat metastases. It will likely be important to biopsy more metastatic tissue to provide the type of designer therapeutics aimed at pathways known to be targetable at the site of the metastasis as we currently do with the primary tumour. Currently, biopsies of metastases are rare. As stroma is known to be an active contributor to the metastasis we also need to develop therapeutic approaches aimed at targeting the stroma. The recent development of new technologies for capture and analysis of circulating tumour cells may help to improve our understanding.

5. Conclusions

Breast cancer is a complicated disease and progression to metastasis may occur by clonal expansion or parallel progression. Changes in gene expression may occur between the primary tumour and the site of metastasis and development of therapeutics aimed at either the breast or stromal cells at the site of the metastasis will likely be needed to develop better therapeutics against breast cancer metastasis. Some of these new therapeutics may be aimed at reconstituting the expression of breast cancer metastasis inhibitor genes and much research is being done in this field. *In vivo* and *in vitro* model systems have contributed in many ways to our understanding of breast cancer metastasis and will surely continue to do so.

6. Acknowledgements

The authors would like to acknowledge the Alberta Cancer Board and the Canadian Breast Cancer Foundation for research funding. We also thank Brant Pohorelic for careful reading of this material.

7. References

(1983). "The World Health Organization. Histological typing of breast tumors." Neoplasma 30(1): 113-123.

Albanese, I., A. G. Scibetta, et al. (2004). "Heterogeneity within and between primary colorectal carcinomas and matched metastases as revealed by analysis of Ki-ras and p53 mutations." Biochem Biophys Res Commun 325(3): 784-791.

Andrechek, E. R. and J. R. Nevins (2010). "Mouse models of cancers: opportunities to address heterogeneity of human cancer and evaluate therapeutic strategies." J Mol Med 88(11): 1095-1100.

Baker, L., P. R. Quinlan, et al. (2010). "p53 mutation, deprivation and poor prognosis in primary breast cancer." Br J Cancer 102(4): 719-726.

Bauer, M., G. Su, et al. (2010). "3D microchannel co-culture: method and biological validation." Integr Biol (Camb) 2(7-8): 371-378.

Belev, B., I. Aleric, et al. (2002). "Nm23 gene product expression in invasive breast cancer--immunohistochemical analysis and clinicopathological correlation." Acta Oncol 41(4): 355-361.

Bhujwalla, Z. M., E. O. Aboagye, et al. (1999). "Nm23-transfected MDA-MB-435 human breast carcinoma cells form tumors with altered phospholipid metabolism and pH: a 31P nuclear magnetic resonance study in vivo and in vitro." Magn Reson Med 41(5): 897-903.

Bordeleau, L. J., J. E. Lipa, et al. (2007). "Management of the BRCA mutation carrier or high-risk patient." Clin Plast Surg 34(1): 15-27; abstract v.

Bosco, E. E. and E. S. Knudsen (2007). "RB in breast cancer: at the crossroads of tumorigenesis and treatment." Cell Cycle 6(6): 667-671.

Brooks, B., N. J. Bundred, et al. (1997). "Investigation of mammary epithelial cell-bone marrow stroma interactions using primary human cell culture as a model of metastasis." Int J Cancer 73(5): 690-696.

Cappelletti, V., C. Ruedl, et al. (1993). "Paracrine interaction in co-culture of hormone-dependent and independent breast cancer cells." Breast Cancer Res Treat 26(3): 275-281.

Chabottaux, V., S. Ricaud, et al. (2009). "Membrane-type 4 matrix metalloproteinase (MT4-MMP) induces lung metastasis by alteration of primary breast tumour vascular architecture." J Cell Mol Med 13(9B): 4002-4013.

Chakraborty, G., S. Jain, et al. (2008). "Down-regulation of osteopontin attenuates breast tumour progression in vivo." J Cell Mol Med 12(6A): 2305-2318.

Charpin, C., S. Garcia, et al. (1998). "Prognostic significance of Nm23/NDPK expression in breast carcinoma, assessed on 10-year follow-up by automated and quantitative immunocytochemical assays." J Pathol 184(4): 401-407.

Christgen, M., H. Christgen, et al. (2009). "Expression of KAI1/CD82 in distant metastases from estrogen receptor-negative breast cancer." Cancer Sci 100(9): 1767-1771.

Debnath, J. and J. S. Brugge (2005). "Modelling glandular epithelial cancers in three-dimensional cultures." Nat Rev Cancer 5(9): 675-688.

Dhurjati, R., V. Krishnan, et al. (2008). "Metastatic breast cancer cells colonize and degrade three-dimensional osteoblastic tissue in vitro." Clin Exp Metastasis 25(7): 741-752.

Dittmer, A., K. Hohlfeld, et al. (2009). "Human mesenchymal stem cells induce E-cadherin degradation in breast carcinoma spheroids by activating ADAM10." Cell Mol Life Sci 66(18): 3053-3065.

El-Haibi, C. P. and A. E. Karnoub (2010). "Mesenchymal stem cells in the pathogenesis and therapy of breast cancer." J Mammary Gland Biol Neoplasia 15(4): 399-409.

Engel, J., R. Eckel, et al. (2003). "The process of metastasisation for breast cancer." Eur J Cancer 39(12): 1794-1806.

Ferrari, G., G. Cusella-De Angelis, et al. (1998). "Muscle regeneration by bone marrow-derived myogenic progenitors." Science 279(5356): 1528-1530.

Fidler, I. J. (1970). "Metastasis: guantitative analysis of distribution and fate of tumor embolilabeled with 125 I-5-iodo-2'-deoxyuridine." J Natl Cancer Inst 45(4): 773-782.

Fidler, I. J. and G. L. Nicolson (1977). "Fate of recirculating B16 melanoma metastatic variant cells in parabiotic syngeneic recipients." J Natl Cancer Inst 58(6): 1867-1872.

Fierro, F. A., W. D. Sierralta, et al. (2004). "Marrow-derived mesenchymal stem cells: role in epithelial tumor cell determination." Clin Exp Metastasis 21(4): 313-319.

Fridlyand, J., A. M. Snijders, et al. (2006). "Breast tumor copy number aberration phenotypes and genomic instability." BMC Cancer 6: 96.

Friedenstein, A. J., J. F. Gorskaja, et al. (1976). "Fibroblast precursors in normal and irradiated mouse hematopoietic organs." Exp Hematol 4(5): 267-274.

Fuhrmann, C., O. Schmidt-Kittler, et al. (2008). "High-resolution array comparative genomic hybridization of single micrometastatic tumor cells." Nucleic Acids Res 36(7): e39.

Galani, E., J. Sgouros, et al. (2002). "Correlation of MDR-1, nm23-H1 and H Sema E gene expression with histopathological findings and clinical outcome in ovarian and breast cancer patients." Anticancer Res 22(4): 2275-2280.

Glinsky, V. V., M. E. Huflejt, et al. (2000). "Effects of Thomsen-Friedenreich antigen-specific peptide P-30 on beta-galactoside-mediated homotypic aggregation and adhesion to the endothelium of MDA-MB-435 human breast carcinoma cells." Cancer Res 60(10): 2584-2588.

Gow, C. H., Y. L. Chang, et al. (2009). "Comparison of epidermal growth factor receptor mutations between primary and corresponding metastatic tumors in tyrosine kinase inhibitor-naive non-small-cell lung cancer." Ann Oncol 20(4): 696-702.

Hall, B., J. Dembinski, et al. (2007). "Mesenchymal stem cells in cancer: tumor-associated fibroblasts and cell-based delivery vehicles." Int J Hematol 86(1): 8-16.

Harms, J. F., D. R. Welch, et al. (2003). "KISS1 metastasis suppression and emergent pathways." Clin Exp Metastasis 20(1): 11-18.

Hebner, C., V. M. Weaver, et al. (2008). "Modeling morphogenesis and oncogenesis in three-dimensional breast epithelial cultures." Annu Rev Pathol 3: 313-339.

Hedley, B. D., K. S. Vaidya, et al. (2008). "BRMS1 suppresses breast cancer metastasis in multiple experimental models of metastasis by reducing solitary cell survival and inhibiting growth initiation." Clin Exp Metastasis 25(7): 727-740.

Hedley, B. D., D. R. Welch, et al. (2008). "Downregulation of osteopontin contributes to metastasis suppression by breast cancer metastasis suppressor 1." Int J Cancer 123(3): 526-534.

Hicks, D. G., B. J. Yoder, et al. (2006). "Loss of breast cancer metastasis suppressor 1 protein expression predicts reduced disease-free survival in subsets of breast cancer patients." Clin Cancer Res 12(22): 6702-6708.

Hombauer, H. and J. J. Minguell (2000). "Selective interactions between epithelial tumour cells and bone marrow mesenchymal stem cells." Br J Cancer 82(7): 1290-1296.

Horak, C. E., J. H. Lee, et al. (2007). "Nm23-H1 suppresses tumor cell motility by down-regulating the lysophosphatidic acid receptor EDG2." Cancer Res 67(15): 7238-7246.

Hurst, D. R., Y. Xie, et al. (2008). "Alterations of BRMS1-ARID4A interaction modify gene expression but still suppress metastasis in human breast cancer cells." J Biol Chem 283(12): 7438-7444.

Husemann, Y., J. B. Geigl, et al. (2008). "Systemic spread is an early step in breast cancer." Cancer Cell 13(1): 58-68.

Husemann, Y. and C. A. Klein (2009). "The analysis of metastasis in transgenic mouse models." Transgenic Res 18(1): 1-5.

Jemal, A., F. Bray, et al. (2011). "Global cancer statistics." CA Cancer J Clin.

Kaplan, R. N., B. Psaila, et al. (2006). "Bone marrow cells in the 'pre-metastatic niche': within bone and beyond." Cancer Metastasis Rev 25(4): 521-529.

Kelly, L. M., Y. Buggy, et al. (2005). "Expression of the breast cancer metastasis suppressor gene, BRMS1, in human breast carcinoma: lack of correlation with metastasis to axillary lymph nodes." Tumour Biol 26(4): 213-216.

Kim, I. S. and S. H. Baek (2010). "Mouse models for breast cancer metastasis." Biochem Biophys Res Commun 394(3): 443-447.

Kim, J. B., R. Stein, et al. (2004). "Three-dimensional in vitro tissue culture models of breast cancer-- a review." Breast Cancer Res Treat 85(3): 281-291.

Klein, C. A. (2003). "The systemic progression of human cancer: a focus on the individual disseminated cancer cell--the unit of selection." Adv Cancer Res 89: 35-67.

Klein, C. A. (2009). "Parallel progression of primary tumours and metastases." Nat Rev Cancer 9(4): 302-312.

Klein, C. A., S. Seidl, et al. (2002). "Combined transcriptome and genome analysis of single micrometastatic cells." Nat Biotechnol 20(4): 387-392.

Klein, C. A. and N. H. Stoecklein (2009). "Lessons from an aggressive cancer: evolutionary dynamics in esophageal carcinoma." Cancer Res 69(13): 5285-5288.

Klein, G. (1998). "Foulds' dangerous idea revisited: the multistep development of tumors 40 years later." Adv Cancer Res 72: 1-23.

Koro, K., S. Parkin, et al. (2010). "Interactions between breast cancer cells and bone marrow derived cells in vitro define a role for osteopontin in affecting breast cancer cell migration." Breast Cancer Res Treat.

Krishnan, V., L. A. Shuman, et al. (2010). ""Dynamic interaction between breast cancer cells and osteoblastic tissue: comparison of two and three dimensional cultures."." J Cell Physiol.

Kumar, S., V. Walia, et al. (2007). "p53 in breast cancer: mutation and countermeasures." Front Biosci 12: 4168-4178.

Kunz-Schughart, L. A., P. Heyder, et al. (2001). "A heterologous 3-D coculture model of breast tumor cells and fibroblasts to study tumor-associated fibroblast differentiation." Exp Cell Res 266(1): 74-86.

Langlois, A. J., W. D. Holder, Jr., et al. (1979). "Morphological and biochemical properties of a new human breast cancer cell line." Cancer Res 39(7 Pt 1): 2604-2613.

Lefkovits, I. and H. Waldmann (1999). Limiting dilution analysis of cells of the immune system. Oxford ; New York, Oxford University Press.

Leone, A., U. Flatow, et al. (1993). "Transfection of human nm23-H1 into the human MDA-MB-435 breast carcinoma cell line: effects on tumor metastatic potential, colonization and enzymatic activity." Oncogene 8(9): 2325-2333.

Lombardi, G., C. Di Cristofano, et al. (2007). "High level of messenger RNA for BRMS1 in primary breast carcinomas is associated with poor prognosis." Int J Cancer 120(6): 1169-1178.

MacDonald, N. J., J. M. Freije, et al. (1996). "Site-directed mutagenesis of nm23-H1. Mutation of proline 96 or serine 120 abrogates its motility inhibitory activity upon transfection into human breast carcinoma cells." J Biol Chem 271(41): 25107-25116.

Malik, F. A., A. J. Sanders, et al. (2009). "Transcriptional and translational modulation of KAI1 expression in ductal carcinoma of the breast and the prognostic significance." Int J Mol Med 23(2): 273-278.

Malik, F. A., A. J. Sanders, et al. (2009). "Effect of expressional alteration of KAI1 on breast cancer cell growth, adhesion, migration and invasion." Cancer Genomics Proteomics 6(4): 205-213.

Martin, F. T., R. M. Dwyer, et al. (2010). "Potential role of mesenchymal stem cells (MSCs) in the breast tumour microenvironment: stimulation of epithelial to mesenchymal transition (EMT)." Breast Cancer Res Treat 124(2): 317-326.

Mastro, A. M. and E. A. Vogler (2009). "A three-dimensional osteogenic tissue model for the study of metastatic tumor cell interactions with bone." Cancer Res 69(10): 4097-4100.

Morgan, T. M., P. H. Lange, et al. (2009). "Disseminated tumor cells in prostate cancer patients after radical prostatectomy and without evidence of disease predicts biochemical recurrence." Clin Cancer Res 15(2): 677-683.

Neve, R. M., K. Chin, et al. (2006). "A collection of breast cancer cell lines for the study of functionally distinct cancer subtypes." Cancer Cell 10(6): 515-527.

Nguyen, D. X., P. D. Bos, et al. (2009). "Metastasis: from dissemination to organ-specific colonization." Nat Rev Cancer 9(4): 274-284.

Oh, H. S., A. Moharita, et al. (2004). "Bone marrow stroma influences transforming growth factor-beta production in breast cancer cells to regulate c-myc activation of the preprotachykinin-I gene in breast cancer cells." Cancer Res 64(17): 6327-6336.

Paget (1889). "The Distribution of Secondary Growths in Cancer of the Breast." Cancer Metastasis Reviews 8: 98.

Pantel, K., G. Schlimok, et al. (1993). "Differential expression of proliferation-associated molecules in individual micrometastatic carcinoma cells." J Natl Cancer Inst 85(17): 1419-1424.

Parr, C. and W. G. Jiang (2009). "Metastasis suppressor 1 (MTSS1) demonstrates prognostic value and anti-metastatic properties in breast cancer." Eur J Cancer 45(9): 1673-1683.

Patani, N., F. Jouhra, et al. (2008). "Osteopontin expression profiles predict pathological and clinical outcome in breast cancer." Anticancer Res 28(6B): 4105-4110.

Peihong, S. and F. Perry (2007). "Expression of nm23, MMP-2, TIMP-2 in breast neoplasm in Zhengzhou Center Hospital, China." Ethiop Med J 45(1): 79-83.

Phadke, P. A., K. S. Vaidya, et al. (2008). "BRMS1 suppresses breast cancer experimental metastasis to multiple organs by inhibiting several steps of the metastatic process." Am J Pathol 172(3): 809-817.

Pittenger, M. F., A. M. Mackay, et al. (1999). "Multilineage potential of adult human mesenchymal stem cells." Science 284(5411): 143-147.

Rabbani, S. A. and A. P. Mazar (2007). "Evaluating distant metastases in breast cancer: from biology to outcomes." Cancer Metastasis Rev 26(3-4): 663-674.

Rakha, E. A., J. S. Reis-Filho, et al. (2010). "Breast cancer prognostic classification in the molecular era: the role of histological grade." Breast Cancer Res 12(4): 207.

Ramirez, N. E., Z. Zhang, et al. (2011). "The alphabeta integrin is a metastasis suppressor in mouse models and human cancer." J Clin Invest 121(1): 226-237.

Rhodes, L. V. and M. E. Burow (2010). "Human mesenchymal stem cells as mediators of breast carcinoma tumorigenesis and progression." ScientificWorldJournal 10: 1084-1087.

Ribeiro-Silva, A. and J. P. Oliveira da Costa (2008). "Osteopontin expression according to molecular profile of invasive breast cancer: a clinicopathological and immunohistochemical study." Int J Biol Markers 23(3): 154-160.

Riethdorf, S., H. Wikman, et al. (2008). "Review: Biological relevance of disseminated tumor cells in cancer patients." Int J Cancer 123(9): 1991-2006.

Roetger, A., A. Merschjann, et al. (1998). "Selection of potentially metastatic subpopulations expressing c-erbB-2 from breast cancer tissue by use of an extravasation model." Am J Pathol 153(6): 1797-1806.

Ronnov-Jessen, L., O. W. Petersen, et al. (1995). "The origin of the myofibroblasts in breast cancer. Recapitulation of tumor environment in culture unravels diversity and implicates converted fibroblasts and recruited smooth muscle cells." J Clin Invest 95(2): 859-873.

Rose, A. A. and P. M. Siegel (2010). "Emerging therapeutic targets in breast cancer bone metastasis." Future Oncol 6(1): 55-74.

Ross, J. S. and J. A. Fletcher (1999). "The HER-2/neu oncogene: prognostic factor, predictive factor and target for therapy." Semin Cancer Biol 9(2): 125-138.

Russell, R. L., A. N. Pedersen, et al. (1998). "Relationship of nm23 to proteolytic factors, proliferation and motility in breast cancer tissues and cell lines." Br J Cancer 78(6): 710-717.

Sgouros, J., E. Galani, et al. (2007). "Correlation of nm23-H1 gene expression with clinical outcome in patients with advanced breast cancer." In Vivo 21(3): 519-522.

Sharp, J. A., V. Sung, et al. (1999). "Tumor cells are the source of osteopontin and bone sialoprotein expression in human breast cancer." Lab Invest 79(7): 869-877.

Slamon, D. J., G. M. Clark, et al. (1987). "Human breast cancer: correlation of relapse and survival with amplification of the HER-2/neu oncogene." Science 235(4785): 177-182.

Smith, S. C. and D. Theodorescu (2009). "Learning therapeutic lessons from metastasis suppressor proteins." Nat Rev Cancer 9(4): 253-264.

Stafford, L. J., K. S. Vaidya, et al. (2008). "Metastasis suppressors genes in cancer." Int J Biochem Cell Biol 40(5): 874-891.

Steeg, P. S., T. Ouatas, et al. (2003). "Metastasis suppressor genes: basic biology and potential clinical use." Clin Breast Cancer 4(1): 51-62.

Stoecklein, N. H. and C. A. Klein (2010). "Genetic disparity between primary tumours, disseminated tumour cells, and manifest metastasis." Int J Cancer 126(3): 589-598.

Terasaki-Fukuzawa, Y., H. Kijima, et al. (2002). "Decreased nm23 expression, but not Ki-67 labeling index, is significantly correlated with lymph node metastasis of breast invasive ductal carcinoma." Int J Mol Med 9(1): 25-29.

Tortola, S., R. Steinert, et al. (2001). "Discordance between K-ras mutations in bone marrow micrometastases and the primary tumor in colorectal cancer." J Clin Oncol 19(11): 2837-2843.

Tseng, Y. H., D. Vicent, et al. (2001). "Regulation of growth and tumorigenicity of breast cancer cells by the low molecular weight GTPase Rad and nm23." Cancer Res 61(5): 2071-2079.

Vernon, A. E., S. J. Bakewell, et al. (2007). "Deciphering the molecular basis of breast cancer metastasis with mouse models." Rev Endocr Metab Disord 8(3): 199-213.

Wagner, W. and A. D. Ho (2007). "Mesenchymal stem cell preparations--comparing apples and oranges." Stem Cell Rev 3(4): 239-248.

Wagner, W., C. Roderburg, et al. (2007). "Molecular and secretory profiles of human mesenchymal stromal cells and their abilities to maintain primitive hematopoietic progenitors." Stem Cells 25(10): 2638-2647.

Weaver, V. M., A. H. Fischer, et al. (1996). "The importance of the microenvironment in breast cancer progression: recapitulation of mammary tumorigenesis using a unique human mammary epithelial cell model and a three-dimensional culture assay." Biochem Cell Biol 74(6): 833-851.

Welch, D. R. (1997). "Technical considerations for studying cancer metastasis in vivo." Clin Exp Metastasis 15(3): 272-306.

Yang, X., L. L. Wei, et al. (2001). "Overexpression of KAI1 suppresses in vitro invasiveness and in vivo metastasis in breast cancer cells." Cancer Res 61(13): 5284-5288.

Yang, X., D. R. Welch, et al. (1997). "KAI1, a putative marker for metastatic potential in human breast cancer." Cancer Lett 119(2): 149-155.

11

Breast Cancer Metastases to Bone: Role of the Microenvironment

Jenna E. Fong and Svetlana V. Komarova

Faculty of Dentistry, McGill University, Montreal

Canada

1. Introduction

Bone is the preferred site for breast cancer metastasis, which leads to altered mineral metabolism, disruption of bone architecture, and considerable pain burden. Prior to homing to the bone, the primary breast tumour releases soluble factors that lead to the creation of a pre-metastatic niche in the bone, which then serves to attract and maintain invading breast cancer cells. Breast cancer cells actively influence resident bone cells, altering both the action of and cross-talk between bone forming osteoblasts and bone-destroying osteoclasts. Breast cancer cells inhibit osteoblast differentiation and prevent them from creating and mineralizing new bone. Immature osteoblasts act as part of a hematopoietic stem cell niche and provide an attachment site for breast cancer cells. Breast cancer cells also produce factors, such as parathyroid hormone-related protein (PTHrP), which induce osteoblasts to stimulate the production of the pro-resorptive cytokine RANKL and to inhibit the production of RANKL inhibitor, OPG. RANKL, together with other osteoclastogenic factors released from breast cancer cells, promotes the fusion and differentiation of osteoclasts, resulting in bone destruction. As a result of bone resorption, growth factors stored in the bone matrix, such as TGFβ, are released and can further stimulate the proliferation and survival of tumour cells. Thus, the complex interactions between breast cancer cells and the bone microenvironment underlie the homing of the breast cancer to bone and the subsequent progression of osteolytic lesions. Current therapeutics against bone metastases aim to prevent osteoclastic bone resorption by blocking osteoclast differentiation or stimulating their apoptosis. The osteoblast provides a valuable potential target, as a source of osteoclastic differentiation factors, and a platform for cancer cell attachment. Recent results from basic and clinical research provide new targets to prevent the interactions between breast cancer cells and the bone microenvironment at different stages of the metastatic cascade.

2. Chapter outline

- Physiological regulation of breast and bone
  - Breast Growth and Development
    - Interactions of normal breast tissue with bone
    - Breast carcinoma
  - Bone Microenvironment

- Bone structure and composition
- Bone functions
- Osteoclasts, osteoblasts and osteocytes: origins, differentiation, function, physiology, pathology
- Bone marrow and hematopoietic stem cell niche
- Bone cell communications during normal bone remodelling
- Homing of breast cancer cells to bone
  - Creation of pre-metastatic niche
  - Migration of breast cancer cells to bone
  - Attachment proteins between breast cancer cells and the bone
  - Osteomimicry
- Establishing of a metastatic tumor in the bone microenvironment
  - Interactions with osteoblasts
    - Inhibition of osteoblasts by breast cancer cells
    - Contribution of osteoblasts to the creation of an osteolytic environment
    - Role of osteoblasts in supporting breast cancer cells
  - Interactions with osteoclasts
    - Stimulation of osteoclasts by breast cancer cells
    - Role of osteoclasts in supporting breast cancer cells
- Therapeutic targets in the bone microenvironment
- Conclusions
- References

3. Physiological regulation of breast and bone

3.1 Breast growth and development

Interactions of normal breast tissue with bone

The interactions of normal breast tissue with bone arise during childbearing and breastfeeding. A normal human fetus needs approximately 30 g of calcium to mineralize its skeleton during gestation (1), that leads to significant changes in calcium homeostasis during pregnancy, including adjustments in levels of parathyroid hormone (PTH), calcitonin and 1,25 dihydroxy-vitamin D [1,25[OH]D] (2). These hormones exhibit their effects through three main target tissues – the intestines, kidneys and bone (3). Parathyroid hormone related peptide (PTHrP) is a hormone closely related to PTH, but which is produced by local tissues, such as breast, and is important for its differentiation (4). In addition to its role in local tissue development, PTHrP can substitute for PTH in the tissues expressing their common receptor, and thus participate in calcium homeostasis by elevating 1,25(OH)D and suppressing PTH, regulating placental calcium transport, and affecting bone resorption in the maternal skeleton (3). The regulation of calcium homeostasis by the lactating mammary gland may be of critical importance, since nursing humans secrete 300-400 mg of calcium into milk each day (5). The hormonal balance changes again during lactation, with still-reduced PTH levels, but normalized calcitonin and 1,25(OH)D, and increased PTHrP (2). During this time, increased prolactin concentrations allow for the release of breast milk, and also act to enhance bone turnover (6,7). Suckling stimulates prolactin secretion and inhibits GnRH production, both of which reduce estradiol levels, leading to bone resorption (8). Bone resorption has been shown to increase during lactation, and bone formation to decrease, resulting in a loss of 5-10% of trabecular mineral content per month (9). Lactation-induced fragility fractures have been reported as a result, but are not common (10). Of interest, other important molecular mediators for the developing of lactating mammary gland are receptor activator of nuclear factor κB (RANK) and its ligand RANKL, which are better known for their key role in regulating the formation of osteoclasts. Expression of RANKL in the mammary epithelium is induced by hormones increased during pregnancy, such as prolactin, progesterone, and PTHrP, and mice lacking RANKL or RANK cannot form lobuloalveolar mammary gland structures, resulting in complete inability to develop a lactating mammary gland (11). Thus, normal breast tissue can interact with bone through a system of hormonal regulators that are important during lactation, and it expresses molecular machinery that employs the same mediators to perform locally distinct functions (Figure 1).

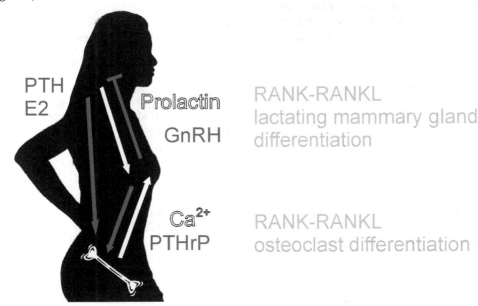

Fig. 1. Physiological interactions between the functions of breast and bone. Lactation involves secretion of large amounts of calcium. Bone is a key participant in calcium homeostasis. PTH is reduced during lactation while PTHrP production by the breast tissue is increased. Suckling stimulates prolactin secretion and inhibits GnRH production, both of which reduce estradiol levels, leading to bone resorption. Prolactin and PTHrP induce breast expression of RANKL, necessary for normal lactating mammary gland function. In the bone tissue, osteoblast-produced RANKL is key regulator of osteoclastogenesis.

Breast carcinoma

Breast carcinomas may arise from the inner lining of the milk ducts or from the lobules, known, respectively, as ductal carcinomas or lobular carcinomas (12). Once a tumour exceeds 1-2 mm in diameter, it requires extensive vascularization in order to survive (13), but the speed of cancer growth often exceeds its capability to form normal vascular organization. Poor angiogenesis results in an under-vascularized microenvironment, which leads to hypoxia, acidic pH and nutrient depletion in the tumour (14). Some cancer cells may develop the ability to detach from the primary tumour and invade other areas to form secondary tumours, in a process called metastasis. Breast cancer cells favour regional lymph nodes as well as the liver, lungs, brain and bone as sites of metastasis (15). The metastatic process occurs in a complex series of interrelated steps. An epithelial-to-mesenchymal-transition (EMT) may occur whereby epithelial breast cancer cells take on a mesenchymal phenotype of reduced attachment to neighbouring cells and increased migratory capabilities (16). This may assist in their intravasation process, where the cell breaks through the epithelium into a blood vessel (17). From here, the cell migrates to a distant site, which is driven by chemotaxis and the communication between the cancer cell and a secondary site where it aims to establish (18-20). Instead of combating cancer cells, tumor-associated macrophages and T-cells may assist in the survival and dissemination of cancer cells by mitigating the immune response and promoting cancer progression (21,22). When the cell has reached its destination, it will then undergo extravasation to exit the blood vessel and establish in a new tissue (23). Bone is a preferred site for breast cancer metastases, therefore specific interactions are likely to establish between breast cancer cells and bone cells.

3.2 Bone microenvironment

Bone is a dynamic tissue that provides support and protection for organs and maintains body mineral homeostasis. All 213 bones are constantly remodelled by the coordinated action of specialized bone cells—osteoclasts that destroy bone and osteoblasts that build bone. Bone remodelling contributes to the many functions that bones provide and occurs at different rates in different areas. Higher rates of bone turnover are observed in trabecular bone compared to cortical bone (24), and at bone sites adjacent to actively hematopoietic bone marrow in the axial skeleton, where bone metastases also commonly occur (25). High bone turnover has been found to correlate to poor prognosis in patients with bone metastases (26), and prostate cancer cells have been shown to preferentially metastasize to sites of active bone turnover (27), making bone homeostasis an essential part of understanding cancer progression.

Structure

The adult skeleton is composed of 80% solid and dense cortical bone, surrounding the remaining 20% trabecular bone, a network of plates and rods through the bone marrow (28). Bone is composed of an organic phase of extracellular matrix containing collagen-1 triple-helical chains and non-collagenous proteins, and mineral phase of hydroxyapatite crystals $[Ca_{10}(PO_4)_6(OH)_2]$. Osteogenesis occurs by two distinct mechanisms – endochondral ossification, and intramembranous bone formation. Endochondral ossification occurs in most bones of mesodermal origin that form the axial skeleton, including long bones, skull, ribs and vertebrae, and involves the formation of initial mineralized cartilage template, which is first degraded by osteoclasts and then replaced with bone matrix by osteoblasts (29,30). Intramembranous ossification occurs in the flat bones and the mandible, maxilla and clavicle, where an ossification centre is created when mesenchymal stem cells condense, and directly differentiate into bone-forming osteoblasts (31).

Functions

The mechanical functions of bone are probably their best recognized. Bones protect internal organs from damage and support the structure of the body. Bones provide anchorage for muscles, ligaments and tendons to allow movement in three-dimensional space. Hearing is also attributed to the mechanics of bones, with several of the body's smallest bones involved in the transmission of sound in the ear. Bone is the body's major reservoir of calcium, storing approximately 99% of it in the bone's mineral phase. Plasma calcium levels are strictly regulated in the range of 2.2-2.6 mmol/L total calcium. Such regulation is achieved by regulating calcium exchange with the environment through the kidney and intestine, and, in the absence or insufficiency of environmental sources, by regulating calcium exchange between plasma and bone through osteoblastic bone formation and osteoclastic bone destruction (32). The coordination of calcium fluxes is achived through complex hormonal regulation. Parathyroid hormone and 1,25 dihydroxy-vitamin D act to increase calcium by increasing calcium reabsorption from the kidneys and small intestine, respectively, and both act by enhancing the mobilization of calcium from bone through resorption (33). Calcitonin acts to reduce blood calcium by suppressing renal calcium reabsorption and inhibiting the mobilization from bone by preventing bone resorption (34). The combined work of these systems ensures that hypo- or hyper-calcemia is corrected, and ingested calcium is stored or eliminated as waste.

Bone tissue also interacts with other functionally diverse systems in the body. The endosteal surface of the medullary cavity of bones houses the haematopoietic stem cell niche, the specific location where blood stem cells best differentiate. Osteoblasts are well known to support the haematopoietic stem cell niche directly (35), and haematopoietic cells in turn regulate osteogenesis (36). Adipocyte-derived leptin regulates both appetite and bone mass accrual (37), and osteoblast-derived osteocalcin affects insulin secretion and sensitivity, as well as energy expenditure (38,39). It has most recently been shown that the skeleton regulates male fertility through osteocalcin (40), extending the breadth of bone's influence into reproduction as well.

Bone cells

The three cell types critical to bone's structure and function are the bone-resorbing osteoclast, the bone forming osteoblast, and the mechanosensory osteocyte. These cells work in concert to build bones, maintain mechanically sound bone tissue by replacing it on average every 10 years, and repair bones in the incidence of trauma.

Osteoclasts: The destruction of bone, both physiological in the case of morphogenesis and replacing old or damaged bone, and pathological in the case of osteolytic diseases such as osteoporosis, breast cancer metastasis to bone and rheumatoid arthritis, occurs through the activity of the osteoclast. Osteoclasts are cells of hematopoietic origin. The key molecular mediators of osteoclast formation from monocytic precursors are macrophage colony-stimulating factor (M-SCF) acting through its receptor c-fms, and RANKL which binds to its receptor RANK (41-43). Osteoprotegerin (OPG) is the high affinity decoy receptor for RANKL and is able to prevent osteoclast differentiation by inhibiting RANK-RANKL interactions (44). RANKL binding to RANK in the presence of M-CSF induces the recruitment of adaptor molecules including TRAF6 by RANK (45), resulting in the activation of transcription factor NFκB. One of the early targets of NFκB is another transcription factor essential for osteoclastogenesis, nuclear factor of activated T-cells c1 (NFATc1), which later undergoes auto-amplification with the assistance of an activator protein-1 complex containing c-Fos (46-48). NFATc1 nuclear localization is regulated by calcium signalling, which also activates calmodulin-dependent kinase, critical for further osteoclast differentiation (49). These events lead to the expression of osteoclast-specific genes including tartrate-resistant acid phosphatase (TRAP), cathepsin K, and b3 integrin (50), which are important for the degradation of bone tissue. Osteoclasts resorb bone by creating a unique microenvironment localized between this cell and bone tissue. Osteoclasts first recognize and bind to the bone matrix with integrin receptors β1 that bind collagen, fibronectin and laminin, and αvβ3 that binds osteopontin and bone sialoprotein (51). This border forms a sealing zone over the area of bone to be resorbed, and the polarization of osteoclasts results in the formation of a ruffled border between the osteoclast and matrix (52). Targeted secretion of H^+ ions through the ruffled border H^+ ATPase, accompanied by movement of Cl^- through chloride channels, acidifies the sealed space to a pH of approximately 4.5 (53,54), resulting in dissolution of the mineral phase of bone, and proteolytic enzymes cathepsin K and matrix metalloproteinase-9 (MMP-9) are released and activated to digest the organic matrix (55).

Osteoblasts: Osteoblasts are differentiated from the mesenchymal stem cells (MSC) that can also give rise to progenitors of myoblasts, adipocytes and chondrocytes (56). Commitment of MSC to become osteoprogenitors results in the upregulation of receptors for hormones, cytokines and growth factors, including PTH, prostaglandin, interleukin-11, insulin-like growth factor-1 and transforming growth factor-β (57). Next, osteoprogenitor cells differentiate into preosteoblasts, cells that exhibit limited proliferation and start to express extracellular matrix proteins, such as collagen type I, bone sialoprotein and osteopontin. Preosteoblasts are also active in the production of pro-resorptive cytokine RANKL (58). Finally, mature osteoblasts do not proliferative, but actively produce and secrete collagen type I, bone sialoprotein and osteopontin as well as osteocalcin. In addition, mature osteoblasts switch to produce the RANKL inhibitor, OPG (58). Osteoblastogenesis commitment is driven by the downstream activities of Wingless-ints (Wnt) singling, the closely associated Hedgehog signalling pathway (Sonic Hedgehog, Indian Hedgehog) and bone morphogenetic proteins (BMPs), which determine where mesenchymal stem cells condense during embryonic patterning and cross-talk to induce osteoblast differentiation (59,60). Another developmentally important pathway, Notch signalling, has been shown to negatively regulate osteoblast differentiation (61-63). Important signalling events during osteoblast differentiation include the activation of the runt-related transcription factor 2 (Runx2) transcription factor, which regulates the expression of the zinc finger-containing transcription factor Osterix (64). Osterix interacts with nuclear factor for activated T cells 2 (NFATc2), and in collaboration, controls the transcription of osteoblastic target genes osteocalcin, osteopontin, osteonectin and collagen-1 (65,66). Osteoblasts anchor to newly formed bone matrix by cadherin-11 and N-cadherin, and secrete type 1 collagen and non-collagenous matrix proteins (57). The osteoblasts then regulate the subsequent mineralization of extracellular matrix (67-69).

Osteocytes: While each cell type is essential for the maintenance of bone homeostasis, osteocytes are the most populous and account for over 95% of all cells in the skeleton, covering 94% of all bone surface (70). Osteocytes are differentiated from osteoblasts embedded in the bone matrix. During differentiation, the osteocyte cell body size decreases, and the number of long dendrite-like cell processes increases and they extend, connecting the cell with other osteocytes (70,71). Osteocyte-specific genes are activated, including phosphate-regulating gene with homologies to endopeptidases on the X chromosome

(PHEX), matrix extracellular phosphoglycoprotein (MEPE), dentin matrix protein 1 (DMP1), and fibroblast growth factor-23 (FGF23) (72,73). Osteocyte networks in the bone tissue are implicated in regulating the maintenance and mineralization of bone tissue (70,74), through expression of sclerostin, a negative regulator of bone formation (75), as well as in sensing mechanical load in part through sheer stress generated by interstitial fluid moving through the lacuno-canalicular network (76). It has also been suggested that osteocytes participate in mineral homeostasis by resorbing the lacunar walls in which they are embedded (77-79).

Communication between bone cells during normal bone remodelling

Osteoblasts, osteoclasts and osteocytes must work in concert to maintain bone homeostasis (Figure 2). In normal bone physiology, the osteoclast will resorb worn or damaged bone, and then the osteoblast will form new bone in its place. The best studied example of the crosstalk between bone cells involves the RANK-RANKL-OPG triangle, where osteoblasts and osteocytes produce RANKL to promote osteoclast differentiation and survival, and OPG to prevent it, while osteoclasts express RANK, allowing them to respond to these regulatory cues. Many hormonal regulators of bone remodelling, such as PTH and estrogen, were demonstrated to act through changing the ratio of RANKL and OPG expression by osteoblasts (80). Interestingly, production of RANKL and OPG by osteoblasts is also regulated by their developmental stage, with immature osteoblasts producing more RANKL and mature osteoblasts produce more OPG, (58). Osteocytes also, at least in part, affect osteoclastogenesis through production of RANKL, which is induced in mechanically-stimulated osteocytes (81). Osteoclasts are in turn able to influence osteoblast activity. The concept of osteoclast-mediated osteoblastogenesis arose from the finding that 97% of new bone formation occurs in resorption pits (82). Several studies where osteoclasts have been genetically altered to have impaired function demonstrated diminished bone formation (83), and studies have begun to find mediators of this reversal coupling. Cardiotrophin-1 is among the first identified, and is expressed by osteoclasts and increases osteoblast activity (84). Sphingosine-1-phosphate has been shown to act earlier and induce osteoblast precursor recruitment and subsequent mature cell survival (85). Ephrin-B2/EphB4 bidirectional signaling between osteoclasts and osteoblasts, has also been identified as a key mediator of contact-dependent communication. Forward signalling by ephrin-B2 on osteoclasts to EphB4 on osteoblasts activates bone formation, whereas reverse signalling from EphB4 on osteoblasts binding to ephrin-B2 on osteoclasts inhibits osteoclastogenesis (86). Since the ability for bone cells to communicate is essential for the maintenance of bone homeostasis, it can be anticipated that disruptions in these the complex networks would lead to profound consequences. Indeed, the RANKL/OPG ratio represents one of the key mediators of pathological bone destruction (87).

4. Homing of breast cancer cells to bone

4.1 Creation of the pre-metastatic niche

Recent evidence has led to the idea that the bone marrow supports a pre-metastatic niche - a site that receives signals from the primary tumour mass before dissemination, and changes the landscape of the target tissue to be conducive to tumour growth. It has been shown in mice treated with medium conditioned by tumour cells of different origin, the potential to home to different organs of subsequently injected cancer cells can be altered (88). In particular, in bone, bone marrow derived hematopoietic stem cells have been implicated in mediating the establishment of pre-metastatic niche (19,88). Molecular mediators such as vascular endothelial growth factor (VEGF) receptor 1 (VEGFR1) and integrin α4β1 have been implicated in this process. VEGFR1 positive haematopoietic progenitor cells are recruited to sites of future metastasis (88). VEGF receptors are expressed by breast cancer cells as well as osteoclasts and osteoclast precursors, and VEGF expression correlates to increased tumour size and grade in humans (89). In addition, we have shown that breast cancer cells secrete factors that support the subsequent attachment of breast cancer cells acting at least in part through γ-secretase-mediated Notch signalling (20).

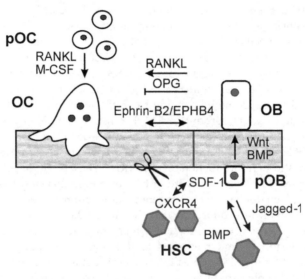

Fig. 2. Cell-cell interactions in the bone microenvironment. Osteoclast differentiation from monocytic precursors is induced by M-CSF, RANKL produced by osteoblastic cells. Osteoblasts are derived from mesenchymal stem cells through Wnt and BMP signalling pathways. Osteoblasts and osteoclasts communicate through osteoblast-derived RANKL/OPG and bidirectional Ephrin-B2/EphB4 signalling. Haematopoietic stem cells (HSC) support osteoblasts in the HSC niche through BMPs, while osteoblasts support HSCs through upregulated Notch signalling through Jagged-1. Osteoclasts cleave SDF-1 to mobilize HSCs from the endosteal niche.

4.2 Migration of breast cancer cells to bone

Breast cancer cells express receptors that direct their movement towards fertile sites where they may establish into secondary tumors. These proteins are generally expressed in normal cells, and are often involved in developmental pathways. Several chemokines have been suggested to be released from the bone microenvironment, implicating chemoattraction through G-protein-coupled chemokine receptors in driving the movement of tumour cells towards bone (90). Interactions between stromal-derived factor-1 (SDF-1) and CXCR4 are essential for the correct localization of lymphocytes and haematopoietic cells in physiological states. Breast cancer cells express higher levels of CXCR4 compared to normal breast tissue (15), and SDF-1 is strongly expressed in lung, liver, bone marrow and lymph nodes, the primary sites of secondary breast tumours, leading to the identification of the role of the SDF-1/CXCR4 in promoting breast cancer metastasis to bone (91). In addition to directional migration, chemokines have been shown to promote cancer cell survival, proliferation, and adhesion (92). In keeping, the inhibition of CXCR4 limited breast cancer metastases in mice (93), and the overexpression of CXCR4 indicates poor prognosis in both human and murine breast cancer (92,94). Another chemokine implicated in metastases of breast cancer cells expressing high levels of CCL21, is CCR7 that is expressed highly in metastatic sites, such as lymph nodes (15). Since haematopoietic stem cells (HSCs) use these chemokine and receptor interactions to home to the HSC niche in the bone marrow, it has been suggested that cancer cells use this same mechanism to parasitize these microenvironments and harvest the resources of HSCs (95). Another pertinent means of cancer cell migration towards bone relies on the cancer cell expression of RANK (96), which mediates directional migration of breast, melanoma and prostate cancer cells towards RANKL, produced in bone by osteoblasts (97,98).

Breast cancer cells may also stimulate the action of matrix metalloproteinases that support cancer cell migration and invasion. The murine orthologue of Glycogen Nonmetastatic Melanoma Protein B (GPNMB) is called osteoactivin and has been identified as a key modulator of osteolysis. Its forced expression leads to increased tumour grade and enhanced bone metastasis by upregulated MMP3 through ERK signaling (99,100). Furthermore, GPNMB was identified as a poor prognostic marker in patients with breast cancer (101). Most recently, this group has identified ADAM10 as a sheddase that releases osteoactivin from the cell, which induces endothelial cell migration and subsequent angiogenesis (102). ADAMTS1 and MMP1 are also tumour-derived metalloproteinases able to degrade the matrix. The stimulated action of these enzymes by breast cancer cells enhances osteoclast differentiation by suppressing OPG expression, and their expression in human samples correlates to a greater incidence of bone metastases (103).

4.3 Attachment proteins between breast cancer cells and the bone

Cancer cells express or induce the expression of adhesion molecules that may facilitate their interactions with the bone microenvironment. The best studied family of proteins that bind cancer cells to bone cells are integrins, heterodimeric transmembrane glycoproteins whose α and β subunits combine to form 24 known combinations with unique specificity for binding, signaling and regulatory mechanisms (104). Integrins have been demonstrated to be involved in several stages of cancer dissemination, with highly metastatic cancer cells displaying a different integrin profile than cells from the primary tumour (105). Several integrins have been shown to interact with extracellular matrix proteins during bone metastasis, with the most important being αvβ3, a receptor for osteopontin, fibronectin and vitronectin (106). Adhesion molecules engaged between breast cancer cells and bone cells may overlap with those that bind haematopoietic stem cells (HSC) to osteoblasts. HSC preferentially home to areas with more fibronectin (88). Breast cancer cells can attach to fibronectin, in an integrin-dependent manner (107). The interaction of cancer cells with fibronectin increases the production of matrix metalloproteinase-2 from fibroblasts to facilitate invasion (108). Another molecule involved the adhesion of HSC to the endosteal niche is annexin II (95). By serving as an anchor for SDF-1/CXCL12, it has been shown to regulate the homing of HSC as well as prostate cancer cells to the HSC niche (109,110).

Blocking annexin II or its receptor limited the localization of prostate cancer cells to osteoblasts and endothelial cells (111). In keeping, the inhibition of the SDF-1/CXCL12 and annexin II signaling was shown to inhibit breast cancer progression (112,113). Bone matrix proteins, such as bone sialoprotein (BSP) or osteopontin (OPN) have been shown to exhibit a potential to regulate the attachment of breast cancer cells to bone (114). Early reports have argued that BSP inhibits breast cancer cell binding to bone cells (115). However, breast cancer cells have been shown to express both BSP and OPN, and to upregulate BSP expression in pre-osteoblasts through BMP signalling; and OPN was found localized between cancer cells and bone cells at sites of metastasis (116,117). Moreover, the expression of BSP has been found to correlate with bone metastasis development (118), and OPN expression and serum concentrations have been shown to be poor prognosis markers in breast cancer patients (119,120). As osteopontin is also a mediator of the hematopoietic stem cell niche, directing migration and acting as an adhesion molecule to HSC via β1 integrin (121), it represents a potentially valuable therapeutic target against bone metastases.

4.4 Osteomimicry

Osteomimicry describes the phenomenon where osteotropic cancer cells express proteins and receptors found on bone cells and the bone matrix. It was speculated that such measures allow cancer cells to evade the immune system and/or establish in the bone microenvironment (122,123). These proteins include but are not limited to osteocalcin, osteopontin, alkaline phopsphatase and Runx2 (124). Osteoblast transcription factor Runx2 is ectopically expressed by breast cancer cells and stimulates their proliferation, motility, and invasion through increased MMP9 expression from both cancer cells and osteoblasts (125,126). Runx2 has also been shown to regulate TGFβ-influenced PTHrP levels, as well as upregulate Indian hedgehog (127). Breast cancer cells express Hedgehog ligands that activate osteopontin expression in osteoclasts, promoting osteoclast maturation and resorptive activity through upregulated Cathepsin K and MMP9 (128,129). Of interest, expression of anti-resorptive OPG has been demonstrated to correlate with increased bone-specific homing and colonization potential in breast cancer cells (122), and to promote cancer cell survival (130,131). Osteoclastic intergrin αvβ3 (54), has been shown to be upregulated in metastatic versus primary tumour cells, and has been identified as a critical mediator of breast cancer metastasis to bone (107,132). It is unclear whether cells from the primary tumour display osteomimetic features that allow their metastasis to bone, or whether secondary tumour cells established in the bone marrow and matrix receive environmental factors that give them their osteomimetic features. Regardless, the ability of cancer cells to produce many of these factors has been beneficial to thrive in the bone microenvironment.

5. Establishing of a metastatic tumour in the bone microenvironment

5.1 Interactions of breast cancer cells with osteoblasts

Inhibition of osteoblasts by breast cancer cells

Breast cancer metastasis to bone is associated with a reduction in bone formation markers in patients with bone metastases (133). In vitro, breast cancer cells have been shown to produce soluble factors able to inhibit osteoblast differentiation (20,134), the effect that may be mediated at least in part by the dysregulation of Notch and Wnt developmental signalling pathways. Notch signalling is essential in embryogenesis but has distinct roles in bone homeostasis, regulating the proliferation of immature osteoblasts (135) and suppressing osteoblast differentiation (62,63). Upregulated Notch signalling in breast cancer, through ligand Jagged-1, has been shown to correlate with increased bone metastases (136), and breast cancer cells have been shown to induce Jagged-1 expression and upregulate Notch signalling by osteoblasts (20). Wnt signaling is also a highly conserved developmental pathway, well studied in bone and essential for osteoblast and osteoclast differentiation, as well as for the production of pro-resorptive cytokine RANKL and anti-resorptive OPG (137). Wnt inhibitor DKK-1 has been shown to be upregulated in diseases associated with bone destruction, such as osteoarthritis (138), myeloma (139), and potentially in Paget's disease (140). Blocking DKK-1 in a breast cancer metastasis model has also been shown to reverse breast cancer-mediated suppression of osteoblast differentiation and reinstate OPG expression (141). Breast cancer cells have also been shown to induce osteoblast apoptosis, through increased Bax/Bcl-2 ratio and caspase expression in osteoblasts (142,143). In addition to preventing the formation of new bone, breast cancer-induced inhibition of osteoblast differentiation likely indirectly contributes to the change in production of cytokines regulating osteoclast formation and function.

Contribution of osteoblasts to the creation of an osteolytic environment

The formation of an osteoclast-supportive microenvironment is critical for the successful establishment of an osteolytic lesion during breast cancer metastasis to bone. It has been previously shown that an increase in the ratio between a pro-resorptive RANKL and anti-resorptive OPG is a key change induced by breast cancer cells (reviewed in (144,145)). Since osteoblasts are the primary source of both pro-resorptive and anti-resorptive cytokines, they represent a critical target for cancer-derived factors. Osteoblast production of RANKL is stimulated by tumour-derived PTHrP, Il-8 , Il-6 and Monocyte Chemoattractant Protein (MCP-1) (reviewed in (146)). Moreover, under the influence of breast cancer cells, undifferentiated osteoblasts express higher levels of RANKL and lower OPG, resulting in an increase in osteoblast-mediated osteoclastogenesis (20), an effect that was reversed when osteoblastic cultures were treated with the inhibitors of γ-secretase – an enzyme implicated in Notch signalling (20,136). One of the mediators of these changes was shown to be the tumour-overexpressed CCN3, that can inhibit osteoblast differentiation and shift the RANKL/OPG ratio to favour osteolysis (147). Another osteoblast-produced osteoclastogenic factor, MCSF, has also been implicated in breast cancer metastases to bone (148).

Role of osteoblasts in supporting breast cancer cells

An emerging area of interest is the role of osteoblasts in supporting the haematopoietic stem cell niche and how cancer cells parasitize this relationship. Haematopoiesis occurs on the endosteal surface of the bone marrow, where haematopoietic stem cells (HSCs) are maintained by the supporting cells, including osteoblasts. The main functions of the interaction between these cell types are *i*) the maintenance of HSC quiescence through osteoblast-derived osteopontin, and *ii*) modification to expand the progenitor population through Notch signaling (35,121). Several osteoblast-expressed receptors, cytokines and growth factors have been found to regulate an haematopoietic stem cell niche (149,150), including PTH/PTHrP receptors and BMPs acting to expand the osteoblast population, and Notch ligand Jagged-1 to expand the population of HSCs (35,151). Cancer cells disseminated from the primary tumour may also lay dormant for long periods of time before being activated to form metastases (152), so it is plausible that cancer cells harvest resources from the HSCs niche to maintain their survival and to induce expansion at the right environmental cues.

5.2 Interactions of breast cancer cells with osteoclasts

Stimulation of osteoclasts by breast cancer cells

Breast cancer cells have been found to produce many factors capable of simulating osteoclastogenesis, both by inducing RANKL expression by osteoblasts and stromal cells, and by producing osteoclastogenic factors themselves. PTHrP was one of the first factors identified to be secreted by breast cancer cells and to promote osteolysis through the stimulation of RANKL by stromal cells (153). Although the expression of PTHrP in primary tumours has been associated with a lower incidence of bone metastasis (154,155), it was shown that increased PTHrP expression by cancer cells present in the bone metastatic lesion positively correlates with increasing osteoclast activity and subsequent osteolysis (155), suggesting that the expression pattern of the cancer cells can change during metastasis, and implicating local factors, such as TGFβ derived from osteoclastic bone resorption in affecting metastasizing breast cancer cells. Osteoclastogenesis may also be stimulated by IL-8 secreted from breast cancer cells and acting both directly on osteoclasts and through osteoblastic RANKL signalling (156,157). Although the mechanisms of IL-8 action are not fully understood, the expression of IL-8 correlated with a higher incidence of bone metastasis in mice *in vivo* (158).

It has also been shown that during differentiation osteoclast precursors may acquire sensitivity to cancer-derived factors that are ineffective in inducing osteoclast formation from naive monocytes (159). Several signalling pathways in osteoclast precursors have been implicated in these effects, including calcium signalling, NFATc1 activation and MAPKs ERK1/2 and p38 (159,160). Tumour-produced CCN3 was demonstrated to stimulate osteoclast formation from RANKL-primed osteoclast precursors (147). These effects can be relevant to the propensity of cancer cells to metastasize to bone sites undergoing active bone remodelling, and thus containing increased numbers of RANKL-primed osteoclast precursors. At such sites, breast cancer cells can promote further osteoclast formation, and can affect the survival of mature osteoclasts, increasing their resorptive capacity. In this regard, M-CSF secreted from breast cancer cells was shown to be responsible for the delayed apoptosis in osteoclasts (146,161). Anti-apoptotic effects of breast cancer-derived factors included PLCγ-mediated suppression of pro-apoptotic protein BIM, and M-CSF-mediated inhibition of caspase cleavage (146).

Role of osteoclasts in supporting breast cancer cells

During osteoclastic resorption, the bone matrix components, including many growth factors stored in the bone, such as TGFβ, BMPs, IGFs, fibroblast growth factors (FGFs), and platelet-derived growth factors (PDGF) are released into extracellular space, where they are free to act on surrounding cells, including metastasizing cancer cells (162). Matrix released- TGFβ activated by osteoclastic resorption (163), is one of the most commonly studied matrix-derived growth factors, which was shown to stimulate cancer cell growth, modify cell invasion, and affect immune regulation (164,165). Considerable research has linked increased TGF-β in the microenvironment to the progression of metastasis, with TGFβ altering both the growth and phenotype of breast cancer cells (166), and increasing their expression of CTGF, CXCL11 and PTHrP (167) via Smad and MAPK signalling in breast cancer cells (153,168,169). PTHrP increases VEGF production, leading to stimulated osteoclastogenesis through the ERK1/2 and p38 signalling pathways (170). TGFβ also acts on other cells present in the bone microenvironment, such as osteoclasts themselves by sensitizing them to other breast cancer derived factors (159), through the ERK1/2, p38 and c-Jun-NH$_2$ kinase signalling pathways (160,171). In keeping with a key role of TGFβ in bone metastases, pharmacological inhibition of TGFβ signalling through the TβRI kinase inhibitor SD-208 resulted in decreased bone metastasis and tumour burden, and improved bone quality (172). The self-accelerating cycle of osteoclast stimulation by breast cancer cells, resulting in release of matrix growth factors due to osteoclastic resorption, leading to further stimulation of breast cancer cells and further increase in osteoclastic resorption was coined the name of "vicious cycle" (173), underlying the strong rationale for the use of anti-resorptive drugs for the treatment of cancer metastases to bone.

6. Therapeutic targets in the bone microenvironment

The bone microenvironment presents multiple targets for developing therapeutic treatments targeting the homing of breast cancer cells to bone, as well as progression of bone metastatic lesions (Figure 3). Molecular mediators of critical events underlying the stimulation of bone resorption and inhibition of bone formation, as well as tumour supportive environmental changes and cellular targets have been explored for their benefits in treatment of osteolytic bone metastases.

Since its discovery, the RANKL pathway has been considered to be of important therapeutic value given its role in osteoclastogenesis mediating osteolysis and subsequently discovered breast cancer cell migration, underlying pre-metastatic homing. Fully human monoclonal antibody against RANKL, Denosumab, was approved for major North American and European markets in 2010 for the prevention of osteoporosis and skeletal related events in patients with bone metastases from solid tumours. Compared to the most potent osteoclast-targeting drug in the market, bisphosphonate zoledronic acid, Denosumab treatment further delayed the occurrence of the first skeletal related event (SRE), and provided a further reduction in bone turnover markers in breast cancer patients (174). In non-metastatic breast cancer patients additionally receiving adjuvant aromatase inhibitors, bone mineral density gains were greater with Denosumab treatment (175). Bisphosphonate-resistant patients with bone metastases from breast or prostate cancer also benefitted from Denosumab treatment, with most having normalized serum markers of bone resorption after 13 weeks of treatment (176). Although Denosumab proves an effective treatment option, long-term use and toxicity data remains unknown.

DKK-1 was identified as a key mediator of myeloma-induced inhibition of bone formation, and was demonstrated to play important role in breast cancer induced inhibition of osteoblastogenesis. Neutralizing anti-DKK-1 antibodies have demonstrated significant benefits in preclinical studies in mouse models of myeloma-induced bone disease, resulting in increased osteoblast numbers, reduced osteoclast numbers and increased bone volume, and stimulating interest in further development of this approach (177). Bortezomib, a proteasome inhibitor that among other proteins affects DKK-1 and BIM (a pro-apoptotic protein that mediates osteoclast apoptosis) (178,179), was shown to inhibit osteoclastogenesis (180) and has been successful in combating the osteolytic effects of multiple myeloma (181), making it an attractive candidate for the prevention and treatment of breast cancer-induced osteolysis.

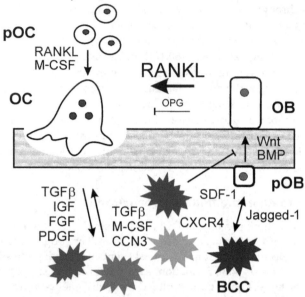

Fig. 3. Breast cancer cells alter normal bone homeostasis. Breast cancer cells maintain osteoblasts in an immature state and stimulate RANKL production by osteoblasts, while inhibiting OPG. Breast cancer cells stimulate osteoclastogenesis directly through TGFβ, M-CSF and CCN3 production. Increased bone resorption by activated osteoclasts releases matrix-derived growth factors TGFβ, IGF, FGF, PDGF, which act back on breast cancer cells to stimulate their growth and survival.

VEGF represents an interesting target potentially affecting breast cancer cell homing, development of pre-metastatic niche and new vasculature formation. Many anti-VEGF therapies exist to prevent vascularization of tumours and inhibit their growth (182). There have been several hindrances in the progress of this therapy due to drug resistance and toxicity (183), and the increased incidence of osteonecrosis of the jaw in combined bisphosphonate-antiangiogenic agent therapy (184). Notwithstanding, the use of VEGF-A monoclonal antibody Bevacizumab in combination with chemotherapy has proven beneficial in reducing breast cancer growth (185) and osteolysis (186). Other targets based on the in vitro and in vivo studies, such as TGFβ, GPNMB, and CXCR4 are being explored in preclinical and clinical studies, providing the basis for the next generation of treatments.

Osteoclasts are commonly targeted therapeutically for osteolytic disease, with one of the most widely used drugs being bisphosphonates. Analogs of mineralization-inhibiting pyrophosphate (187), bisphosphonates are a class of synthetic compounds composed of two phosphate groups covalently linked to carbon with a P-C-P backbone and side groups that vary their properties and pharmacokinetics. Bisphosphonates attach selectively to bone and induce osteoclast apoptosis when they are ingested during resorption. In osteoporosis studies, all bisphosphonates given daily have been shown to reduce osteoporotic vertebral fracture rates by 40-50% (188), and zoledronic acid and risedronate have been shown to significantly reduce non-vertebral fracture risk in pivotal trials (189). Bisphosphonates are widely used in prevention and treatment of breast cancer metastases to bone, resulting in delay and reduction in skeletal related events (190). In addition to their effects on osteoclasts, bisphosphonates have been shown to inhibit tumour growth, induce tumour cell apoptosis, and stimulate the immune response against tumour cells (191). However, some patients do not tolerate bisphosphonates well, and low but significant incidences of osteonecrosis of the jaw have been observed in patients that have undergone dental extraction procedures while treated with bisphosohonates (192). In addition, significant proportion of patients failed to normalize bone resorptive indices in response to bisphosphonate treatment (176), demonstrating the need for new therapeutic approaches.

7. Conclusion

Breast cancer is the most commonly diagnosed cancer in women, which may lead to bone metastasis resulting in altered mineral homeostasis, the disruption of bone microarchitecture, pain and pathological fractures. Recent studies have demonstrated that breast cancer cells start affecting the bone microenvironment prior to their dissemination from the primary tumour by secreting circulating soluble factors that prepare bone for the future arrival of metastasizing cancer cells, a process that likely involves mediators of the hematopoietic stem cell niche. Multiple mediators of directional migration of breast cancer cells have been identified, as well as mediators of breast cancer cells anti-osteoblastic and pro-osteoclastic actions. Breast cancer-stimulated RANKL, M-CSF, PTHrP, TGFβ, GPNMB, Runx2 and CXCR4 remain among the most critical mediators of cancer-induced osteoclastic bone resorption. Yet, they are not the whole picture, and new players are being identified, providing more complex and comprehensive description of the events leading from the formation of primary tumour to the establishment of progressive osteolytic bone lesions. However, while considering the multitude of molecular mediators, it is important to remember the heterogeneity of breast cancer disease in patients, suggesting that treatments targeting different molecular mediators should develop in parallel with the testing capabilities able to implicate a particular mediator in disease progression in a specific patient. An alternative approach is to target the processes and cellular targets similarly altered through different molecular mediators. An example of such approach is the clinical success of bisphosphonates, which broadly target osteoclast formation and activity. Nevertheless, both approaches need to be developed to provide clinicians with the set of tools for broad preventive measures, as well as for targeted personalized medicine for non-responsive or atypical cases.

8. References

[1] Mitchell DM, Juppner H 2010 Regulation of calcium homeostasis and bone metabolism in the fetus and neonate. Current opinion in endocrinology, diabetes, and obesity 17(1):25-30.
[2] Kovacs CS, Kronenberg HM 1997 Maternal-fetal calcium and bone metabolism during pregnancy, puerperium, and lactation. Endocrine reviews 18(6):832-72.

[3] Kovacs CS 2008 Vitamin D in pregnancy and lactation: maternal, fetal, and neonatal outcomes from human and animal studies. The American journal of clinical nutrition 88(2):520S-528S.

[4] Hens JR, Wysolmerski JJ 2005 Key stages of mammary gland development: molecular mechanisms involved in the formation of the embryonic mammary gland. Breast cancer research: BCR 7(5):220-4.

[5] Thomas M, Weisman SM 2006 Calcium supplementation during pregnancy and lactation: effects on the mother and the fetus. American journal of obstetrics and gynecology 194(4):937-45.

[6] Seriwatanachai D, Thongchote K, Charoenphandhu N, Pandaranandaka J, Tudpor K, Teerapornpuntakit J, Suthiphongchai T, Krishnamra N 2008 Prolactin directly enhances bone turnover by raising osteoblast-expressed receptor activator of nuclear factor kappaB ligand/osteoprotegerin ratio. Bone 42(3):535-46.

[7] Coss D, Yang L, Kuo CB, Xu X, Luben RA, Walker AM 2000 Effects of prolactin on osteoblast alkaline phosphatase and bone formation in the developing rat. American journal of physiology. Endocrinology and metabolism 279(6):E1216-25.

[8] Wysolmerski JJ 2010 Interactions between breast, bone, and brain regulate mineral and skeletal metabolism during lactation. Annals of the New York Academy of Sciences 1192:161-9.

[9] Kovacs CS, Fuleihan Gel H 2006 Calcium and bone disorders during pregnancy and lactation. Endocrinology and metabolism clinics of North America 35(1):21-51, v.

[10] Michalakis K, Peitsidis P, Ilias I 2011 Pregnancy- and lactation-associated osteoporosis: a narrative mini-review. Endocrine regulations 45(1):43-7.

[11] Fata JE, Kong YY, Li J, Sasaki T, Irie-Sasaki J, Moorehead RA, Elliott R, Scully S, Voura EB, Lacey DL, Boyle WJ, Khokha R, Penninger JM 2000 The osteoclast differentiation factor osteoprotegerin-ligand is essential for mammary gland development. Cell 103(1):41-50.

[12] Sariego J 2010 Breast cancer in the young patient. The American surgeon 76(12):1397-400.

[13] Folkman J 1986 How is blood vessel growth regulated in normal and neoplastic tissue? G.H.A. Clowes memorial Award lecture. Cancer research 46(2):467-73.

[14] Vaupel P 2004 The role of hypoxia-induced factors in tumor progression. The oncologist 9 Suppl 5:10-7.

[15] Muller A, Homey B, Soto H, Ge N, Catron D, Buchanan ME, McClanahan T, Murphy E, Yuan W, Wagner SN, Barrera JL, Mohar A, Verastegui E, Zlotnik A 2001 Involvement of chemokine receptors in breast cancer metastasis. Nature 410(6824):50-6.

[16] Vincent-Salomon A, Thiery JP 2003 Host microenvironment in breast cancer development: epithelial-mesenchymal transition in breast cancer development. Breast cancer research : BCR 5(2):101-6.

[17] Thiery JP 2002 Epithelial-mesenchymal transitions in tumour progression. Nature reviews. Cancer 2(6):442-54.

[18] Karnoub AE, Dash AB, Vo AP, Sullivan A, Brooks MW, Bell GW, Richardson AL, Polyak K, Tubo R, Weinberg RA 2007 Mesenchymal stem cells within tumour stroma promote breast cancer metastasis. Nature 449(7162):557-63.

[19] Psaila B, Kaplan RN, Port ER, Lyden D 2006 Priming the 'soil' for breast cancer metastasis: the pre-metastatic niche. Breast disease 26:65-74.

[20] Fong JE, Le Nihouannen D, Komarova SV 2010 Tumor-supportive and osteoclastogenic changes induced by breast cancer-derived factors are reversed by inhibition of {gamma}-secretase. The Journal of biological chemistry 285(41):31427-34.

[21] Mukhtar RA, Nseyo O, Campbell MJ, Esserman LJ 2011 Tumor-associated macrophages in breast cancer as potential biomarkers for new treatments and diagnostics. Expert review of molecular diagnostics 11(1):91-100.

[22] Watanabe MA, Oda JM, Amarante MK, Cesar Voltarelli J 2010 Regulatory T cells and breast cancer: implications for immunopathogenesis. Cancer metastasis reviews 29(4):569-79.

[23] McSherry EA, Donatello S, Hopkins AM, McDonnell S 2007 Molecular basis of invasion in breast cancer. Cellular and molecular life sciences : CMLS 64(24):3201-18.

[24] Silverberg SJ, Gartenberg F, Jacobs TP, Shane E, Siris E, Staron RB, McMahon DJ, Bilezikian JP 1995 Increased bone mineral density after parathyroidectomy in primary hyperparathyroidism. The Journal of clinical endocrinology and metabolism 80(3):729-34.

[25] Coleman RE 2006 Clinical features of metastatic bone disease and risk of skeletal morbidity. Clinical cancer research : an official journal of the American Association for Cancer Research 12(20 Pt 2):6243s-6249s.

[26] Brown JE, Cook RJ, Major P, Lipton A, Saad F, Smith M, Lee KA, Zheng M, Hei YJ, Coleman RE 2005 Bone turnover markers as predictors of skeletal complications in prostate cancer, lung cancer, and other solid tumors. Journal of the National Cancer Institute 97(1):59-69.

[27] Schneider A, Kalikin LM, Mattos AC, Keller ET, Allen MJ, Pienta KJ, McCauley LK 2005 Bone turnover mediates preferential localization of prostate cancer in the skeleton. Endocrinology 146(4):1727-36.

[28] Eriksen EF AD, Melsen F 1994 Bone Histomorphometry. Raven Press, New York.

[29] Olsen BR, Reginato AM, Wang W 2000 Bone development. Annual review of cell and developmental biology 16:191-220.

[30] Chung UI, Kawaguchi H, Takato T, Nakamura K 2004 Distinct osteogenic mechanisms of bones of distinct origins. Journal of orthopaedic science : official journal of the Japanese Orthopaedic Association 9(4):410-4.

[31] Ferguson CM, Miclau T, Hu D, Alpern E, Helms JA 1998 Common molecular pathways in skeletal morphogenesis and repair. Annals of the New York Academy of Sciences 857:33-42.

[32] Favus MJ GD 2008 Regulation of Calcium and Magnesium. In: Rosen CJ (ed.) Primer on the Metabolic Bone Diseases and Disorders of Mineral Metabolism, vol. Seventh Edition. American Society for Bone and Mineral Reserach, Washington, DC, pp 104-108.

[33] Poole KE, Reeve J 2005 Parathyroid hormone - a bone anabolic and catabolic agent. Current opinion in pharmacology 5(6):612-7.

[34] Boden SD, Kaplan FS 1990 Calcium homeostasis. The Orthopedic clinics of North America 21(1):31-42.

[35] Calvi LM, Adams GB, Weibrecht KW, Weber JM, Olson DP, Knight MC, Martin RP, Schipani E, Divieti P, Bringhurst FR, Milner LA, Kronenberg HM, Scadden DT 2003 Osteoblastic cells regulate the haematopoietic stem cell niche. Nature 425(6960):841-6.

[36] Shiozawa Y, Jung Y, Ziegler AM, Pedersen EA, Wang J, Wang Z, Song J, Lee CH, Sud S, Pienta KJ, Krebsbach PH, Taichman RS 2010 Erythropoietin couples hematopoiesis with bone formation. PloS one 5(5):e10853.

[37] Yadav VK, Oury F, Suda N, Liu ZW, Gao XB, Confavreux C, Klemenhagen KC, Tanaka KF, Gingrich JA, Guo XE, Tecott LH, Mann JJ, Hen R, Horvath TL, Karsenty G 2009 A serotonin-dependent mechanism explains the leptin regulation of bone mass, appetite, and energy expenditure. Cell 138(5):976-89.

[38] Ferron M, Wei J, Yoshizawa T, Del Fattore A, DePinho RA, Teti A, Ducy P, Karsenty G 2010 Insulin signaling in osteoblasts integrates bone remodeling and energy metabolism. Cell 142(2):296-308.

[39] Fulzele K, Riddle RC, DiGirolamo DJ, Cao X, Wan C, Chen D, Faugere MC, Aja S, Hussain MA, Bruning JC, Clemens TL 2010 Insulin receptor signaling in osteoblasts regulates postnatal bone acquisition and body composition. Cell 142(2):309-19.

[40] Oury F, Sumara G, Sumara O, Ferron M, Chang H, Smith CE, Hermo L, Suarez S, Roth BL, Ducy P, Karsenty G 2011 Endocrine regulation of male fertility by the skeleton. Cell 144(5):796-809.

[41] Quinn JM, Gillespie MT 2005 Modulation of osteoclast formation. Biochemical and biophysical research communications 328(3):739-45.

[42] Pixley FJ, Stanley ER 2004 CSF-1 regulation of the wandering macrophage: complexity in action. Trends in cell biology 14(11):628-38.

[43] Lacey DL, Timms E, Tan HL, Kelley MJ, Dunstan CR, Burgess T, Elliott R, Colombero A, Elliott G, Scully S, Hsu H, Sullivan J, Hawkins N, Davy E, Capparelli C, Eli A, Qian YX, Kaufman S, Sarosi I, Shalhoub V, Senaldi G, Guo J, Delaney J, Boyle WJ 1998 Osteoprotegerin ligand is a cytokine that regulates osteoclast differentiation and activation. Cell 93(2):165-76.

[44] Yasuda H, Shima N, Nakagawa N, Yamaguchi K, Kinosaki M, Mochizuki S, Tomoyasu A, Yano K, Goto M, Murakami A, Tsuda E, Morinaga T, Higashio K, Udagawa N, Takahashi N, Suda T 1998 Osteoclast differentiation factor is a ligand for osteoprotegerin/osteoclastogenesis-inhibitory factor and is identical to TRANCE/RANKL. Proceedings of the National Academy of Sciences of the United States of America 95(7):3597-602.

[45] Kiviranta R, Morko J, Alatalo SL, NicAmhlaoibh R, Risteli J, Laitala-Leinonen T, Vuorio E 2005 Impaired bone resorption in cathepsin K-deficient mice is partially compensated for by enhanced osteoclastogenesis and increased expression of other proteases via an increased RANKL/OPG ratio. Bone 36(1):159-72.

[46] Takayanagi H, Kim S, Koga T, Nishina H, Isshiki M, Yoshida H, Saiura A, Isobe M, Yokochi T, Inoue J, Wagner EF, Mak TW, Kodama T, Taniguchi T 2002 Induction and activation of the transcription factor NFATc1 (NFAT2) integrate RANKL signaling in terminal differentiation of osteoclasts. Developmental cell 3(6):889-901.

[47] Ishida N, Hayashi K, Hoshijima M, Ogawa T, Koga S, Miyatake Y, Kumegawa M, Kimura T, Takeya T 2002 Large scale gene expression analysis of osteoclastogenesis in vitro and elucidation of NFAT2 as a key regulator. The Journal of biological chemistry 277(43):41147-56.

[48] Asagiri M, Takayanagi H 2007 The molecular understanding of osteoclast differentiation. Bone 40(2):251-64.

[49] Sato K, Takayanagi H 2006 Osteoclasts, rheumatoid arthritis, and osteoimmunology. Current opinion in rheumatology 18(4):419-26.

[50] Takayanagi H 2007 The role of NFAT in osteoclast formation. Annals of the New York Academy of Sciences 1116:227-37.

[51] Ross FP, Teitelbaum SL 2005 alphavbeta3 and macrophage colony-stimulating factor: partners in osteoclast biology. Immunological reviews 208:88-105.

[52] Nakamura I, Gailit J, Sasaki T 1996 Osteoclast integrin alphaVbeta3 is present in the clear zone and contributes to cellular polarization. Cell and tissue research 286(3):507-15.

[53] Teitelbaum SL, Abu-Amer Y, Ross FP 1995 Molecular mechanisms of bone resorption. Journal of cellular biochemistry 59(1):1-10.

[54] Teitelbaum SL, Ross FP 2003 Genetic regulation of osteoclast development and function. Nature reviews. Genetics 4(8):638-49.

[55] Stenbeck G 2002 Formation and function of the ruffled border in osteoclasts. Seminars in cell & developmental biology 13(4):285-92.

[56] Aubin JE 2001 Regulation of osteoblast formation and function. Rev Endocr Metab Disord 2(1):81-94.

[57] Zaidi M 2007 Skeletal remodeling in health and disease. Nature medicine 13(7):791-801.

[58] Gori F, Hofbauer LC, Dunstan CR, Spelsberg TC, Khosla S, Riggs BL 2000 The expression of osteoprotegerin and RANK ligand and the support of osteoclast formation by stromal-osteoblast lineage cells is developmentally regulated. Endocrinology 141(12):4768-76.

[59] Yuasa T, Kataoka H, Kinto N, Iwamoto M, Enomoto-Iwamoto M, Iemura S, Ueno N, Shibata Y, Kurosawa H, Yamaguchi A 2002 Sonic hedgehog is involved in osteoblast differentiation by cooperating with BMP-2. Journal of cellular physiology 193(2):225-32.

[60] Nakashima A, Katagiri T, Tamura M 2005 Cross-talk between Wnt and bone morphogenetic protein 2 (BMP-2) signaling in differentiation pathway of C2C12 myoblasts. The Journal of biological chemistry 280(45):37660-8.

[61] de Jong DS, Steegenga WT, Hendriks JM, van Zoelen EJ, Olijve W, Dechering KJ 2004 Regulation of Notch signaling genes during BMP2-induced differentiation of osteoblast precursor cells. Biochemical and biophysical research communications 320(1):100-7.

[62] Hilton MJ, Tu X, Wu X, Bai S, Zhao H, Kobayashi T, Kronenberg HM, Teitelbaum SL, Ross FP, Kopan R, Long F 2008 Notch signaling maintains bone marrow mesenchymal progenitors by suppressing osteoblast differentiation. Nature medicine 14(3):306-14.

[63] Zanotti S, Smerdel-Ramoya A, Stadmeyer L, Durant D, Radtke F, Canalis E 2008 Notch inhibits osteoblast differentiation and causes osteopenia. Endocrinology 149(8):3890-9.

[64] Nishio Y, Dong Y, Paris M, O'Keefe RJ, Schwarz EM, Drissi H 2006 Runx2-mediated regulation of the zinc finger Osterix/Sp7 gene. Gene 372:62-70.

[65] Nakashima K, Zhou X, Kunkel G, Zhang Z, Deng JM, Behringer RR, de Crombrugghe B 2002 The novel zinc finger-containing transcription factor osterix is required for osteoblast differentiation and bone formation. Cell 108(1):17-29.

[66] Schroeder TM, Jensen ED, Westendorf JJ 2005 Runx2: a master organizer of gene transcription in developing and maturing osteoblasts. Birth defects research. Part C, Embryo today : reviews 75(3):213-25.

[67] Hessle L, Johnson KA, Anderson HC, Narisawa S, Sali A, Goding JW, Terkeltaub R, Millan JL 2002 Tissue-nonspecific alkaline phosphatase and plasma cell membrane

glycoprotein-1 are central antagonistic regulators of bone mineralization. Proceedings of the National Academy of Sciences of the United States of America 99(14):9445-9.

[68] Xu L, Anderson AL, Lu Q, Wang J 2007 Role of fibrillar structure of collagenous carrier in bone sialoprotein-mediated matrix mineralization and osteoblast differentiation. Biomaterials 28(4):750-61.

[69] Murshed M, McKee MD 2010 Molecular determinants of extracellular matrix mineralization in bone and blood vessels. Current opinion in nephrology and hypertension 19(4):359-65.

[70] Franz-Odendaal TA, Hall BK, Witten PE 2006 Buried alive: how osteoblasts become osteocytes. Developmental dynamics : an official publication of the American Association of Anatomists 235(1):176-90.

[71] Bonewald LF 2011 The amazing osteocyte. Journal of bone and mineral research : the official journal of the American Society for Bone and Mineral Research 26(2):229-38.

[72] Bonewald LF 2007 Osteocytes as dynamic multifunctional cells. Annals of the New York Academy of Sciences 1116:281-90.

[73] Bonewald LF, Johnson ML 2008 Osteocytes, mechanosensing and Wnt signaling. Bone 42(4):606-15.

[74] Palumbo C, Palazzini S, Zaffe D, Marotti G 1990 Osteocyte differentiation in the tibia of newborn rabbit: an ultrastructural study of the formation of cytoplasmic processes. Acta anatomica 137(4):350-8.

[75] Dallas SL, Bonewald LF 2010 Dynamics of the transition from osteoblast to osteocyte. Annals of the New York Academy of Sciences 1192:437-43.

[76] Kamel MA, Picconi JL, Lara-Castillo N, Johnson ML 2010 Activation of beta-catenin signaling in MLO-Y4 osteocytic cells versus 2T3 osteoblastic cells by fluid flow shear stress and PGE2: Implications for the study of mechanosensation in bone. Bone 47(5):872-81.

[77] Krempien B, Manegold C, Ritz E, Bommer J 1976 The influence of immobilization on osteocyte morphology: osteocyte differential count and electron microscopical studies. Virchows Archiv. A, Pathological anatomy and histology 370(1):55-68.

[78] Tazawa K, Hoshi K, Kawamoto S, Tanaka M, Ejiri S, Ozawa H 2004 Osteocytic osteolysis observed in rats to which parathyroid hormone was continuously administered. Journal of bone and mineral metabolism 22(6):524-9.

[79] Teti A, Zallone A 2009 Do osteocytes contribute to bone mineral homeostasis? Osteocytic osteolysis revisited. Bone 44(1):11-6.

[80] Locklin RM, Khosla S, Turner RT, Riggs BL 2003 Mediators of the biphasic responses of bone to intermittent and continuously administered parathyroid hormone. Journal of cellular biochemistry 89(1):180-90.

[81] Verborgt O, Tatton NA, Majeska RJ, Schaffler MB 2002 Spatial distribution of Bax and Bcl-2 in osteocytes after bone fatigue: complementary roles in bone remodeling regulation? Journal of bone and mineral research : the official journal of the American Society for Bone and Mineral Research 17(5):907-14.

[82] Takahashi H, Epker B, Frost HM 1964 Resorption Precedes Formative Activity. Surgical forum 15:437-8.

[83] Martin TJ, Sims NA 2005 Osteoclast-derived activity in the coupling of bone formation to resorption. Trends in molecular medicine 11(2):76-81.

[84] Walker EC, McGregor NE, Poulton IJ, Pompolo S, Allan EH, Quinn JM, Gillespie MT, Martin TJ, Sims NA 2008 Cardiotrophin-1 is an osteoclast-derived stimulus of bone

formation required for normal bone remodeling. Journal of bone and mineral research : the official journal of the American Society for Bone and Mineral Research 23(12):2025-32.

[85] Pederson L, Ruan M, Westendorf JJ, Khosla S, Oursler MJ 2008 Regulation of bone formation by osteoclasts involves Wnt/BMP signaling and the chemokine sphingosine-1-phosphate. Proceedings of the National Academy of Sciences of the United States of America 105(52):20764-9.

[86] Zhao C, Irie N, Takada Y, Shimoda K, Miyamoto T, Nishiwaki T, Suda T, Matsuo K 2006 Bidirectional ephrinB2-EphB4 signaling controls bone homeostasis. Cell metabolism 4(2):111-21.

[87] Boyce BF, Xing L 2008 Functions of RANKL/RANK/OPG in bone modeling and remodeling. Archives of biochemistry and biophysics 473(2):139-46.

[88] Kaplan RN, Riba RD, Zacharoulis S, Bramley AH, Vincent L, Costa C, MacDonald DD, Jin DK, Shido K, Kerns SA, Zhu Z, Hicklin D, Wu Y, Port JL, Altorki N, Port ER, Ruggero D, Shmelkov SV, Jensen KK, Rafii S, Lyden D 2005 VEGFR1-positive haematopoietic bone marrow progenitors initiate the pre-metastatic niche. Nature 438(7069):820-7.

[89] Aldridge SE, Lennard TW, Williams JR, Birch MA 2005 Vascular endothelial growth factor acts as an osteolytic factor in breast cancer metastases to bone. British journal of cancer 92(8):1531-7.

[90] Wilson TJ, Singh RK 2008 Proteases as modulators of tumor-stromal interaction: primary tumors to bone metastases. Biochimica et biophysica acta 1785(2):85-95.

[91] Zlotnik A 2006 Involvement of chemokine receptors in organ-specific metastasis. Contributions to microbiology 13:191-9.

[92] Dewan MZ, Ahmed S, Iwasaki Y, Ohba K, Toi M, Yamamoto N 2006 Stromal cell-derived factor-1 and CXCR4 receptor interaction in tumor growth and metastasis of breast cancer. Biomedicine & pharmacotherapy = Biomedecine & pharmacotherapie 60(6):273-6.

[93] Liang Z, Wu T, Lou H, Yu X, Taichman RS, Lau SK, Nie S, Umbreit J, Shim H 2004 Inhibition of breast cancer metastasis by selective synthetic polypeptide against CXCR4. Cancer research 64(12):4302-8.

[94] Rhodes LV, Short SP, Neel NF, Salvo VA, Zhu Y, Elliott S, Wei Y, Yu D, Sun M, Muir SE, Fonseca JP, Bratton MR, Segar C, Tilghman SL, Sobolik-Delmaire T, Horton LW, Zaja-Milatovic S, Collins-Burow BM, Wadsworth S, Beckman BS, Wood CE, Fuqua SA, Nephew KP, Dent P, Worthylake RA, Curiel TJ, Hung MC, Richmond A, Burow ME 2011 Cytokine receptor CXCR4 mediates estrogen-independent tumorigenesis, metastasis, and resistance to endocrine therapy in human breast cancer. Cancer research 71(2):603-13.

[95] Jung Y, Wang J, Song J, Shiozawa Y, Havens A, Wang Z, Sun YX, Emerson SG, Krebsbach PH, Taichman RS 2007 Annexin II expressed by osteoblasts and endothelial cells regulates stem cell adhesion, homing, and engraftment following transplantation. Blood 110(1):82-90.

[96] Mori K, Ando K, Heymann D, Redini F 2009 Receptor activator of nuclear factor-kappa B ligand (RANKL) stimulates bone-associated tumors through functional RANK expressed on bone-associated cancer cells? Histology and histopathology 24(2):235-42.

[97] Armstrong AP, Miller RE, Jones JC, Zhang J, Keller ET, Dougall WC 2008 RANKL acts directly on RANK-expressing prostate tumor cells and mediates migration and expression of tumor metastasis genes. The Prostate 68(1):92-104.

[98] Jones DH, Nakashima T, Sanchez OH, Kozieradzki I, Komarova SV, Sarosi I, Morony S, Rubin E, Sarao R, Hojilla CV, Komnenovic V, Kong YY, Schreiber M, Dixon SJ, Sims SM, Khokha R, Wada T, Penninger JM 2006 Regulation of cancer cell migration and bone metastasis by RANKL. Nature 440(7084):692-6.

[99] Rose AA, Pepin F, Russo C, Abou Khalil JE, Hallett M, Siegel PM 2007 Osteoactivin promotes breast cancer metastasis to bone. Molecular cancer research : MCR 5(10):1001-14.

[100] Furochi H, Tamura S, Mameoka M, Yamada C, Ogawa T, Hirasaka K, Okumura Y, Imagawa T, Oguri S, Ishidoh K, Kishi K, Higashiyama S, Nikawa T 2007 Osteoactivin fragments produced by ectodomain shedding induce MMP-3 expression via ERK pathway in mouse NIH-3T3 fibroblasts. FEBS letters 581(30):5743-50.

[101] Rose AA, Grosset AA, Dong Z, Russo C, Macdonald PA, Bertos NR, St-Pierre Y, Simantov R, Hallett M, Park M, Gaboury L, Siegel PM 2010 Glycoprotein nonmetastatic B is an independent prognostic indicator of recurrence and a novel therapeutic target in breast cancer. Clinical cancer research : an official journal of the American Association for Cancer Research 16(7):2147-56.

[102] Rose AA, Annis MG, Dong Z, Pepin F, Hallett M, Park M, Siegel PM 2010 ADAM10 releases a soluble form of the GPNMB/Osteoactivin extracellular domain with angiogenic properties. PloS one 5(8):e12093.

[103] Lu X, Wang Q, Hu G, Van Poznak C, Fleisher M, Reiss M, Massague J, Kang Y 2009 ADAMTS1 and MMP1 proteolytically engage EGF-like ligands in an osteolytic signaling cascade for bone metastasis. Genes & development 23(16):1882-94.

[104] Schwartz MA, Schaller MD, Ginsberg MH 1995 Integrins: emerging paradigms of signal transduction. Annual review of cell and developmental biology 11:549-99.

[105] Edlund M, Miyamoto T, Sikes RA, Ogle R, Laurie GW, Farach-Carson MC, Otey CA, Zhau HE, Chung LW 2001 Integrin expression and usage by prostate cancer cell lines on laminin substrata. Cell growth & differentiation : the molecular biology journal of the American Association for Cancer Research 12(2):99-107.

[106] Schneider JG, Amend SR, Weilbaecher KN 2011 Integrins and bone metastasis: integrating tumor cell and stromal cell interactions. Bone 48(1):54-65.

[107] van der P, Vloedgraven H, Papapoulos S, Lowick C, Grzesik W, Kerr J, Robey PG 1997 Attachment characteristics and involvement of integrins in adhesion of breast cancer cell lines to extracellular bone matrix components. Laboratory investigation; a journal of technical methods and pathology 77(6):665-75.

[108] Saad S, Gottlieb DJ, Bradstock KF, Overall CM, Bendall LJ 2002 Cancer cell-associated fibronectin induces release of matrix metalloproteinase-2 from normal fibroblasts. Cancer research 62(1):283-9.

[109] Shiozawa Y, Pedersen EA, Havens AM, Jung Y, Mishra A, Joseph J, Kim JK, Patel LR, Ying C, Ziegler AM, Pienta MJ, Song J, Wang J, Loberg RD, Krebsbach PH, Pienta KJ, Taichman RS 2011 Human prostate cancer metastases target the hematopoietic stem cell niche to establish footholds in mouse bone marrow. The Journal of clinical investigation.

[110] Jung Y, Shiozawa Y, Wang J, Patel LR, Havens AM, Song J, Krebsbach PH, Roodman GD, Taichman RS 2011 Annexin-2 is a regulator of stromal cell-derived factor-

1/CXCL12 function in the hematopoietic stem cell endosteal niche. Experimental hematology 39(2):151-166 e1.

[111] Shiozawa Y, Havens AM, Jung Y, Ziegler AM, Pedersen EA, Wang J, Lu G, Roodman GD, Loberg RD, Pienta KJ, Taichman RS 2008 Annexin II/annexin II receptor axis regulates adhesion, migration, homing, and growth of prostate cancer. Journal of cellular biochemistry 105(2):370-80.

[112] Singh S, Srivastava SK, Bhardwaj A, Owen LB, Singh AP 2010 CXCL12-CXCR4 signalling axis confers gemcitabine resistance to pancreatic cancer cells: a novel target for therapy. British journal of cancer 103(11):1671-9.

[113] Sharma MR, Koltowski L, Ownbey RT, Tuszynski GP, Sharma MC 2006 Angiogenesis-associated protein annexin II in breast cancer: selective expression in invasive breast cancer and contribution to tumor invasion and progression. Experimental and molecular pathology 81(2):146-56.

[114] Takayama T, Suzuki N, Narukawa M, Goldberg HA, Otsuka K, Ito K 2005 Enamel matrix derivative is a potent inhibitor of breast cancer cell attachment to bone. Life sciences 76(11):1211-21.

[115] van der Pluijm G, Vloedgraven HJ, Ivanov B, Robey FA, Grzesik WJ, Robey PG, Papapoulos SE, Lowik CW 1996 Bone sialoprotein peptides are potent inhibitors of breast cancer cell adhesion to bone. Cancer research 56(8):1948-55.

[116] Ibrahim T, Leong I, Sanchez-Sweatman O, Khokha R, Sodek J, Tenenbaum HC, Ganss B, Cheifetz S 2000 Expression of bone sialoprotein and osteopontin in breast cancer bone metastases. Clinical & experimental metastasis 18(3):253-60.

[117] Bunyaratavej P, Hullinger TG, Somerman MJ 2000 Bone morphogenetic proteins secreted by breast cancer cells upregulate bone sialoprotein expression in preosteoblast cells. Experimental cell research 260(2):324-33.

[118] Bellahcene A, Kroll M, Liebens F, Castronovo V 1996 Bone sialoprotein expression in primary human breast cancer is associated with bone metastases development. Journal of bone and mineral research : the official journal of the American Society for Bone and Mineral Research 11(5):665-70.

[119] Bramwell VH, Doig GS, Tuck AB, Wilson SM, Tonkin KS, Tomiak A, Perera F, Vandenberg TA, Chambers AF 2006 Serial plasma osteopontin levels have prognostic value in metastatic breast cancer. Clinical cancer research : an official journal of the American Association for Cancer Research 12(11 Pt 1):3337-43.

[120] Patani N, Jouhra F, Jiang W, Mokbel K 2008 Osteopontin expression profiles predict pathological and clinical outcome in breast cancer. Anticancer research 28(6B):4105-10.

[121] Nilsson SK, Johnston HM, Whitty GA, Williams B, Webb RJ, Denhardt DT, Bertoncello I, Bendall LJ, Simmons PJ, Haylock DN 2005 Osteopontin, a key component of the hematopoietic stem cell niche and regulator of primitive hematopoietic progenitor cells. Blood 106(4):1232-9.

[122] Kapoor P, Suva LJ, Welch DR, Donahue HJ 2008 Osteoprotegrin and the bone homing and colonization potential of breast cancer cells. Journal of cellular biochemistry 103(1):30-41.

[123] Garcia T, Jackson A, Bachelier R, Clement-Lacroix P, Baron R, Clezardin P, Pujuguet P 2008 A convenient clinically relevant model of human breast cancer bone metastasis. Clinical & experimental metastasis 25(1):33-42.

[124] Rucci N, Teti A 2010 Osteomimicry: how tumor cells try to deceive the bone. Frontiers in bioscience 2:907-15.

[125] Pratap J, Javed A, Languino LR, van Wijnen AJ, Stein JL, Stein GS, Lian JB 2005 The Runx2 osteogenic transcription factor regulates matrix metalloproteinase 9 in bone metastatic cancer cells and controls cell invasion. Molecular and cellular biology 25(19):8581-91.

[126] Leong DT, Lim J, Goh X, Pratap J, Pereira BP, Kwok HS, Nathan SS, Dobson JR, Lian JB, Ito Y, Voorhoeve PM, Stein GS, Salto-Tellez M, Cool SM, van Wijnen AJ 2010 Cancer-related ectopic expression of the bone-related transcription factor RUNX2 in non-osseous metastatic tumor cells is linked to cell proliferation and motility. Breast cancer research : BCR 12(5):R89.

[127] Pratap J, Wixted JJ, Gaur T, Zaidi SK, Dobson J, Gokul KD, Hussain S, van Wijnen AJ, Stein JL, Stein GS, Lian JB 2008 Runx2 transcriptional activation of Indian Hedgehog and a downstream bone metastatic pathway in breast cancer cells. Cancer research 68(19):7795-802.

[128] Das S, Samant RS, Shevde LA 2011 Hedgehog signaling induced by breast cancer cells promotes osteoclastogenesis and osteolysis. The Journal of biological chemistry 286(11):9612-22.

[129] Mi Z, Guo H, Wai PY, Gao C, Wei J, Kuo PC 2004 Differential osteopontin expression in phenotypically distinct subclones of murine breast cancer cells mediates metastatic behavior. The Journal of biological chemistry 279(45):46659-67.

[130] Holen I, Cross SS, Neville-Webbe HL, Cross NA, Balasubramanian SP, Croucher PI, Evans CA, Lippitt JM, Coleman RE, Eaton CL 2005 Osteoprotegerin (OPG) expression by breast cancer cells in vitro and breast tumours in vivo--a role in tumour cell survival? Breast cancer research and treatment 92(3):207-15.

[131] Fisher JL, Thomas-Mudge RJ, Elliott J, Hards DK, Sims NA, Slavin J, Martin TJ, Gillespie MT 2006 Osteoprotegerin overexpression by breast cancer cells enhances orthotopic and osseous tumor growth and contrasts with that delivered therapeutically. Cancer research 66(7):3620-8.

[132] Takayama S, Ishii S, Ikeda T, Masamura S, Doi M, Kitajima M 2005 The relationship between bone metastasis from human breast cancer and integrin alpha(v)beta3 expression. Anticancer research 25(1A):79-83.

[133] Mountzios G, Dimopoulos MA, Bamias A, Papadopoulos G, Kastritis E, Syrigos K, Pavlakis G, Terpos E 2007 Abnormal bone remodeling process is due to an imbalance in the receptor activator of nuclear factor-kappaB ligand (RANKL)/osteoprotegerin (OPG) axis in patients with solid tumors metastatic to the skeleton. Acta oncologica 46(2):221-9.

[134] Mercer RR, Miyasaka C, Mastro AM 2004 Metastatic breast cancer cells suppress osteoblast adhesion and differentiation. Clinical & experimental metastasis 21(5):427-35.

[135] Engin F, Yao Z, Yang T, Zhou G, Bertin T, Jiang MM, Chen Y, Wang L, Zheng H, Sutton RE, Boyce BF, Lee B 2008 Dimorphic effects of Notch signaling in bone homeostasis. Nature medicine 14(3):299-305.

[136] Sethi N, Dai X, Winter CG, Kang Y 2011 Tumor-derived JAGGED1 promotes osteolytic bone metastasis of breast cancer by engaging notch signaling in bone cells. Cancer cell 19(2):192-205.

[137] Goldring SR, Goldring MB 2007 Eating bone or adding it: the Wnt pathway decides. Nature medicine 13(2):133-4.

[138] Diarra D, Stolina M, Polzer K, Zwerina J, Ominsky MS, Dwyer D, Korb A, Smolen J, Hoffmann M, Scheinecker C, van der Heide D, Landewe R, Lacey D, Richards WG,

Schett G 2007 Dickkopf-1 is a master regulator of joint remodeling. Nature medicine 13(2):156-63.

[139] Qiang YW, Walsh K, Yao L, Kedei N, Blumberg PM, Rubin JS, Shaughnessy J, Jr., Rudikoff S 2005 Wnts induce migration and invasion of myeloma plasma cells. Blood 106(5):1786-93.

[140] McCarthy HS, Marshall MJ 2010 Dickkopf-1 as a potential therapeutic target in Paget's disease of bone. Expert opinion on therapeutic targets 14(2):221-30.

[141] Bu G, Lu W, Liu CC, Selander K, Yoneda T, Hall C, Keller ET, Li Y 2008 Breast cancer-derived Dickkopf1 inhibits osteoblast differentiation and osteoprotegerin expression: implication for breast cancer osteolytic bone metastases. International journal of cancer. Journal international du cancer 123(5):1034-42.

[142] Fromigue O, Kheddoumi N, Lomri A, Marie PJ, Body JJ 2001 Breast cancer cells release factors that induced apoptosis in human bone marrow stromal cells. Journal of bone and mineral research : the official journal of the American Society for Bone and Mineral Research 16(9):1600-10.

[143] Mastro AM, Gay CV, Welch DR, Donahue HJ, Jewell J, Mercer R, DiGirolamo D, Chislock EM, Guttridge K 2004 Breast cancer cells induce osteoblast apoptosis: a possible contributor to bone degradation. Journal of cellular biochemistry 91(2):265-76.

[144] Roodman GD, Dougall WC 2008 RANK ligand as a therapeutic target for bone metastases and multiple myeloma. Cancer Treat Rev 34(1):92-101.

[145] Santini D, Galluzzo S, Vincenzi B, Zoccoli A, Ferraro E, Lippi C, Altomare V, Tonini G, Bertoldo F 2010 Longitudinal evaluation of vitamin D plasma levels during anthracycline- and docetaxel-based adjuvant chemotherapy in early-stage breast cancer patients. Annals of oncology : official journal of the European Society for Medical Oncology / ESMO 21(1):185-6.

[146] Hussein O, Tiedemann K, Komarova SV 2011 Breast cancer cells inhibit spontaneous and bisphosphonate-induced osteoclast apoptosis. Bone 48(2):202-11.

[147] Ouellet V, Tiedemann K, Mourskaia A, Fong JE, Tran-Thanh D, Amir E, Clemons M, Perbal B, Komarova SV, Siegel PM 2011 CCN3 impairs osteoblast and stimulates osteoclast differentiation to favor breast cancer metastasis to bone. American Journal of Pathology (in press).

[148] Blouin S, Basle MF, Chappard D 2008 Interactions between microenvironment and cancer cells in two animal models of bone metastasis. British journal of cancer 98(4):809-15.

[149] Taichman RS, Emerson SG 1994 Human osteoblasts support hematopoiesis through the production of granulocyte colony-stimulating factor. The Journal of experimental medicine 179(5):1677-82.

[150] Taichman RS 2005 Blood and bone: two tissues whose fates are intertwined to create the hematopoietic stem-cell niche. Blood 105(7):2631-9.

[151] Zhang J, Niu C, Ye L, Huang H, He X, Tong WG, Ross J, Haug J, Johnson T, Feng JQ, Harris S, Wiedemann LM, Mishina Y, Li L 2003 Identification of the haematopoietic stem cell niche and control of the niche size. Nature 425(6960):836-41.

[152] Nash KT, Phadke PA, Navenot JM, Hurst DR, Accavitti-Loper MA, Sztul E, Vaidya KS, Frost AR, Kappes JC, Peiper SC, Welch DR 2007 Requirement of KISS1 secretion for multiple organ metastasis suppression and maintenance of tumor dormancy. Journal of the National Cancer Institute 99(4):309-21.

[153] Yin JJ, Selander K, Chirgwin JM, Dallas M, Grubbs BG, Wieser R, Massague J, Mundy GR, Guise TA 1999 TGF-beta signaling blockade inhibits PTHrP secretion by breast cancer cells and bone metastases development. The Journal of clinical investigation 103(2):197-206.

[154] Powell GJ, Southby J, Danks JA, Stillwell RG, Hayman JA, Henderson MA, Bennett RC, Martin TJ 1991 Localization of parathyroid hormone-related protein in breast cancer metastases: increased incidence in bone compared with other sites. Cancer research 51(11):3059-61.

[155] Henderson M, Danks J, Moseley J, Slavin J, Harris T, McKinlay M, Hopper J, Martin T 2001 Parathyroid hormone-related protein production by breast cancers, improved survival, and reduced bone metastases. Journal of the National Cancer Institute 93(3):234-7.

[156] Bendre MS, Montague DC, Peery T, Akel NS, Gaddy D, Suva LJ 2003 Interleukin-8 stimulation of osteoclastogenesis and bone resorption is a mechanism for the increased osteolysis of metastatic bone disease. Bone 33(1):28-37.

[157] Bendre MS, Margulies AG, Walser B, Akel NS, Bhattacharrya S, Skinner RA, Swain F, Ramani V, Mohammad KS, Wessner LL, Martinez A, Guise TA, Chirgwin JM, Gaddy D, Suva LJ 2005 Tumor-derived interleukin-8 stimulates osteolysis independent of the receptor activator of nuclear factor-kappaB ligand pathway. Cancer research 65(23):11001-9.

[158] Bendre MS, Gaddy-Kurten D, Mon-Foote T, Akel NS, Skinner RA, Nicholas RW, Suva LJ 2002 Expression of interleukin 8 and not parathyroid hormone-related protein by human breast cancer cells correlates with bone metastasis in vivo. Cancer research 62(19):5571-9.

[159] Guo Y, Tiedemann K, Khalil JA, Russo C, Siegel PM, Komarova SV 2008 Osteoclast precursors acquire sensitivity to breast cancer derived factors early in differentiation. Bone 43(2):386-93.

[160] Tiedemann K, Hussein O, Sadvakassova G, Guo Y, Siegel PM, Komarova SV 2009 Breast cancer-derived factors stimulate osteoclastogenesis through the Ca2+/protein kinase C and transforming growth factor-beta/MAPK signaling pathways. The Journal of biological chemistry 284(48):33662-70.

[161] Gallet M, Mentaverri R, Sevenet N, Brazier M, Kamel S 2006 Ability of breast cancer cell lines to stimulate bone resorbing activity of mature osteoclasts correlates with an anti-apoptotic effect mediated by macrophage colony stimulating factor. Apoptosis: an international journal on programmed cell death 11(11):1909-21.

[162] Mohan S, Baylink DJ 1991 Bone growth factors. Clinical orthopaedics and related research (263):30-48.

[163] Wilson TJ, Nannuru KC, Singh RK 2009 Cathepsin G-mediated activation of pro-matrix metalloproteinase 9 at the tumor-bone interface promotes transforming growth factor-beta signaling and bone destruction. Molecular cancer research : MCR 7(8):1224-33.

[164] Massague J 2008 TGFbeta in Cancer. Cell 134(2):215-30.

[165] Mourskaia AA, Northey JJ, Siegel PM 2007 Targeting aberrant TGF-beta signaling in pre-clinical models of cancer. Anti-cancer agents in medicinal chemistry 7(5):504-14.

[166] Kingsley LA, Fournier PG, Chirgwin JM, Guise TA 2007 Molecular biology of bone metastasis. Molecular cancer therapeutics 6(10):2609-17.

[167] Nannuru KC, Singh RK 2010 Tumor-stromal interactions in bone metastasis. Current osteoporosis reports 8(2):105-13.

[168] Lindemann RK, Ballschmieter P, Nordheim A, Dittmer J 2001 Transforming growth factor beta regulates parathyroid hormone-related protein expression in MDA-MB-231 breast cancer cells through a novel Smad/Ets synergism. The Journal of biological chemistry 276(49):46661-70.

[169] Kakonen SM, Selander KS, Chirgwin JM, Yin JJ, Burns S, Rankin WA, Grubbs BG, Dallas M, Cui Y, Guise TA 2002 Transforming growth factor-beta stimulates parathyroid hormone-related protein and osteolytic metastases via Smad and mitogen-activated protein kinase signaling pathways. The Journal of biological chemistry 277(27):24571-8.

[170] Isowa S, Shimo T, Ibaragi S, Kurio N, Okui T, Matsubara K, Hassan NM, Kishimoto K, Sasaki A 2010 PTHrP regulates angiogenesis and bone resorption via VEGF expression. Anticancer research 30(7):2755-67.

[171] Derynck R, Zhang YE 2003 Smad-dependent and Smad-independent pathways in TGF-beta family signalling. Nature 425(6958):577-84.

[172] Dunn LK, Mohammad KS, Fournier PG, McKenna CR, Davis HW, Niewolna M, Peng XH, Chirgwin JM, Guise TA 2009 Hypoxia and TGF-beta drive breast cancer bone metastases through parallel signaling pathways in tumor cells and the bone microenvironment. PloS one 4(9):e6896.

[173] Mundy GR 2002 Metastasis to bone: causes, consequences and therapeutic opportunities. Nat Rev Cancer 2(8):584-93.

[174] Stopeck AT, Lipton A, Body JJ, Steger GG, Tonkin K, de Boer RH, Lichinitser M, Fujiwara Y, Yardley DA, Viniegra M, Fan M, Jiang Q, Dansey R, Jun S, Braun A 2010 Denosumab compared with zoledronic acid for the treatment of bone metastases in patients with advanced breast cancer: a randomized, double-blind study. Journal of clinical oncology : official journal of the American Society of Clinical Oncology 28(35):5132-9.

[175] Ellis GK, Bone HG, Chlebowski R, Paul D, Spadafora S, Fan M, Kim D 2009 Effect of denosumab on bone mineral density in women receiving adjuvant aromatase inhibitors for non-metastatic breast cancer: subgroup analyses of a phase 3 study. Breast cancer research and treatment 118(1):81-7.

[176] Fizazi K, Lipton A, Mariette X, Body JJ, Rahim Y, Gralow JR, Gao G, Wu L, Sohn W, Jun S 2009 Randomized phase II trial of denosumab in patients with bone metastases from prostate cancer, breast cancer, or other neoplasms after intravenous bisphosphonates. Journal of clinical oncology : official journal of the American Society of Clinical Oncology 27(10):1564-71.

[177] Gavriatopoulou M, Dimopoulos MA, Christoulas D, Migkou M, Iakovaki M, Gkotzamanidou M, Terpos E 2009 Dickkopf-1: a suitable target for the management of myeloma bone disease. Expert opinion on therapeutic targets 13(7):839-48.

[178] Terpos E, Heath DJ, Rahemtulla A, Zervas K, Chantry A, Anagnostopoulos A, Pouli A, Katodritou E, Verrou E, Vervessou EC, Dimopoulos MA, Croucher PI 2006 Bortezomib reduces serum dickkopf-1 and receptor activator of nuclear factor-kappaB ligand concentrations and normalises indices of bone remodelling in patients with relapsed multiple myeloma. Br J Haematol 135(5):688-92.

[179] Li C, Li R, Grandis JR, Johnson DE 2008 Bortezomib induces apoptosis via Bim and Bik up-regulation and synergizes with cisplatin in the killing of head and neck squamous cell carcinoma cells. Mol Cancer Ther 7(6):1647-55.

[180] von Metzler I, Krebbel H, Hecht M, Manz RA, Fleissner C, Mieth M, Kaiser M, Jakob C, Sterz J, Kleeberg L, Heider U, Sezer O 2007 Bortezomib inhibits human

osteoclastogenesis. Leukemia : official journal of the Leukemia Society of America, Leukemia Research Fund, U.K 21(9):2025-34.

[181] Heider U, Kaiser M, Muller C, Jakob C, Zavrski I, Schulz CO, Fleissner C, Hecht M, Sezer O 2006 Bortezomib increases osteoblast activity in myeloma patients irrespective of response to treatment. European journal of haematology 77(3):233-8.

[182] Rosen LS 2005 VEGF-targeted therapy: therapeutic potential and recent advances. The oncologist 10(6):382-91.

[183] Koutras AK, Fountzilas G, Makatsoris T, Peroukides S, Kalofonos HP 2010 Bevacizumab in the treatment of breast cancer. Cancer treatment reviews 36(1):75-82.

[184] Christodoulou C, Pervena A, Klouvas G, Galani E, Falagas ME, Tsakalos G, Visvikis A, Nikolakopoulou A, Acholos V, Karapanagiotidis G, Batziou E, Skarlos DV 2009 Combination of bisphosphonates and antiangiogenic factors induces osteonecrosis of the jaw more frequently than bisphosphonates alone. Oncology 76(3):209-11.

[185] Ortholan C, Durivault J, Hannoun-Levi JM, Guyot M, Bourcier C, Ambrosetti D, Safe S, Pages G 2010 Bevacizumab/docetaxel association is more efficient than docetaxel alone in reducing breast and prostate cancer cell growth: a new paradigm for understanding the therapeutic effect of combined treatment. European journal of cancer 46(16):3022-36.

[186] Bauerle T, Hilbig H, Bartling S, Kiessling F, Kersten A, Schmitt-Graff A, Kauczor HU, Delorme S, Berger MR 2008 Bevacizumab inhibits breast cancer-induced osteolysis, surrounding soft tissue metastasis, and angiogenesis in rats as visualized by VCT and MRI. Neoplasia 10(5):511-20.

[187] Addison WN, Azari F, Sorensen ES, Kaartinen MT, McKee MD 2007 Pyrophosphate inhibits mineralization of osteoblast cultures by binding to mineral, up-regulating osteopontin, and inhibiting alkaline phosphatase activity. The Journal of biological chemistry 282(21):15872-83.

[188] Keller MI 2004 Treating osteoporosis in post-menopausal women: a case approach. Cleveland Clinic journal of medicine 71(10):829-37.

[189] Rizzoli R 2011 Bisphosphonates for post-menopausal osteoporosis: are they all the same? QJM : monthly journal of the Association of Physicians 104(4):281-300.

[190] Aft R 2011 Bisphosphonates in breast cancer: clinical activity and implications of preclinical data. Clinical advances in hematology & oncology : H&O 9(3):194-205.

[191] Sun M, Iqbal J, Singh S, Sun L, Zaidi M 2010 The crossover of bisphosphonates to cancer therapy. Annals of the New York Academy of Sciences 1211:107-12.

[192] Bamias A, Kastritis E, Bamia C, Moulopoulos LA, Melakopoulos I, Bozas G, Koutsoukou V, Gika D, Anagnostopoulos A, Papadimitriou C, Terpos E, Dimopoulos MA 2005 Osteonecrosis of the jaw in cancer after treatment with bisphosphonates: incidence and risk factors. Journal of clinical oncology : official journal of the American Society of Clinical Oncology 23(34):8580-7.

12

Junctional Adhesion Molecules (JAMs) - New Players in Breast Cancer?

Gozie Offiah, Kieran Brennan and Ann M. Hopkins
Royal College of Surgeons in Ireland, Beaumont Hospital, Dublin
Ireland

1. Introduction

1.1 Global incidence of breast cancer

Worldwide, breast cancer remains a leading cause of death amongst women. Annually, it is estimated that breast cancer is diagnosed in over a million women (Kasler *et al.*, 2009) with over 450,000 deaths worldwide (Tirona *et al.*, 2010). The incidence of the disease is highest in economically-developed countries, with lower rates in developing countries. Despite continual advances in breast cancer care which have led to reduced mortality, however, the incidence of the disease is still rising. The decrease in breast cancer-specific mortality has been attributed to improvements in screening techniques which permit earlier detection, surgical and radiotherapy interventions, better understanding of disease pathogenesis and utilization of traditional chemotherapies in a more efficacious manner. Consequently, early stage breast cancer is now a curable disease while advanced breast cancer remains a significant clinical problem.

Breast cancer is a heterogeneous disease encompassing many subtypes, which differ both in terms of their molecular backgrounds and clinical prognosis. These breast cancer subtypes range from pre-invasive early stage disease to advanced invasive disease. The simplest classifications of disease subdivide breast cancer into pre-invasive and invasive forms; with the pre-invasive forms being ductal carcinoma *in situ* (DCIS) and lobular carcinoma *in situ* (LCIS). Carcinoma *in situ* is proliferation of cancer cells within the epithelial tissue without invasion of the surrounding stromal tissue (Bland & Copeland, 1998). DCIS arises in the terminal ductal lobular units (TDLU) and in extra-lobular ducts while LCIS occurs in the breast lobules, and is recognisable histopathologically by the presence of populations of aberrant cells with small nuclei (Hanby & Hughes, 2008). Invasive breast cancers are sub-classified into invasive ductal breast cancer, invasive lobular breast cancer, inflammatory breast cancer and Paget's disease. Invasive ductal carcinoma (IDC) is the most common form of invasive breast cancer, accounting for around 85% of all cases.

DCIS is frequently considered as an obligate precursor to IDC, progressing from lower to higher grades and then onto invasive cancer with progressive accumulation of genomic changes (Farabegoli *et al.*, 2002). However it has alternately been suggested that there exist genetically-distinct subgroups of DCIS, only some of which have the potential to progress to invasion (Shackney & Silverman, 2003). Long-term natural history studies of DCIS have provided supportive evidence for both possibilities (Page *et al.*, 1995; Collins *et al.*, 2005; Sanders *et al.*, 2005). Despite such controversies, the large extent to which the genome is altered in DCIS strongly suggests that genomic instability precedes phenotypic evidence of invasion (Hwang *et al.*, 2004). This serves to underline the fact that malignant transformation in a heterogeneous disease like breast cancer is a dynamic process evolving through multiple multi-step pathway models.

Many factors are thought to be responsible for the development of breast cancer. Genetic factors play a vital role in the predisposition to breast cancer, with mutations of *BRCA1* and *BRCA2* genes accounting for 5–10% of breast cancer cases and being responsible for 80% of inherited breast cancers (Nathanson *et al.*, 2001). On a more complex level, much insight has been gained from the genetic profiling of thousands of tumours to generate gene signatures of prognostic value (Sorlie *et al.*, 2001; van 't Veer *et al.*, 2002; van de Vijver *et al.*, 2002), which have spurred the development of commercially-available diagnostic tests. The importance of reproductive factors in the aetiology of breast cancer is also well recognised with early onset of menarche, nulliparity, late menopause, endogenous and exogenous hormones representing the main risk factors (Reeves *et al.*, 2000; Key *et al.*, 2001; Howell & Evans, 2011). Several other studies have reported an increased risk of breast cancer with lack of physical activity (especially in pre menopausal women), as well as increasing age and obesity (Clarke *et al.*, 2006; Walker & Martin, 2007; Harrison *et al.*, 2009; Rod *et al.*, 2009; Awatef *et al.*, 2011). These risk factors accentuate the abnormal growth control of cells by increasing the circulating levels of oestrogen thereby promoting tumourigenesis within the breast microenvironment. A proper understanding of the breast cancer microenvironment is essential for understanding breast cancer, and will be explored in detail in the next sections.

1.2 Breast structure and breast cancer microenvironment

The breasts are modified sweat glands with a specialized function to produce milk. In the adult, the mature breast extends from the second ribs to the seventh rib and from the lateral border of the sternum to the midaxillary line and projects into the axilla at the axillary tail of Spence (Monkhouse, 2007). The breast is located within the superficial fascia of the anterior thoracic wall and is made up of 15-20 lobes of glandular tissue (Bland & Copeland, 1998). Fibrous connective tissue forms the framework that supports the lobes and adipose tissue which fills the space between the lobes. Each lobe of the mammary gland terminates in a lactiferous duct which opens onto the nipple and is lined with breast epithelial tissue. These ducts have a sinus at the base beneath the areola called the lactiferous sinus (Figure 1).

Breast cancers are characterised by abnormal proliferation of breast epithelial cells and mostly originate in milk ducts (Sainsbury *et al.*, 2000). Normal milk ducts consist of an outer myoepithelial cell layer and an inner luminal epithelial layer. Myoepithelial cells, which are of ectodermal origin, lie between the surface epithelial cells and the basal lamina. Both the epithelial and myoepithelial cells of the breast duct lie on a basement membrane composed of extracellular matrix factors secreted by those cells (Figure 2). The basement membrane is important for defining the barriers of the normal duct, and thus alterations in the basement membrane have been implicated in abnormal cell differentiation and the formation of metastases (Kleinman *et al.*, 2001).

Proliferation of cells within the breast ducts is controlled by growth-promoting proto-oncogenes and growth-inhibiting tumour suppressor genes. In most cases, normal cells divide as many times as needed and then stop. Carcinogenic mutations in either (or both) oncogenes and tumour suppressor genes (along with subsequent interactions between defective genes and the breast microenvironment) alter not just cell proliferation, but also differentiation, survival and genome stability (Hahn & Weinberg, 2002) of breast cells, leading to abnormal cell growth and potentially cancer.

Much evidence supports the contention that the pathogenesis of breast cancer is influenced by complex interactions between ductal epithelial cells and the cells that compose the tumour microenvironment (Weaver *et al.*, 1996; Polyak & Hu, 2005; Hu *et al.*, 2008). The next section will focus on the cells of the microenvironment with respect to normal breast tissue structure and also their possible involvement in breast tumourigenesis.

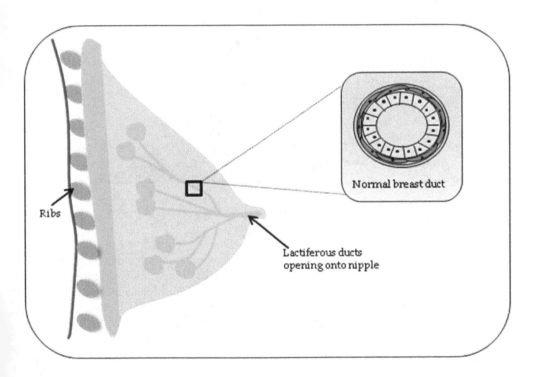

Fig. 1. Structure of the breast showing lobules and lactiferous ducts terminating at the nipple

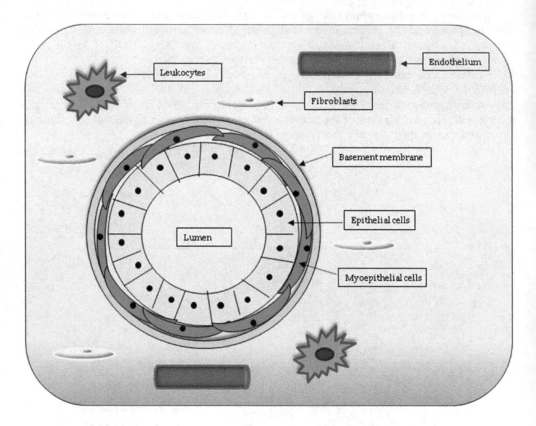

Fig. 2. Diagram of a normal breast duct depicting cells of the microenvironment.

1.2.1 Cells of the breast microenvironment

The abnormal epithelial cells composing a breast carcinoma form only one component of a complex microenvironment which influences the success or failure of a developing tumour. In fact the breast tumour microenvironment consists also of multiple cell types; including myoepithelial cells, fibroblasts, endothelial cells and immune cells such as macrophages (Figure 2). In terms of their likely contributions to breast tumourigenesis, fibroblasts and macrophages are often considered as tumour promoters through downstream signalling from various secreted factors, while the endothelial cells which develop in tumour-associated blood vessels also support cancer development. In contrast, myoepithelial cells exert functions broadly considered as tumour-suppressive.

Fibroblasts are an important structural component of the extracellular environment in the normal breast, where they help control the development of the breast epithelium (McCave *et al.* 2010). Their secretion of extracellular matrix components and cytokines has also implicated them in tumorigenic growth associated with invasive breast cancer (Orimo *et al.*, 2005), and differences in cellular responsiveness to normal versus tumour-derived fibroblasts have been noted (Sadlonova *et al.*, 2005). Many studies have highlighted the potential involvement of fibroblasts in promoting tumour progression both at genomic and transcriptomic levels, with reports of altered genetic signatures between normal and tumour-associated fibroblasts supporting a complex role for fibroblasts in influencing tumour progression (Hu et al., 2005; Hu et al., 2008; Ma et al., 2009).

Macrophages within the breast cancer microenvironment have been shown to enhance tumour growth through the secretion of pro-angiogenic factors like vascular endothelial growth factor (VEGF); (Murdoch et al., 2004; Lamagna et al., 2005 ; Lewis & Hughes, 2007). They have also been implicated in promoting a metastatic phenotype, via the secretion of pro-migratory factors such as EGF (Wyckoff et al., 2004) which enhance cellular dissemination from a primary tumour. Accordingly, the enhanced physical juxtaposition of macrophages, tumour cells and endothelial cells has been proposed as a new prognostic histopathological marker associated with increased risk of metastases in human breast cancer (Robinson et al., 2009).

Endothelial cells which line the blood vessels are derived from angioblasts forming the vascular network. Enhanced vessel density occurring as a result of tumour-associated angiogenesis is a major contributor to both the survival of primary breast tumours (via the delivery of systemic growth factors) and the risk of metastasis (via increased access of disseminated tumour cells to a circulatory source). Expression of pro-angiogenic factors such as VEGF has been shown to increase in haematological malignancies (Fiedler et al., 1997; Molica et al., 1999) in addition to solid tumours including breast, renal, ovarian, gastric and lung cancer (Patel et al., 2009; Burger, 2011; Gou et al., 2011; Sharma et al., 2011). VEGF promotes neovascularisation via mitogenic and pro-migratory effects on endothelial cells (Asahara et al., 1999).

Finally, myoepithelial cells are known to play a role in the formation of the basement membrane and thereby assist in maintaining polarity of the breast ductal epithelium. They also interact with epithelial cells to regulate the cell cycle and suppress breast cancer cell growth, invasion and angiogenesis (Weaver et al., 1996; Alpaugh et al., 2000; Barsky, 2003). Tumour and non-tumour primary myoepithelial cells have been described to differ in functional properties relating to the secretion of extracellular matrix components such as laminin-1 (Gudjonsson et al., 2002), and accordingly myoepithelial cells reportedly lose their established tumour-suppressive properties during tumour progression (Polyak & Hu, 2005). Taken together, the many cell types within the breast tumour microenvironment can both individually and coordinately regulate several functions relevant to tumour progression. In order to better understand their relative contributions to breast cancer, it is necessary to dissect the signals that regulate their own functions. Since adhesive functions are central to the behaviour of all of these cell types, the remainder of this chapter will focus on their potential regulation by a family of adhesion proteins termed the Junction Adhesion Molecules (JAMs), whose role in breast cancer initiation and progression is just emerging.

2. Cell-cell adhesion and the functional roles of JAMs in epithelial/endothelial cells

2.1 Introduction to cell-cell adhesion complexes and JAMs

Cells within the breast tumour microenvironment physically interact with each other and with the extracellular matrix through a range of cell adhesion proteins. Cell adhesion proteins play fundamental roles in normal physiology (such as the control of cell polarity and epithelial barrier function), but their dysregulation has been shown to participate in tumour cell migration, invasion and adhesion (for review, see Brennan et al.,2010). Adhesion proteins rarely exist in isolation from each other on the cell membrane, rather they form components of multi-cellular adhesion complexes containing a network of adhesion, scaffolding and signalling proteins. Breast epithelial cells express various types of adhesion complexes, namely hemidesmosomes and focal adhesions at the cell-matrix interface, with tight junctions, adherens junctions, desmosomes and gap junctions at the cell-cell interface. Collectively, adhesion complexes are composed of integral membrane proteins and cytoplasmic scaffolding proteins that organise signalling complexes and anchor cell-cell contacts to intermediate filaments (at desmosomes and hemidesmosomes) or to actin filaments (at adherens junctions, tight junctions and focal adhesions).

Tight junctions (TJs) play a vital role in regulating the paracellular flux of ions, small molecules and inflammatory cells as well as defining distinctly-polarized membrane domains and facilitating bi-directional signalling between the intracellular and extracellular compartments. These functions of the TJ are regulated by the balance of three different types of integral membrane proteins; (1) Occludins and Tricellulin, (2) Claudins and (3) Immunoglobulin Superfamily (IgSF) members. Of most interest in this chapter is the Junctional Adhesion Molecule (JAM) subfamily of the IgSF, and its potential contribution to cancer initiation and progression.

The JAM family consists of 5 proteins (JAM-A, -B, -C, -4, -L) which are major components of TJs in endothelial and epithelial cells in a variety of vertebrate and invertebrate tissues (Martin-Padura et al., 1998; Liang et al., 2000; Liu et al., 2000; Arrate et al., 2001; Aurrand-Lions et al., 2001; Itoh et al., 2001; Hirabayashi et al., 2003; Tajima et al., 2003). JAM proteins are also expressed on the surface of haematopoetic cells such as platelets, neutrophils, monocytes, lymphocytes, leukocytes and erythrocytes; in addition to connective tissue cells such as fibroblasts and smooth muscle cells (Azari et al., 2010; Kornecki et al., 1990; Naik et al., 1995; Malergue et al., 1998; Williams et al., 1999; Cunningham et al., 2000; Palmeri et al., 2000; Arrate et al., 2001; Aurrand-Lions et al., 2001; Moog-Lutz et al., 2003; Morris et al., 2006). JAMs are type I transmembrane proteins consisting of an N-terminal signal peptide, an extracellular domain (consisting of two immunoglobulin-like domains), a single membrane-spanning domain and a short cytoplasmic tail (Martin-Padura et al., 1998; Liu et al., 2000; Sobocka et al., 2000; Aurrand-Lions et al., 2001; Naik et al., 2001; Santoso et al., 2002). The cytoplasmic tail is thought to play a major role in the assembly of adhesion signalling complexes, since it has been reported to bind to PDZ domain-containing scaffold proteins such as ZO-1 (Bazzoni et al., 2000; Ebnet et al., 2000), AF-6 (Ebnet et al., 2000) and MUPP1 (Hamazaki et al., 2002).

JAMs -A, -B and -C exhibit a short cytoplasmic tail of 45–50 residues that ends with a type II PDZ binding motif, while JAM-4 and JAM-L have longer cytoplasmic tails (of 105 and 98 residues respectively). JAM-4 and JAM-L differ in that the cytoplasmic tail of the former ends in a canonical type I PDZ binding motif, while that of the latter lacks a PDZ-binding motif (Mandell & Parkos, 2005). The cytoplasmic tails of JAM proteins also contain consensus phosphorylation sites that may serve as substrates for protein kinase C, protein kinase A and Casein Kinase II (Naik et al., 1995; Cunningham et al., 2000; Ozaki et al., 2000; Sobocka et al., 2000; Arrate et al., 2001; Naik et al., 2001). Indeed, evidence suggests that specific phosphorylation sites may be critical for targeting of JAMs to intercellular junctions (Ozaki et al., 2000; Ebnet et al., 2003).

JAM proteins have been implicated in a diverse array of physiological functions involving cell–cell adhesion/barrier function (Liang *et al.*, 2000; Liu *et al.*, 2000; Mandell *et al.*, 2004), leukocyte migration (Martin-Padura *et al.*, 1998; Palmeri *et al.*, 2000; Johnson-Leger *et al.*, 2002; Ostermann *et al.*, 2002), platelet activation (Kornecki *et al.*, 1990; Naik *et al.*, 1995; Gupta *et al.*, 2000; Ozaki *et al.*, 2000; Sobocka *et al.*, 2000; Naik *et al.*, 2001; Babinska *et al.*, 2002; Babinska *et al.*, 2002) and angiogenesis (Naik *et al.*, 2003; Naik *et al.*, 2003). These functions will be further discussed in the next sections.

2.2 JAM proteins regulate epithelial/endothelial cell–cell adhesion and barrier function

JAM proteins are well-known to be important for cell-cell adhesion in both epithelial and endothelial cells (for review see Mandell & Parkos, 2005), but emerging evidence supports the possibility that they also regulate cell-matrix adhesion complexes. Interestingly, JAM-A knockdown in endothelial cells and MCF7 breast cancer cells has been shown to reduce adhesion to fibronectin and vitronectin (McSherry *et al.*, 2011; Naik & Naik, 2006), while JAM-C overexpression in endothelial cells reportedly decreases attachment to fibronectin, vitronectin, and laminin (Li *et al.*, 2009). This apparent incongruity may relate to the fact that JAM-A may activate β1 integrins (McSherry *et al.*, 2011), while JAM-C has conversely been described to inactivate β1 integrins (Li *et al.*, 2009). An inverse relationship between JAMs – A and –C has also been observed in terms of tight junction function, with JAM-A promoting tight junction sealing while phosphorylated JAM-C increases paracellular leakiness due to its redistribution away from TJs (Li *et al.*, 2009). Furthermore, adhesion of the lung carcinoma cell line NCI-H522 to endothelial cells was significantly blocked by soluble JAM-C (Santoso *et al.*, 2005).

The contribution of JAM proteins to cell-cell adhesion and the assembly of epithelial/endothelial TJs relates to their ability to promote the localization of ZO-1, AF-6, CASK and occludin at points of cell-cell contact. Evidence suggests that both homophilic and heterophilic interactions, as well as an intact PDZ binding motif, are important for such protein functions of JAMs. Accordingly, JAMs have been shown to physically interact with the PDZ proteins, ZO-1 (Bazzoni *et al.*, 2000; Ebnet *et al.*, 2000), AF-6 (Ebnet *et al.*, 2000), CASK (Martinez-Estrada *et al.*, 2001), PAR-3 (Ebnet *et al.*, 2001; Itoh *et al.*, 2001) and MUPP-1 (Hamazaki *et al.*, 2002); which are involved in actin cytoskeletal rearrangement (Fanning *et al.*, 2002), cell signalling (McSherry *et al.*, 2011; Boettner *et al.*, 2000) and the control of cell polarity. However JAMs can also bind to non-PDZ proteins such as cingulin (Bazzoni *et al.*, 2000), and indirectly bind occludin (Bazzoni *et al.*, 2000) and claudin 1 via their interactions with ZO-1 (Hamazaki *et al.*, 2002). Although the manner in which JAMs interact with some of these proteins is incompletely understood, it appears that homo-dimerisation of JAM proteins is important for regulating some key downstream functions. This has been illustrated by the fact that dimerisation-blocking anti-JAM-A antibodies (Liu *et al.*, 2000) and soluble Fc-JAM-A (Liang *et al.*, 2000) delay the recovery of electrical resistance (a marker of TJ function) in epithelial cells following transient depletion of extracellular calcium.

2.3 JAM proteins regulate epithelial/endothelial migration

In general cell adhesion and cell migration are inversely related, and serve to control important physiological functions and pathophysiological events. However, in the case of JAM family members, close functional associations with cell polarity proteins may act as a switch between increased adhesion (predisposing to slow, directional migration) and decreased adhesion (predisposing to faster, more random motility). For example, JAM-A re-expression in JAM-A-/- mouse endothelial cells has been shown to reduce the occurrence of spontaneous and random motility. This ability of JAM-A to influence the polarised movement of cells was reliant on its interaction with polarity proteins through its PDZ binding motif (Bazzoni & Dejana, 2004). JAM-A deletion mutants lacking their PDZ-binding residues have been shown to have increased availability of Par3 (Ebnet *et al.*, 2001), resulting in PKCζ inactivation and the loss of contact-dependent inhibition of cell motility (Mishima *et al.*, 2002; Bazzoni & Dejana, 2004). These data show that loss of functional JAM-A results in faster random motility with reduced cell-cell contact inhibition of migration. Interestingly, JAM-C redistribution away from TJs stimulates β1 and β3 integrin activation, resulting in increased cell migration and adhesion (Aurrand-Lions *et al.*, 2001). Furthermore, JAM-A and JAM-4 have been found to induce the formation of actin-based membrane protrusions, an essential part of cell migration, in endothelial and COS-7 cells (Mori *et al.*, 2004). Together these data suggest loss of JAM-A promotes random motility, while JAM-A, JAM-C and JAM-4 promote directional cell migration through their effects on integrin function and cytoskeletal reorganization.

In the context of cancer, knockdown of JAM-A has been shown to enhance invasiveness of the breast cancer cell lines MDA-MB-231 and T47D, and the renal cancer cell line RCC4 (Naik *et al.*, 2008; Gutwein *et al.*, 2009). Conversely, the overexpression of JAM-A in MDA-MB-231 cells reportedly inhibits both migration and invasion through collagen gels (Naik *et al.*, 2008), suggesting that loss of JAM-A expression increases cancer cell dissemination and invasion. However, the specific contribution of JAM-A to breast cancer progression remains controversial. McSherry *et al* showed a significant association between *high* JAM-A gene or protein expression and poor survival in 2 large cohorts of patients with invasive breast cancer, and concurrently a decrease in the migratory abilities of high JAM-A-expressing MCF-7 cells upon knockdown or functional inhibition of JAM-A (McSherry *et al.*, 2009). Reduced motility after JAM-A loss was subsequently linked to reduced interactions between JAM-A, AF-6 and the Rap1 activator PDZ-GEF2, resulting in reduced activity of Rap1 GTPase (McSherry *et al.*, 2011), a known activator of β1-integrins (Sebzda *et al.*, 2002) and a regulator of breast tumourigenesis (Itoh *et al.*, 2007). Complementary evidence in a recent publication by Gotte *et al.* has also supported the theory that JAM-A overexpression is of more functional relevance in breast cancer than JAM-A loss, since over-expression of micro RNA (miR)-145 in breast cancer cells led to a decrease in cellular migration and invasion via downregulation of JAM-A expression (Gotte *et al.*, 2010). Still more recently (during the proofing stage of this chapter), additional histopathological evidence has been provided for a link between JAM-A over-expression and poor prognosis in breast cancer patients (Murakami *et al.*, 2011). This, along with the finding that JAM-A promotes the survival of mammary cancer cells (Murakami *et al.*, 2011), strongly suggests that JAM-A depletion or antagonism could offer promise in reducing breast tumour progression. Furthermore, depletion of JAM-A has been found to inhibit bFGF-induced migration of human umbilical vein endothelial cells (HUVEC) on vitronectin, through effects on integrin function (Naik & Naik, 2006). In other cell systems, silencing of the JAM-A gene has been shown to block the migration of inflamed smooth muscle cells (Azari *et al.*, 2010) and to increase the random motility of dendritic cells (Cera *et al.*, 2004). JAM-A has also been shown to be required for neutrophil directional motility (Corada *et al.*, 2005), and to promote neutrophil chemotaxis by controlling integrin internalization and recycling (Cera *et al.*, 2009). Thus while the area remains controversial, increasing evidence is suggesting that JAMs promote migration and invasion through the regulation of integrin expression and activation (McSherry *et al.*, 2011; Naik & Naik, 2006; Li *et al.*, 2009; McSherry *et al.*, 2009).

In breast cancer, the formation of metastases at distant sites is the leading cause of cancer-related death. In order for breast cancer cells to metastasize, they must first migrate out of the primary tumour before ever reaching a distant organ and potentially proliferating into a secondary tumour. While JAMs are already known to regulate migration, the possibility that they are also involved in the regulation of proliferation will be referred to in section 3.3 of this chapter.

All together these data highlight the role of JAM family members in controlling the balance between cell adhesion and migration. Although much remains to be understood about the exact role of JAMs in breast cancer cell migration, the classic description of tumours as "wounds which do not heal" (Riss *et al.*, 2006) suggests that the migratory mechanisms employed by JAMs in physiological responses (such as wound healing) may also be utilised by cancer cells to promote tumour progression or survival.

2.4 Potential role of JAM proteins in epithelial/endothelial differentiation

In previous sections we discussed the biphasic role of JAM family members in regulating cell adhesion and migration. In this section we will outline the emerging contribution of the JAM family to cellular differentiation. Cell differentiation in the context of normal tissue usually involves the transition from an undifferentiated stem/progenitor cell to a terminally-differentiated cell such as an epithelial, muscle or nerve cell.

JAM-A, JAM-B, JAM-C and JAM-4 have been found to be highly expressed on hematopoietic stem cells (HSCs) in the bone marrow, with their expression decreasing during the acquisition of a more differentiated state (Nagamatsu *et al.*, 2006; Sakaguchi *et al.*, 2006; Sugano *et al.*, 2008; Praetor *et al.*, 2009). Furthermore JAM-A expression has been reported to be high on undifferentiated HC11 mammary epithelial cells relative to differentiated cells (Perotti *et al.*, 2009). In support of a potential association between high JAM-A and poor differentiation status, high JAM-A gene or protein expression has been associated with a poorer grade of differentiation in tissues from patients with invasive breast cancer (McSherry *et al.*, 2009). Conversely, JAM-A has been found to mediate the differentiation of CD34+ progenitor cells to endothelial progenitor cells and to facilitate CD34+ cell-induced re-endothelialization *in vitro* (Stellos *et al.*, 2010). This suggests that JAM-A is required for circulating CD34+ progenitor cells to recognise a site of injury, differentiate into endothelial cells and proliferate to repair the injured endothelium. In addition, JAM-A is reportedly upregulated during the differentiation of pancreatic AR42J cells (Yoshikumi *et al.*, 2008), while JAM-A mRNA and protein levels have been shown to be increased during differentiation of human monocytic cell THP-1 into mature dendritic cells (Ogasawara *et al.*, 2009). JAM-L is also induced during differentiation of myeloid leukaemia cells, with expression of JAM-L in myeloid leukaemia cells resulting in enhanced cell adhesion to endothelial cells (Moog-Lutz *et al.*, 2003). This upregulation of JAM-A during differentiation is reportedly followed by increased expression of the polarity proteins par3 and PKCλ (Yoshikumi *et al.*, 2008), which have been previously shown to affect cell polarity and migration. While these data suggest conflicting roles for JAMs in stem cell populations versus their role in differentiation, at this early stage the exact role(s) of JAMs in stem cell renewal or differentiation can only be speculated upon. Fundamentally, it is also unknown whether the expression of JAMs is actively required or passively upregulated in stem cell populations. However, based on the increased expression of JAM-A in poorly-differentiated breast cancers (McSherry *et al.*, 2009) and the emerging role of JAM-A in regulating proliferation and apoptosis (Azari *et al.*, 2010; Nava *et al.*, 2011; Naik *et al.*, 2003; Murakami *et al.*, 2011), it will be interesting to determine if JAM-A is upregulated on cancer stem cell populations and whether its expression promotes self-renewal.

3. Functional regulation of cells in the breast cancer microenvironment by JAMs

3.1 JAM proteins regulate endothelial angiogenesis

As already alluded to, JAM proteins are highly expressed on endothelial cells and have been crucially implicated in the control of barrier function and cell motility. In the context of cancer, however, endothelial cells assume a new importance via the development of neovascularisation sites to support growing tumours (Hanahan & Folkman, 1996). This section will review the evidence currently linking JAM proteins to angiogenesis as a contributory mechanism to cancer progression.

Angiogenesis in response to enhanced growth factor signalling is of particular relevance in tumour microenvironments. A body of work from Naik *et al* has convincingly shown an important role for JAM-A in angiogenesis induced by basic fibroblast growth factor (bFGF). Specifically, bFGF signalling facilitates the disassembly of an inhibitory complex between JAM-A and αvβ3 integrin, permitting JAM-A-dependent activation of MAP kinase which leads to endothelial tube formation, a surrogate for angiogenesis (Naik *et al.*, 2003). JAM-A has also been shown to activate extracellular signal-related kinase (ERK) signalling in response to bFGF, facilitating endothelial migration (Naik *et al.*, 2003) in a matrix-specific context (Naik & Naik, 2006). *In vivo*, JAM-A expression has been linked with the very early stages of murine embryonic vasculature development (Parris *et al.*, 2005), and although deletion of JAM-A appears to be dispensable for vascular tree development, homozygous JAM-null mice were found to be incapable of supporting FGF-2-induced angiogenesis in isolated aortic ring assays (Cooke *et al.*, 2006). In the context of tumour neovascularisation, others have reported reduced angiogenesis in a model of pancreatic carcinoma in JAM-A-null mice (Murakami *et al.*, 2010).

Other JAM family members appear to contribute similarly to angiogenesis; with functional blockade of JAM-C being shown to decrease aortic ring angiogenesis and block angiogenesis in hypoxic vessels of the murine retina (Lamagna *et al.*, 2005; Orlova *et al.*, 2006). Furthermore, soluble JAM-C shed into the serum of patients with inflammatory conditions (presumably following cleavage by ADAM enzymes) was noted to induce endothelial tube formation in a Matrigel model (Rabquer *et al.*, 2010). An interesting dichotomy, however, is that amplification of JAM-B in a trisomy-21 mouse model of Down's syndrome has been linked with reductions in VEGF-induced angiogenesis and thus anti-tumour effects in a lung carcinoma model in these mice (Reynolds *et al.*, 2010).

Taken together, these studies illustrate that by influencing angiogenic functions in endothelial cells, JAMs may indirectly influence the ability of tumours to survive and progress. While there appears to be a consensus that JAMs –A and –C activate signalling cascades that promote angiogenesis, it is possible that clear roles for the other family members in the regulation of angiogenesis will also emerge in time. It is tempting to speculate that pharmacological antagonism of JAMs will show promise as an option for blocking tumour progression, similar to the VEGF-A-neutralizing antibody bevacizumab (avastin) (Van Meter & Kim, 2010).

3.2 JAM proteins regulate trafficking of leukocytes

In addition to the potential regulatory roles of JAM proteins on the vascular endothelium, effects exerted on JAM-expressing leukocytes within the breast tumour microenvironment may also have relevance to cancer progression. For instance, JAMs are known to play important roles in the transendothelial migration of monocytes, which differentiate into macrophages once in the breast tissue. Accordingly, a function-blocking monoclonal antibody directed against JAM-A (BV11) has been described to inhibit spontaneous and chemokine-induced monocyte transmigration both *in vitro* and *in vivo* (Martin-Padura et al., 1998). Furthermore, treatment of mice with a monoclonal antibody directed against JAM-C has been shown to reduce macrophage infiltration into a murine lung tumour model (Lamagna et al., 2005), and to promote reverse transmigration of monocytes back into the bloodstream from inflamed tissue sites (Bradfield et al., 2007). Given the existence of a breast tumour-promoting paracrine loop between epidermal growth factor secreted by macrophages and colony-stimulating factor-1 secreted by tumour cells (Goswami et al., 2005), this implies that JAM-based regulation of monocyte transmigration could have a profound and self-amplifying influence on macrophage trafficking and tumour proliferation.

In the context of leukocytes other than monocytes/macrophages, many studies have implicated JAMs in the functional control of neutrophil transmigration across both epithelial (Zen et al., 2004; Zen et al., 2005) and endothelial (Sircar et al., 2007; Woodfin et al., 2007) barriers. As yet nothing is known about JAM-dependent events that might control neutrophil trafficking or activation within the breast tissue, despite the fact that neutrophils accumulate in highly aggressive inflammatory breast cancers. In other tissues, JAM-A has been shown to be required for efficient infiltration of neutrophils into the inflamed peritoneum or into the heart upon ischemia–reperfusion injury; as evidenced by increased adhesion and impaired transmigration in JAM-A-deficient mice (Corada et al., 2005). Interestingly, in this model JAM-A expression on the neutrophil appears to be more important than that on the endothelium; since selective loss of endothelial JAM-A did not phenocopy the transmigration deficits (Corada et al., 2005). In addition, soluble JAM-A shed from cultured endothelial cells has been shown to reduce *in vitro* transendothelial migration of neutrophils and to decrease neutrophil infiltration *in vivo* (Koenen et al., 2009).

Recent evidence also proves that family members other than JAM-A can participate in leukocyte trafficking, with JAM-C over-expressing mice exhibiting an increased accumulation of leukocytes into inflammatory sites or during ischaemia/reperfusion injury, while JAM-C neutralization or loss reduces leukocyte recruitment in models of lung, kidney or muscular inflammation (Aurrand-Lions et al., 2005; Scheiermann et al., 2009). Finally leukocytic expression of JAM-L has been shown to promote attachment to endothelium (Luissint et al., 2008), and functional inhibition of JAM-B is reported to decrease migration of peripheral blood lymphocytes across cultured human umbilical vein endothelial cells (HUVECs) (Johnson-Leger et al., 2002).

Collectively these data highlight an important role for JAMs in the migration of immune cells across endothelia, a mechanism that could be hijacked by JAM-overexpressing cancer cells as they leave the breast and invade into blood vessels.

3.3 JAM proteins and the regulation of stromal cells

The final grouping of breast cancer microenvironmental cells which will be discussed are stromal cells, broadly including fibroblasts and myoepithelial cells. Although little is known about JAM-mediated control of breast stromal cells specifically, insights from other cellular systems may suggest that this multifunctional family of proteins could have a hand in influencing the mesenchymal element of tumourigenic processes.

JAM-C expression has been noted on the surface of primary fibroblasts derived from human lung, skin and cornea (Morris *et al.*, 2006). The same authors observed JAM-A and JAM-C expression on the widely-studied NIH-3T3 fibroblast cell line. Interestingly, high JAM-C expression on synovial fibroblasts has been associated with the pathology of murine experimental arthritis, and JAM-C antagonism shown to have functional benefits in reducing the severity of inflammation (Palmer *et al.*, 2007). An immunohistochemical study in human arthritis has also demonstrated JAM-C expression on the synovial fibroblasts of both osteoarthritis and rheumatoid arthritis patients, in conjunction with JAM-C-dependent adhesion of myeloid cells to these fibroblasts (Rabquer *et al.*, 2008). Enhanced expression of JAM-A has also been described on the skin of patients with the inflammatory disorder systemic sclerosis, in comparison to that on normal dermal fibroblasts (Hou *et al.*, 2009).

Aside from facilitating adhesion of leukocytic cells to stromal elements such as fibroblasts, another way in which JAM family members could influence the breast cancer microenvironment is by altering proliferation of fibroblasts or other accessory cells. JAM-A has been reported to be required for proliferation of vascular smooth muscle cells, since JAM-A gene silencing exerted anti-proliferative effects in this system (Azari *et al.*, 2010). Whether this is through direct or indirect mechanisms remains uncertain, particularly in light of conflicting evidence in intestinal epithelial cells suggesting that JAM-A expression restricts proliferation by inhibiting Akt-dependent Wnt signalling (Nava *et al.*, 2011). However functional inhibition of the extracellular domain of JAM-A has been shown to inhibit bFGF-induced endothelial cell proliferation, and overexpression of JAM-A was also found to increase endothelial cell proliferation (Naik *et al.*, 2003). Accordingly, very recent evidence has suggested that JAM-A expression exerts a negative tone on apoptosis in the mammary epithelium (Murakami *et al.*, 2011). It is likely that processes as crucial as proliferation are strictly regulated in a spatial manner, which could account for tissue-specific differences as observed from the little available evidence to date. Whether or not JAM family members may influence proliferation of breast stromal cells like fibroblasts and the myoepithelium remains to be investigated. However, it is tempting to speculate that the acquisition of a proliferative phenotype in tumours may be co-ordinately linked to the pro-migratory "mesenchymal" phenotypes observed in many aggressive, poorly-differentiated breast cancers, to which evidence has already linked members of the JAM family. Co-culture models which better recapitulate the complexity of the breast cancer microenvironment than mono-cultures (Holliday *et al.*, 2009) may offer promise in dissecting the relative cellular contributions of JAMs to tumour progression at a reductionist level.

4. JAMs as novel potential drug targets in breast cancer

The pleiotrophic roles of JAM family members in regulating both the breast epithelium and cells of the microenvironment may suggest JAMs as novel therapeutic targets for the future management of breast cancer. Whether by aiming to block migratory behaviour, angiogenesis, proliferation or to promote polarisation and differentiation, selective pharmacological targeting of JAM molecules could prove particularly useful in cancers that overexpress one or more JAMs. This naturally pre-supposes that JAMs are causally involved in the disease process rather than simply acting as passive biomarkers, a fact that remains to be solidified. However, irrespective of the last caveat, another facet worth exploring is the potential of targeting JAMs to promote drug delivery. Since tight junctions (TJs) as a whole are primary regulators of paracellular transport across epithelial cells (Gonzalez-Mariscal et al., 2005), successful drug delivery may require modulation of TJ proteins to allow drug molecules to pass (Matsuhisa et al., 2009). However disruption of TJ proteins for drug delivery purposes is a double-edged sword, given the risk of disrupting homeostatic mechanisms of polarity, differentiation and migration which are tightly regulated by TJs in normal tissues and whose dysregulation may themselves promote tumourigenesis.

As yet, there are no cancer therapies on the market which specifically target tight junctions. However several tight junction proteins have been described as receptors for specific molecules or organisms, and as such, these might provide valid and novel targets for drug delivery. A particular precedent exists with the claudin family of TJ proteins; Claudins-3 and -4 having been suggested as drug delivery targets since they act as the receptor for *Clostridium perfringens* enterotoxin (CPE). The ability of CPE to rapidly and specifically lyse cells expressing claudin-3 or -4 could potentially be exploited in the treatment of breast cancers over-expressing these proteins (Katahira et al., 1997; Morin, 2005; Santin et al., 2007; Santin et al., 2007). Sub-lytic doses of CPE could alternatively be used to compromise TJs thus enhancing the influx of drug molecules across the epithelium. This could be of particular benefit in accessing hypoxic tumour cores, around which the tumour cells may be very tightly packed and thus relatively inaccessible to chemotherapeutic drugs. To date CPE administration has been shown to reduce growth of claudin-4 overexpressing pancreatic tumour cells (Michl et al., 2001; Michl et al., 2003), but their potential use in other cancer settings remains an open question.

How JAM molecules might be therapeutically targeted also remains an unanswered question, but one could predict value in using monoclonal antibodies or small molecule inhibitors to block the signalling functions which contribute to processes such as migration and angiogenesis. However, to date, the role of JAMs as chemotherapeutic targets (or even prognostic/predictive biomarkers) in the clinical setting of breast cancer has yet to be elucidated and validated. Following the lead of JAM-A as a potential biomarker and therapeutic target for breast cancer (McSherry et al., 2009; Gotte et al., 2010; McSherry et al., 2011; Murakami et al., 2011), we speculate that this will be a lucrative area of research in the future.

5. Conclusion

To conclude, breast cancer remains a leading cause of cancer worldwide (Jemal et al., 2008), and the search for new targets of prognostic and therapeutic relevance will continue particularly in this era where semi-personalised medicine is becoming more of a likelihood than an aspiration.

This chapter has attempted to summarize the known roles of the JAM family in controlling cell adhesion, polarity and barrier function, and their emerging roles in controlling functional behaviours within cells of the breast tumour microenvironment which promote cancer progression. Finally, it introduced the topic of JAM as a potential drug target in breast cancer; whether to directly influence JAM-dependent oncogenic signalling or indeed to interfere with cell-cell adhesion for the purposes of enhancing drug delivery. Continued expansion in our understanding of the cell and molecular biology of JAMs and their roles in tumour progression may open up new horizons supporting their evaluation as breast cancer biomarkers and drug targets of the future.

6. References

Alpaugh, ML, Lee, MC, Nguyen, M, Deato, M, Dishakjian, L et al. (2000). Myoepithelial-specific CD44 shedding contributes to the anti-invasive and antiangiogenic phenotype of myoepithelial cells. *Exp Cell Res*, Vol. 261, No. 1, (2000), pp 150-8

Arrate, MP, Rodriguez, JM, Tran, TM, Brock, TA & Cunningham, SA (2001). Cloning of human junctional adhesion molecule 3 (JAM3) and its identification as the JAM2 counter-receptor. *J Biol Chem*, Vol. 276, No. 49, (2001), pp 45826-32

Asahara, T, Takahashi, T, Masuda, H, Kalka, C, Chen, D et al. (1999). VEGF contributes to postnatal neovascularization by mobilizing bone marrow-derived endothelial progenitor cells. *EMBO J*, Vol. 18, No. 14, (1999), pp 3964-72

Aurrand-Lions, M, Duncan, L, Ballestrem, C & Imhof, BA (2001). JAM-2, a novel immunoglobulin superfamily molecule, expressed by endothelial and lymphatic cells. *J Biol Chem*, Vol. 276, No. 4, (2001), pp 2733-41

Aurrand-Lions, M, Johnson-Leger, C, Wong, C, Du Pasquier, L & Imhof, BA (2001). Heterogeneity of endothelial junctions is reflected by differential expression and specific subcellular localization of the three JAM family members. *Blood*, Vol. 98, No. 13, (2001), pp 3699-707

Aurrand-Lions, M, Lamagna, C, Dangerfield, JP, Wang, S, Herrera, P et al. (2005). Junctional adhesion molecule-C regulates the early influx of leukocytes into tissues during inflammation. *J Immunol*, Vol. 174, No. 10, (2005), pp 6406-15

Awatef, M, Olfa, G, Rim, C, Asma, K, Kacem, M et al. (2011). Physical activity reduces breast cancer risk: A case-control study in Tunisia. *Cancer Epidemiol*, Vol. No. (2011), 1877-783x

Azari, BM, Marmur, JD, Salifu, MO, Cavusoglu, E, Ehrlich, YH et al. (2010). Silencing of the F11R gene reveals a role for F11R/JAM-A in the migration of inflamed vascular smooth muscle cells and in atherosclerosis. *Atherosclerosis*, Vol. 212, No. 1, (2010), pp 197-205

Babinska, A, Kedees, MH, Athar, H, Ahmed, T, Batuman, O et al. (2002). F11-receptor (F11R/JAM) mediates platelet adhesion to endothelial cells: role in inflammatory thrombosis. *Thromb Haemost*, Vol. 88, No. 5, (2002), pp 843-50

Babinska, A, Kedees, MH, Athar, H, Sobocki, T, Sobocka, MB et al. (2002). Two regions of the human platelet F11-receptor (F11R) are critical for platelet aggregation, potentiation and adhesion. *Thromb Haemost*, Vol. 87, No. 4, (2002), pp 712-21

Barsky, SH (2003). Myoepithelial mRNA expression profiling reveals a common tumor-suppressor phenotype. *Exp Mol Pathol*, Vol. 74, No. 2, (2003), pp 113-22

Bazzoni, G & Dejana, E (2004). Endothelial cell-to-cell junctions: molecular organization and role in vascular homeostasis. *Physiol Rev*, Vol. 84, No. 3, (2004), pp 869-901

Bazzoni, G, Martinez-Estrada, OM, Orsenigo, F, Cordenonsi, M, Citi, S et al. (2000). Interaction of junctional adhesion molecule with the tight junction components ZO-1, cingulin, and occludin. *J Biol Chem*, Vol. 275, No. 27, (2000), pp 20520-6

Bland, KI & Copeland, EM. (1998). *The Breast: Comprehensive Management of Benign and Malignant Diseases* (edition),

Boettner, B, Govek, EE, Cross, J & Van Aelst, L (2000). The junctional multidomain protein AF-6 is a binding partner of the Rap1A GTPase and associates with the actin cytoskeletal regulator profilin. *Proc Natl Acad Sci U S A*, Vol. 97, No. 16, (2000), pp 9064-9

Bradfield, PF, Scheiermann, C, Nourshargh, S, Ody, C, Luscinskas, FW *et al.* (2007). JAM-C regulates unidirectional monocyte transendothelial migration in inflammation. *Blood*, Vol. 110, No. 7, (2007), pp 2545-55

Brennan, K, Offiah, G, McSherry, EA & Hopkins, AM (2010). Tight junctions : a barrier to the initiation and progression of breast cancer? *J Biomed Biotechnol*, 2010; 2010:460607 (2010)

Burger, RA (2011). Overview of anti-angiogenic agents in development for ovarian cancer. *Gynecol Oncol*, Vol. 121, No. 1, (2011), pp 230-8

Cera, MR, Del Prete, A, Vecchi, A, Corada, M, Martin-Padura, I *et al.* (2004). Increased DC trafficking to lymph nodes and contact hypersensitivity in junctional adhesion molecule-A-deficient mice. *J Clin Invest*, Vol. 114, No. 5, (2004), pp 729-38

Cera, MR, Fabbri, M, Molendini, C, Corada, M, Orsenigo, F *et al.* (2009). JAM-A promotes neutrophil chemotaxis by controlling integrin internalization and recycling. *J Cell Sci*, Vol. 122, No. Pt 2, (2009), pp 268-77

Clarke, CA, Purdie, DM & Glaser, SL (2006). Population attributable risk of breast cancer in white women associated with immediately modifiable risk factors. *BMC Cancer*, Vol. 6, No. (2006), pp 170

Collins, LC, Tamimi, RM, Baer, HJ, Connolly, JL, Colditz, GA *et al.* (2005). Outcome of patients with ductal carcinoma in situ untreated after diagnostic biopsy: results from the Nurses' Health Study. *Cancer*, Vol. 103, No. 9, (2005), pp 1778-84

Cooke, VG, Naik, MU & Naik, UP (2006). Fibroblast growth factor-2 failed to induce angiogenesis in junctional adhesion molecule-A-deficient mice. *Arterioscler Thromb Vasc Biol*, Vol. 26, No. 9, (2006), pp 2005-11

Corada, M, Chimenti, S, Cera, MR, Vinci, M, Salio, M *et al.* (2005). Junctional adhesion molecule-A-deficient polymorphonuclear cells show reduced diapedesis in peritonitis and heart ischemia-reperfusion injury. *Proc Natl Acad Sci U S A*, Vol. 102, No. 30, (2005), pp 10634-9

Cunningham, SA, Arrate, MP, Rodriguez, JM, Bjercke, RJ, Vanderslice, P *et al.* (2000). A novel protein with homology to the junctional adhesion molecule. Characterization of leukocyte interactions. *J Biol Chem*, Vol. 275, No. 44, (2000), pp 34750-6

Ebnet, K, Aurrand-Lions, M, Kuhn, A, Kiefer, F, Butz, S *et al.* (2003). The junctional adhesion molecule (JAM) family members JAM-2 and JAM-3 associate with the cell polarity protein PAR-3: a possible role for JAMs in endothelial cell polarity. *J Cell Sci*, Vol. 116, No. Pt 19, (2003), pp 3879-91

Ebnet, K, Schulz, CU, Meyer Zu Brickwedde, MK, Pendl, GG & Vestweber, D (2000). Junctional adhesion molecule interacts with the PDZ domain-containing proteins AF-6 and ZO-1. *J Biol Chem*, Vol. 275, No. 36, (2000), pp 27979-88

Ebnet, K, Suzuki, A, Horikoshi, Y, Hirose, T, Meyer Zu Brickwedde, MK et al. (2001). The cell polarity protein ASIP/PAR-3 directly associates with junctional adhesion molecule (JAM). *EMBO J*, Vol. 20, No. 14, (2001), pp 3738-48

Fanning, AS, Ma, TY & Anderson, JM (2002). Isolation and functional characterization of the actin binding region in the tight junction protein ZO-1. *FASEB J*, Vol. 16, No. 13, (2002), pp 1835-7

Farabegoli, F, Champeme, MH, Bieche, I, Santini, D, Ceccarelli, C et al. (2002). Genetic pathways in the evolution of breast ductal carcinoma in situ. *J Pathol*, Vol. 196, No. 3, (2002), pp 280-6

Fiedler, W, Graeven, U, Ergun, S, Verago, S, Kilic, N et al. (1997). Vascular endothelial growth factor, a possible paracrine growth factor in human acute myeloid leukemia. *Blood*, Vol. 89, No. 6, (1997), pp 1870-5

Gonzalez-Mariscal, L, Nava, P & Hernandez, S (2005). Critical role of tight junctions in drug delivery across epithelial and endothelial cell layers. *J Membr Biol*, Vol. 207, No. 2, (2005), pp 55-68

Goswami, S, Sahai, E, Wyckoff, JB, Cammer, M, Cox, D et al. (2005). Macrophages promote the invasion of breast carcinoma cells via a colony-stimulating factor-1/epidermal growth factor paracrine loop. *Cancer Res*, Vol. 65, No. 12, (2005), pp 5278-83

Gotte, M, Mohr, C, Koo, CY, Stock, C, Vaske, AK et al. (2010). miR-145-dependent targeting of junctional adhesion molecule A and modulation of fascin expression are associated with reduced breast cancer cell motility and invasiveness. *Oncogene*, Vol. 29, No. 50, (2010), pp 6569-80

Gou, HF, Chen, XC, Zhu, J, Jiang, M, Yang, Y et al. (2011). Expressions of COX-2 and VEGF-C in gastric cancer: correlations with lymphangiogenesis and prognostic implications. *J Exp Clin Cancer Res*, Vol. 30, No. (2011), pp 14

Gudjonsson, T, Ronnov-Jessen, L, Villadsen, R, Rank, F, Bissell, MJ et al. (2002). Normal and tumor-derived myoepithelial cells differ in their ability to interact with luminal breast epithelial cells for polarity and basement membrane deposition. *J Cell Sci*, Vol. 115, No. Pt 1, (2002), pp 39-50

Gupta, SK, Pillarisetti, K & Ohlstein, EH (2000). Platelet agonist F11 receptor is a member of the immunoglobulin superfamily and identical with junctional adhesion molecule (JAM): regulation of expression in human endothelial cells and macrophages. *IUBMB Life*, Vol. 50, No. 1, (2000), pp 51-6

Gutwein, P, Schramme, A, Voss, B, Abdel-Bakky, MS, Doberstein, K et al. (2009). Downregulation of junctional adhesion molecule-A is involved in the progression of clear cell renal cell carcinoma. *Biochem Biophys Res Commun*, Vol. 380, No. 2, (2009), pp 387-91

Hahn, WC & Weinberg, RA (2002). Rules for making human tumor cells. *N Engl J Med*, Vol. 347, No. 20, (2002), pp 1593-603

Hamazaki, Y, Itoh, M, Sasaki, H, Furuse, M & Tsukita, S (2002). Multi-PDZ domain protein 1 (MUPP1) is concentrated at tight junctions through its possible interaction with claudin-1 and junctional adhesion molecule. *J Biol Chem*, Vol. 277, No. 1, (2002), pp 455-61

Hanahan, D & Folkman, J (1996). Patterns and emerging mechanisms of the angiogenic switch during tumourigenesis. *Cell*, Vol. 86, No. 3, (1996), pp 353-64

Hanby, AM & Hughes, TA (2008). In situ and invasive lobular neoplasia of the breast. *Histopathology*, Vol. 52, No. 1, (2008), pp 58-66

Harrison, SA, Hayes, SC & Newman, B (2009). Age-related differences in exercise and quality of life among breast cancer survivors. *Med Sci Sports Exerc*, Vol. 42, No. 1, (2009), pp 67-74

Hirabayashi, S, Tajima, M, Yao, I, Nishimura, W, Mori, H *et al*. (2003). JAM4, a junctional cell adhesion molecule interacting with a tight junction protein, MAGI-1. *Mol Cell Biol*, Vol. 23, No. 12, (2003), pp 4267-82

Holliday, DL, Brouilette, KT, Markert, A, Gordon, LA & Jones, JL (2009). Novel multicellular organotypic models of normal and malignant breast: tools for dissecting the role of the microenvironment in breast cancer progression. *Breast Cancer Res*, Vol. 11, No. 1, (2009), pp R3, 1465-542X

Hou, Y, Rabquer, BJ, Gerber, ML, Del Galdo, F, Jimenez, SA *et al*. (2009). Junctional adhesion molecule-A is abnormally expressed in diffuse cutaneous systemic sclerosis skin and mediates myeloid cell adhesion. *Ann Rheum Dis*, Vol. No. (2009), 1468-2060

Howell, A & Evans, GD (2011). Hormone replacement therapy and breast cancer. *Recent Results Cancer Res*, Vol. 188, No. (2011), pp 115-24

Hu, M, Yao, J, Cai, L, Bachman, KE, van den Brule, F *et al*. (2005). Distinct epigenetic changes in the stromal cells of breast cancers. *Nat Genet*, Vol. 37, No. 8, (2005), pp 899-905

Hu, M, Yao, J, Carroll, DK, Weremowicz, S, Chen, H *et al*. (2008). Regulation of in situ to invasive breast carcinoma transition. *Cancer Cell*, Vol. 13, No. 5, (2008), pp 394-406

Hwang, ES, DeVries, S, Chew, KL, Moore, DH, 2nd, Kerlikowske, K *et al*. (2004). Patterns of chromosomal alterations in breast ductal carcinoma in situ. *Clin Cancer Res*, Vol. 10, No. 15, (2004), pp 5160-7

Itoh, M, Nelson, CM, Myers, CA & Bissell, MJ (2007). Rap1 integrates tissue polarity, lumen formation, and tumorigenic potential in human breast epithelial cells. *Cancer Res*, Vol. 67, No. 10, (2007), pp 4759-66

Itoh, M, Sasaki, H, Furuse, M, Ozaki, H, Kita, T *et al*. (2001). Junctional adhesion molecule (JAM) binds to PAR-3: a possible mechanism for the recruitment of PAR-3 to tight junctions. *J Cell Biol*, Vol. 154, No. 3, (2001), pp 491-7

Jemal, A, Siegel, R, Ward, E, Hao, Y, Xu, J *et al*. (2008). Cancer statistics, 2008. *CA Cancer J Clin*, Vol. 58, No. 2, (2008), pp 71-96

Johnson-Leger, CA, Aurrand-Lions, M, Beltraminelli, N, Fasel, N & Imhof, BA (2002). Junctional adhesion molecule-2 (JAM-2) promotes lymphocyte transendothelial migration. *Blood*, Vol. 100, No. 7, (2002), pp 2479-86

Kasler, M, Polgar, C & Fodor, J (2009). [Current status of treatment for early-stage invasive breast cancer.]. *Orv Hetil*, Vol. 150, No. 22, (2009), pp 1013-21, 0030-6002 (Print)

Katahira, J, Sugiyama, H, Inoue, N, Horiguchi, Y, Matsuda, M *et al*. (1997). Clostridium perfringens enterotoxin utilizes two structurally related membrane proteins as functional receptors in vivo. *J Biol Chem*, Vol. 272, No. 42, (1997), pp 26652-8

Key, T, Verkasalo, P & Banks, E (2001). Epidemiology of breast cancer. *Lancet Oncol*, Vol. 2, No. (2001), pp 133-40,

Kleinman, HK, Koblinski, J, Lee, S & Engbring, J (2001). Role of basement membrane in tumor growth and metastasis. *Surg Oncol Clin N Am*, Vol. 10, No. 2, (2001), pp 329-38

Koenen, RR, Pruessmeyer, J, Soehnlein, O, Fraemohs, L, Zernecke, A *et al.* (2009). Regulated release and functional modulation of junctional adhesion molecule A by disintegrin metalloproteinases. *Blood*, Vol. 113, No. 19, (2009), pp 4799-809

Kornecki, E, Walkowiak, B, Naik, UP & Ehrlich, YH (1990). Activation of human platelets by a stimulatory monoclonal antibody. *J Biol Chem*, Vol. 265, No. 17, (1990), pp 10042-8

Lamagna, C, Hodivala-Dilke, KM, Imhof, BA & Aurrand-Lions, M (2005). Antibody against junctional adhesion molecule-C inhibits angiogenesis and tumor growth. *Cancer Res*, Vol. 65, No. 13, (2005), pp 5703-10

Lewis, CE & Hughes, R (2007). Inflammation and breast cancer. Microenvironmental factors regulating macrophage function in breast tumours: hypoxia and angiopoietin-2. *Breast Cancer Res*, Vol. 9, No. 3, (2007), pp 209

Li, X, Stankovic, M, Lee, BP, Aurrand-Lions, M, Hahn, CN *et al.* (2009). JAM-C induces endothelial cell permeability through its association and regulation of {beta}3 integrins. *Arterioscler Thromb Vasc Biol*, Vol. 29, No. 8, (2009), pp 1200-6

Liang, TW, DeMarco, RA, Mrsny, RJ, Gurney, A, Gray, A *et al.* (2000). Characterization of huJAM: evidence for involvement in cell-cell contact and tight junction regulation. *Am J Physiol Cell Physiol*, Vol. 279, No. 6, (2000), pp C1733-43

Liu, Y, Nusrat, A, Schnell, FJ, Reaves, TA, Walsh, S *et al.* (2000). Human junction adhesion molecule regulates tight junction resealing in epithelia. *J Cell Sci*, Vol. 113 (Pt 13), No. (2000), pp 2363-74

Luissint, AC, Lutz, PG, Calderwood, DA, Couraud, PO & Bourdoulous, S (2008). JAM-L-mediated leukocyte adhesion to endothelial cells is regulated in cis by alpha4beta1 integrin activation. *J Cell Biol*, Vol. 183, No. 6, (2008), pp 1159-73

Ma, XJ, Dahiya, S, Richardson, E, Erlander, M & Sgroi, DC (2009). Gene expression profiling of the tumor microenvironment during breast cancer progression. *Breast Cancer Res*, Vol. 11, No. 1, (2009), pp R7

Malergue, F, Galland, F, Martin, F, Mansuelle, P, Aurrand-Lions, M *et al.* (1998). A novel immunoglobulin superfamily junctional molecule expressed by antigen presenting cells, endothelial cells and platelets. *Mol Immunol*, Vol. 35, No. 17, (1998), pp 1111-9

Mandell, KJ, McCall, IC & Parkos, CA (2004). Involvement of the junctional adhesion molecule-1 (JAM1) homodimer interface in regulation of epithelial barrier function. *J Biol Chem*, Vol. 279, No. 16, (2004), pp 16254-62

Mandell, KJ & Parkos, CA (2005). The JAM family of proteins. *Adv Drug Deliv Rev*, Vol. 57, No. 6, (2005), pp 857-67

Martin-Padura, I, Lostaglio, S, Schneemann, M, Williams, L, Romano, M *et al.* (1998). Junctional adhesion molecule, a novel member of the immunoglobulin superfamily that distributes at intercellular junctions and modulates monocyte transmigration. *J Cell Biol*, Vol. 142, No. 1, (1998), pp 117-27

Martinez-Estrada, OM, Villa, A, Breviario, F, Orsenigo, F, Dejana, E *et al.* (2001). Association of junctional adhesion molecule with calcium/calmodulin-dependent serine protein kinase (CASK/LIN-2) in human epithelial caco-2 cells. *J Biol Chem*, Vol. 276, No. 12, (2001), pp 9291-6

Matsuhisa, K, Kondoh, M, Takahashi, A & Yagi, K (2009). Tight junction modulator and drug delivery. *Expert Opin Drug Deliv*, Vol. 6, No. 5, (2009), pp 509-15

McCave, EJ, Cass, CA, Burg, KJ & Booth, BW (2010). The normal microenvironment directs mammary gland development. *J Mammary Gland Biol Neoplasia*, Vol. 15, No. 3, pp 291-9

McSherry, EA, Brennan, K, Hudson, L, Hill, AD & Hopkins, AM (2011). Breast cancer cell migration is regulated through junctional adhesion molecule-A-mediated activation of Rap1 GTPase. *Breast Cancer Res*, Vol. 13, No. 2, (2011), pp R31

McSherry, EA, McGee, SF, Jirstrom, K, Doyle, EM, Brennan, DJ *et al.* (2009). JAM-A expression positively correlates with poor prognosis in breast cancer patients. *Int J Cancer*, Vol. 125, No. 6, (2009), pp 1343-51

Michl, P, Barth, C, Buchholz, M, Lerch, MM, Rolke, M *et al.* (2003). Claudin-4 expression decreases invasiveness and metastatic potential of pancreatic cancer. *Cancer Res*, Vol. 63, No. 19, (2003), pp 6265-71

Michl, P, Buchholz, M, Rolke, M, Kunsch, S, Lohr, M *et al.* (2001). Claudin-4: a new target for pancreatic cancer treatment using Clostridium perfringens enterotoxin. *Gastroenterology*, Vol. 121, No. 3, (2001), pp 678-84

Mishima, A, Suzuki, A, Enaka, M, Hirose, T, Mizuno, K *et al.* (2002). Over-expression of PAR-3 suppresses contact-mediated inhibition of cell migration in MDCK cells. *Genes Cells*, Vol. 7, No. 6, (2002), pp 581-96

Molica, S, Vitelli, G, Levato, D, Gandolfo, GM & Liso, V (1999). Increased serum levels of vascular endothelial growth factor predict risk of progression in early B-cell chronic lymphocytic leukaemia. *Br J Haematol*, Vol. 107, No. 3, (1999), pp 605-10

Monkhouse, S. (2007). *Clinical Anatomy* (edition), Churchill Livingstone Elsevier,

Moog-Lutz, C, Cave-Riant, F, Guibal, FC, Breau, MA, Di Gioia, Y *et al.* (2003). JAML, a novel protein with characteristics of a junctional adhesion molecule, is induced during differentiation of myeloid leukemia cells. *Blood*, Vol. 102, No. 9, (2003), pp 3371-8

Mori, H, Hirabayashi, S, Shirasawa, M, Sugimura, H & Hata, Y (2004). JAM4 enhances hepatocyte growth factor-mediated branching and scattering of Madin-Darby canine kidney cells. *Genes Cells*, Vol. 9, No. 9, (2004), pp 811-9

Morin, PJ (2005). Claudin proteins in human cancer: promising new targets for diagnosis and therapy. *Cancer Res*, Vol. 65, No. 21, (2005), pp 9603-6

Morris, AP, Tawil, A, Berkova, Z, Wible, L, Smith, CW *et al.* (2006). Junctional Adhesion Molecules (JAMs) are differentially expressed in fibroblasts and co-localize with ZO-1 to adherens-like junctions. *Cell Commun Adhes*, Vol. 13, No. 4, (2006), pp 233-47

Murakami, M, Francavilla, C, Torselli, I, Corada, M, Maddaluno, L *et al.* (2010). Inactivation of junctional adhesion molecule-A enhances antitumoral immune response by promoting dendritic cell and T lymphocyte infiltration. *Cancer Res*, Vol. 70, No. 5, (2010), pp 1759-65

Murakami, M, Giampietro, C, Giannotta, M, Corada, M, Torselli, I, Orsenigo, F, Cocito, A, d'Ario, G, Mazzarol, G, Confalonieri, S, Di Fiore, PP & Dejana, E (2011). Abrogation of junctional adhesion molecule-a expression induces cell apoptosis and reduces breast cancer progression. *PLoS One.* Vol. 6, No. 6, (2011), e21242. Epub 2011 Jun 17

Murdoch, C, Giannoudis, A & Lewis, CE (2004). Mechanisms regulating the recruitment of macrophages into hypoxic areas of tumors and other ischemic tissues. *Blood*, Vol. 104, No. 8, (2004), pp 2224-34

Nagamatsu, G, Ohmura, M, Mizukami, T, Hamaguchi, I, Hirabayashi, S *et al.* (2006). A CTX family cell adhesion molecule, JAM4, is expressed in stem cell and progenitor cell populations of both male germ cell and hematopoietic cell lineages. *Mol Cell Biol*, Vol. 26, No. 22, (2006), pp 8498-506

Naik, MU, Mousa, SA, Parkos, CA & Naik, UP (2003). Signaling through JAM-1 and alphavbeta3 is required for the angiogenic action of bFGF: dissociation of the JAM-1 and alphavbeta3 complex. *Blood*, Vol. 102, No. 6, (2003), pp 2108-14

Naik, MU, Naik, TU, Suckow, AT, Duncan, MK & Naik, UP (2008). Attenuation of junctional adhesion molecule-A is a contributing factor for breast cancer cell invasion. *Cancer Res*, Vol. 68, No. 7, (2008), pp 2194-203

Naik, MU & Naik, UP (2006). Junctional adhesion molecule-A-induced endothelial cell migration on vitronectin is integrin alpha v beta 3 specific. *J Cell Sci*, Vol. 119, No. Pt 3, (2006), pp 490-9

Naik, MU, Vuppalanchi, D & Naik, UP (2003). Essential role of junctional adhesion molecule-1 in basic fibroblast growth factor-induced endothelial cell migration. *Arterioscler Thromb Vasc Biol*, Vol. 23, No. 12, (2003), pp 2165-71

Naik, UP, Ehrlich, YH & Kornecki, E (1995). Mechanisms of platelet activation by a stimulatory antibody: cross-linking of a novel platelet receptor for monoclonal antibody F11 with the Fc gamma RII receptor. *Biochem J*, Vol. 310 (Pt 1), No. (1995), pp 155-62

Naik, UP, Naik, MU, Eckfeld, K, Martin-DeLeon, P & Spychala, J (2001). Characterization and chromosomal localization of JAM-1, a platelet receptor for a stimulatory monoclonal antibody. *J Cell Sci*, Vol. 114, No. Pt 3, (2001), pp 539-47

Nathanson, SD, Wachna, DL, Gilman, D, Karvelis, K, Havstad, S *et al.* (2001). Pathways of lymphatic drainage from the breast. *Ann Surg Oncol*, Vol. 8, No. 10, (2001), pp 837-43

Nava, P, Capaldo, CT, Koch, S, Kolegraff, K, Rankin, CR *et al.* JAM-A regulates epithelial proliferation through Akt/beta-catenin signalling. *EMBO Rep*, Vol. 12, No. 4, pp 314-20

Nava, P, Capaldo, CT, Koch, S, Kolegraff, K, Rankin, CR *et al.* (2011). JAM-A regulates epithelial proliferation through Akt/beta-catenin signalling. *EMBO Rep*, Vol. 12, No. 4, (2011), pp 314-20

Ogasawara, N, Kojima, T, Go, M, Fuchimoto, J, Kamekura, R *et al.* (2009). Induction of JAM-A during differentiation of human THP-1 dendritic cells. *Biochem Biophys Res Commun*, Vol. 389, No. 3, (2009), pp 543-9

Orimo, A, Gupta, PB, Sgroi, DC, Arenzana-Seisdedos, F, Delaunay, T *et al.* (2005). Stromal fibroblasts present in invasive human breast carcinomas promote tumor growth and angiogenesis through elevated SDF-1/CXCL12 secretion. *Cell*, Vol. 121, No. 3, (2005), pp 335-48

Orlova, VV, Economopoulou, M, Lupu, F, Santoso, S & Chavakis, T (2006). Junctional adhesion molecule-C regulates vascular endothelial permeability by modulating VE-cadherin-mediated cell-cell contacts. *J Exp Med*, Vol. 203, No. 12, (2006), pp 2703-14

Ostermann, G, Weber, KS, Zernecke, A, Schroder, A & Weber, C (2002). JAM-1 is a ligand of the beta(2) integrin LFA-1 involved in transendothelial migration of leukocytes. *Nat Immunol*, Vol. 3, No. 2, (2002), pp 151-8

Ozaki, H, Ishii, K, Arai, H, Horiuchi, H, Kawamoto, T *et al.* (2000). Junctional adhesion molecule (JAM) is phosphorylated by protein kinase C upon platelet activation. *Biochem Biophys Res Commun*, Vol. 276, No. 3, (2000), pp 873-8

Page, DL, Dupont, WD, Rogers, LW, Jensen, RA & Schuyler, PA (1995). Continued local recurrence of carcinoma 15-25 years after a diagnosis of low grade ductal carcinoma in situ of the breast treated only by biopsy. *Cancer*, Vol. 76, No. 7, (1995), pp 1197-200

Palmer, G, Busso, N, Aurrand-Lions, M, Talabot-Ayer, D, Chobaz-Peclat, V *et al.* (2007). Expression and function of junctional adhesion molecule-C in human and experimental arthritis. *Arthritis Res Ther*, Vol. 9, No. 4, (2007), pp R65

Palmeri, D, van Zante, A, Huang, CC, Hemmerich, S & Rosen, SD (2000). Vascular endothelial junction-associated molecule, a novel member of the immunoglobulin superfamily, is localized to intercellular boundaries of endothelial cells. *J Biol Chem*, Vol. 275, No. 25, (2000), pp 19139-45

Parris, JJ, Cooke, VG, Skarnes, WC, Duncan, MK & Naik, UP (2005). JAM-A expression during embryonic development. *Dev Dyn*, Vol. 233, No. 4, (2005), pp 1517-24

Patel, NS, Muneer, A, Blick, C, Arya, M & Harris, AL (2009). Targeting vascular endothelial growth factor in renal cell carcinoma. *Tumour Biol*, Vol. 30, No. 5-6, (2009), pp 292-9

Perotti, C, Wiedl, T, Florin, L, Reuter, H, Moffat, S *et al.* (2009). Characterization of mammary epithelial cell line HC11 using the NIA 15k gene array reveals potential regulators of the undifferentiated and differentiated phenotypes. *Differentiation*, Vol. 78, No. 5, (2009), pp 269-82

Polyak, K & Hu, M (2005). Do myoepithelial cells hold the key for breast tumor progression? *J Mammary Gland Biol Neoplasia*, Vol. 10, No. 3, (2005), pp 231-47

Praetor, A, McBride, JM, Chiu, H, Rangell, L, Cabote, L *et al.* (2009). Genetic deletion of JAM-C reveals a role in myeloid progenitor generation. *Blood*, Vol. 113, No. 9, (2009), pp 1919-28

Rabquer, BJ, Amin, MA, Teegala, N, Shaheen, MK, Tsou, PS *et al.* (2010). Junctional adhesion molecule-C is a soluble mediator of angiogenesis. *J Immunol*, Vol. 185, No. 3, (2010), pp 1777-85

Rabquer, BJ, Pakozdi, A, Michel, JE, Gujar, BS, Haines, GK, 3rd *et al.* (2008). Junctional adhesion molecule C mediates leukocyte adhesion to rheumatoid arthritis synovium. *Arthritis Rheum*, Vol. 58, No. 10, (2008), pp 3020-9

Reeves, GK, Patterson, J, Vessey, MP, Yeates, D & Jones, L (2000). Hormonal and other factors in relation to survival among breast cancer patients. *Int J Cancer*, Vol. 89, No. 3, (2000), pp 293-9

Reynolds, LE, Watson, AR, Baker, M, Jones, TA, D'Amico, G *et al.* (2010). Tumour angiogenesis is reduced in the Tc1 mouse model of Down's syndrome. *Nature*, Vol. 465, No. 7299, pp 813-7

Riss, J, Khanna, C, Koo, S, Chandramouli, GV, Yang, HH *et al.* (2006). Cancers as wounds that do not heal: differences and similarities between renal regeneration/repair and renal cell carcinoma. *Cancer Res*, Vol. 66, No. 14, (2006), pp 7216-24

Robinson, BD, Sica, GL, Liu, YF, Rohan, TE, Gertler, FB *et al.* (2009). Tumor microenvironment of metastasis in human breast carcinoma: a potential prognostic marker linked to hematogenous dissemination. *Clin Cancer Res*, Vol. 15, No. 7, (2009), pp 2433-41

Rod, NH, Hansen, AM, Nielsen, J, Schnohr, P & Gronbaek, M (2009). Low-risk factor profile, estrogen levels, and breast cancer risk among postmenopausal women. *Int J Cancer*, Vol. 124, No. 8, (2009), pp 1935-40

Sadlonova, A, Novak, Z, Johnson, MR, Bowe, DB, Gault, SR *et al.* (2005). Breast fibroblasts modulate epithelial cell proliferation in three-dimensional in vitro co-culture. *Breast Cancer Res*, Vol. 7, No. 1, (2005), pp R46-59

Sainsbury, JR, Anderson, TJ & Morgan, DA (2000). ABC of breast diseases: breast cancer. *BMJ*, Vol. 321, No. 7263, (2000), pp 745-50

Sakaguchi, T, Nishimoto, M, Miyagi, S, Iwama, A, Morita, Y *et al.* (2006). Putative "stemness" gene jam-B is not required for maintenance of stem cell state in embryonic, neural, or hematopoietic stem cells. *Mol Cell Biol*, Vol. 26, No. 17, (2006), pp 6557-70

Sanders, ME, Schuyler, PA, Dupont, WD & Page, DL (2005). The natural history of low-grade ductal carcinoma in situ of the breast in women treated by biopsy only revealed over 30 years of long-term follow-up. *Cancer*, Vol. 103, No. 12, (2005), pp 2481-4

Santin, AD, Bellone, S, Marizzoni, M, Palmieri, M, Siegel, ER *et al.* (2007). Overexpression of claudin-3 and claudin-4 receptors in uterine serous papillary carcinoma: novel targets for a type-specific therapy using Clostridium perfringens enterotoxin (CPE). *Cancer*, Vol. 109, No. 7, (2007), pp 1312-22

Santin, AD, Bellone, S, Siegel, ER, McKenney, JK, Thomas, M *et al.* (2007). Overexpression of Clostridium perfringens enterotoxin receptors claudin-3 and claudin-4 in uterine carcinosarcomas. *Clin Cancer Res*, Vol. 13, No. 11, (2007), pp 3339-46

Santoso, S, Orlova, VV, Song, K, Sachs, UJ, Andrei-Selmer, CL *et al.* (2005). The homophilic binding of junctional adhesion molecule-C mediates tumor cell-endothelial cell interactions. *J Biol Chem*, Vol. 280, No. 43, (2005), pp 36326-33

Santoso, S, Sachs, UJ, Kroll, H, Linder, M, Ruf, A *et al.* (2002). The junctional adhesion molecule 3 (JAM-3) on human platelets is a counterreceptor for the leukocyte integrin Mac-1. *J Exp Med*, Vol. 196, No. 5, (2002), pp 679-91

Scheiermann, C, Colom, B, Meda, P, Patel, NS, Voisin, MB *et al.* (2009). Junctional adhesion molecule-C mediates leukocyte infiltration in response to ischemia reperfusion injury. *Arterioscler Thromb Vasc Biol*, Vol. 29, No. 10, (2009), pp 1509-15

Sebzda, E, Bracke, M, Tugal, T, Hogg, N & Cantrell, DA (2002). Rap1A positively regulates T cells via integrin activation rather than inhibiting lymphocyte signaling. *Nat Immunol*, Vol. 3, No. 3, (2002), pp 251-8

Shackney, SE & Silverman, JF (2003). Molecular evolutionary patterns in breast cancer. *Adv Anat Pathol*, Vol. 10, No. 5, (2003), pp 278-90

Sharma, PS, Sharma, R & Tyagi, T (2011). VEGF/VEGFR Pathway Inhibitors as Anti-Angiogenic Agents: Present and Future. *Curr Cancer Drug Targets*, Vol. No. (2011), 1873-5576

Sircar, M, Bradfield, PF, Aurrand-Lions, M, Fish, RJ, Alcaide, P et al. (2007). Neutrophil transmigration under shear flow conditions in vitro is junctional adhesion molecule-C independent. *J Immunol*, Vol. 178, No. 9, (2007), pp 5879-87

Sobocka, MB, Sobocki, T, Banerjee, P, Weiss, C, Rushbrook, JI et al. (2000). Cloning of the human platelet F11 receptor: a cell adhesion molecule member of the immunoglobulin superfamily involved in platelet aggregation. *Blood*, Vol. 95, No. 8, (2000), pp 2600-9

Sorlie, T, Perou, CM, Tibshirani, R, Aas, T, Geisler, S et al. (2001). Gene expression patterns of breast carcinomas distinguish tumor subclasses with clinical implications. *Proc Natl Acad Sci U S A*, Vol. 98, No. 19, (2001), pp 10869-74

Stellos, K, Langer, H, Gnerlich, S, Panagiota, V, Paul, A et al. (2010). Junctional adhesion molecule A expressed on human CD34+ cells promotes adhesion on vascular wall and differentiation into endothelial progenitor cells. *Arterioscler Thromb Vasc Biol*, Vol. 30, No. 6, pp 1127-36

Sugano, Y, Takeuchi, M, Hirata, A, Matsushita, H, Kitamura, T et al. (2008). Junctional adhesion molecule-A, JAM-A, is a novel cell-surface marker for long-term repopulating hematopoietic stem cells. *Blood*, Vol. 111, No. 3, (2008), pp 1167-72

Tajima, M, Hirabayashi, S, Yao, I, Shirasawa, M, Osuga, J et al. (2003). Roles of immunoglobulin-like loops of junctional cell adhesion molecule 4; involvement in the subcellular localization and the cell adhesion. *Genes Cells*, Vol. 8, No. 9, (2003), pp 759-68

Tirona, MT, Sehgal, R & Ballester, O (2010). Prevention of breast cancer (part I): epidemiology, risk factors, and risk assessment tools. *Cancer Invest*, Vol. 28, No. 7, (2010), pp 743-50

van 't Veer, LJ, Dai, H, van de Vijver, MJ, He, YD, Hart, AA et al. (2002). Gene expression profiling predicts clinical outcome of breast cancer. *Nature*, Vol. 415, No. 6871, (2002), pp 530-6

van de Vijver, MJ, He, YD, van't Veer, LJ, Dai, H, Hart, AA et al. (2002). A gene-expression signature as a predictor of survival in breast cancer. *N Engl J Med*, Vol. 347, No. 25, (2002), pp 1999-2009

Van Meter, ME & Kim, ES (2010). Bevacizumab: current updates in treatment. *Curr Opin Oncol*, Vol. 22, No. 6, pp 586-91

Walker, RA & Martin, CV (2007). The aged breast. *J Pathol*, Vol. 211, No. 2, (2007), pp 232-40

Weaver, VM, Fischer, AH, Peterson, OW & Bissell, MJ (1996). The importance of the microenvironment in breast cancer progression: recapitulation of mammary tumourigenesis using a unique human mammary epithelial cell model and a three-dimensional culture assay. *Biochem Cell Biol*, Vol. 74, No. 6, (1996), pp 833-51

Williams, C, Ponten, F, Moberg, C, Soderkvist, P, Uhlen, M *et al.* (1999). A high frequency of sequence alterations is due to formalin fixation of archival specimens. *Am J Pathol*, Vol. 155, No. 5, (1999), pp 1467-71

Woodfin, A, Reichel, CA, Khandoga, A, Corada, M, Voisin, MB *et al.* (2007). JAM-A mediates neutrophil transmigration in a stimulus-specific manner in vivo: evidence for sequential roles for JAM-A and PECAM-1 in neutrophil transmigration. *Blood*, Vol. 110, No. 6, (2007), pp 1848-56

Wyckoff, J, Wang, W, Lin, EY, Wang, Y, Pixley, F *et al.* (2004). A paracrine loop between tumor cells and macrophages is required for tumor cell migration in mammary tumors. *Cancer Res*, Vol. 64, No. 19, (2004), pp 7022-9

Yoshikumi, Y, Ohno, H, Suzuki, J, Isshiki, M, Morishita, Y *et al.* (2008). Up-regulation of JAM-1 in AR42J cells treated with activin A and betacellulin and the diabetic regenerating islets. *Endocr J*, Vol. 55, No. 4, (2008), pp 757-65

Zen, K, Babbin, BA, Liu, Y, Whelan, JB, Nusrat, A *et al.* (2004). JAM-C is a component of desmosomes and a ligand for CD11b/CD18-mediated neutrophil transepithelial migration. *Mol Biol Cell*, Vol. 15, No. 8, (2004), pp 3926-37

Zen, K, Liu, Y, McCall, IC, Wu, T, Lee, W *et al.* (2005). Neutrophil migration across tight junctions is mediated by adhesive interactions between epithelial coxsackie and adenovirus receptor and a junctional adhesion molecule-like protein on neutrophils. *Mol Biol Cell*, Vol. 16, No. 6, (2005), pp 2694-703

13

Rho GTPases and Breast Cancer

Xuejing Zhang and Daotai Nie
Department of Medical Microbiology, Immunology, and Cell Biology
Southern Illinois
University School of Medicine and Simmons Cancer Institute
Springfield
USA

1. Introduction

The Rho GTPases is a subfamily of molecular switches that cycle between an inactive GDP-bound state and an active GTP-bound state within the Ras superfamily. In the past, members of the Rho subfamily were mainly thought to be involved in the regulation of cytoskeletal organization in response to extracellular growth factors. However, a number of studies over the past few years have revealed that the Rho GTPases play crucial roles in a wide spectrum of cellular functions related to cell adhesion to the extracellular matrix, cell morphology, cell cycle progression, malignant transformation, invasion and metastasis. Alterations of the expression levels to Rho GTPases have been detected in many types of human tumors and, in some cases, up-regulation and/or overexpression of Rho protein correlates with poor prognosis. This article reviews the evidence of aberrant Rho signaling and the cellular effects elicited by Rho GTPases signaling in human breast tumors.

2. Categorization

Rho GTPases belong to the Ras superfamily of low molecular mass (~21 kDa) proteins that are widely expressed in mammalian cells (DerMardirossian and Bokoch 2001). In mammals, the Rho family of GTPases contains 22 members which can be classified into six groups: Rho (RhoA, RhoB, RhoC), Rac (Rac1, Rac2, Rac3, RhoG), Cdc42 (Cdc42, TC10, TCL, Chp, Wrch-1), Rnd (Rnd1, Rnd2, Rnd3/RhoE), RhoBTB (RhoBTB1, RhoBTB2) and Miro (Miro-1, Miro-2) (Wennerberg and Der 2004). RhoD, Rif and RhoH/TTF have not been grouped yet. RhoA, Rac1 and Cdc42 are the best-characterized family members of Rho family GTPases. Each controls the formation of a distinct cytoskeletal element in mammalian cells. Activation of Rac induces Actin polymerization to form lamellipodia (Ridley, Paterson et al. 1992), whereas activation of CDC42 stimulates the polymerization of actin to filopodia or microspikes (Nobes and Hall 1995). In contrast, Rho regulates bundling of actin filaments into stress fibers and the formation of focal adhesion complexes (Keely, Westwick et al. 1997).

3. Regulators and effectors in Rho GTPases signaling

3.1 Regulators of the Rho GTPases

Like all members of the Ras superfamily, the activity of the Rho GTPases is tightly controlled by the ratio of their GTP/GDP-bound forms in the cell (Fig. 1)(Scheffzek and Ahmadian 2005).

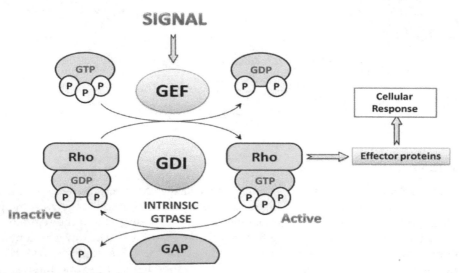

Fig. 1. Regulation of Rho family proteins.

The cycle of activation/inactivation of Rho family GTPases is under the regulation of three distinct families of proteins: GEFs, guanine nucleotide exchange factors catalyze nucleotide exchange when activated by upstream signals; GAPs, GTPase-activating proteins promote the GTP hydrolisis; GDIs, guanine nucleotide dissociation inhibitors block both nucleotide hydrolisis and exchange and participate in Rho GTPase movement between cytosol and membranes.

Rho-specific guanine nucleotide exchange factors (RhoGEFs) activate Rho proteins by facilitating the exchange of GDP for GTP. Rho GTPase activating proteins (RhoGAPs) stimulate the intrinsic rate of hydrolysis of Rho proteins, thus converting them into their inactive state. While Rho-specific guanine nucleotide dissociation inhibitors (RhoGDIs) compete with RhoGEFs for binding to GDP-bound Rho proteins, and sequester Rho in the inactive state (Olofsson 1999).

3.1.1 GEFs

GEFs for Rho GTPases belong to a rapidly growing family of proteins that share common minimal functional units, including a Db1-homolog (DH) domain followed by a pleckstrin homology (PH) domain (Cerione and Zheng 1996). The DH domain is the catalytic site required for GDP-GTP exchange, whereas the PH domain contributes to protein-protein, protein-cytoskeleton, and protein-lipid interactions that help regulate the intracellular localization of GEFs as well as their catalytic activity. Db1 oncogene product is the prototype for the DH domain, and was originally discovered because of its ability to induce focus formation and tumorigesis when expressed in NIH-3T3 cells (Eva and Aaronson 1985). It has 29% sequence identity with the *Saccharomyces cerevisiae* cell division protein Cdc24, which is found upstream of the yeast small GTP-binding protein Cdc42 in the bud assembly pathway (Ron, Zannini et al. 1991). This was the first clue that DB1 functions as a GEF. Biochemical study has confirmed that Db1 is able to release GDP from the human homolog of Cdc42 *in vitro*. Further study suggested that the DH domain is essential and sufficient for the catalytic activity and that this domain was also necessary to induce oncogenicity (Zheng, Zangrilli et al. 1996).

After the discovery of Dbl, a number of mammalian proteins containing DH and PH domain have been studied (Cerione and Zheng 1996). Many of these have been identified as oncogenes in transfection assays. Tiam, however, was first identified as an invasion-inducing gene using proviral tagging and *in vitro* selection for invasiveness (Habets, Scholtes et al. 1994). Two other members of the DH/PH-containing protein family, Fgd1 and Vav, have been shown to be essential for normal embryonic development (Pasteris, Cadle et al. 1994; Tarakhovsky, Turner et al. 1995). Moreover, some members of the DH protein family (such as Dbl) have been shown to exhibit exchange activity *in vitro* for a broad range of Rho-like GTPases, whereas others appear to be more specific. For example, Lbc and oncoproteins Lfc and Lsc, are specific for Rho, whereas Fgd1 is specific for Cdc42 (Glaven, Whitehead et al. 1996). Although Vav was originally identified as an activator of Ras (Gulbins, Coggeshall et al. 1993), it has been demonstrated more recently to function as a GEF for members of the Rho family (Crespo, Schuebel et al. 1997; Han, Das et al. 1997).

3.1.2 GAPs

The first GAP protein specific for the Rho family GTPases was purified from cell extracts using recombinant Rho. This protein, designated p50Rho-GAP, was shown to have GAP activity toward Rho, Cdc42 and Rac *in vitro* (Hall 1990; Lancaster, Taylor-Harris et al. 1994). Since then, a growing number of proteins that present GAP activity for Rho GTPases have been identified in mammalian cells, all of which share a related GAP domain that spans 140 amino acids without significant resemblance to Ras GAP. In addition to accelerating the hydrolysis of GTP, Rho GAPs also mediate other downstream functions of Rho proteins in mammalian systems. For example, it has been reported that the p190GAP plays a role in cytoskeletal rearrangement (Chang, Gill et al. 1995).

3.1.3 GDIs

The ubiquitously expressed protein Rho GDI was the first GDI identified for the members of the Rho family. It was isolated as a cytosolic protein that preferentially associated with the GDP-bound form of RhoA and RhoB and thereby inhibited the dissociation of GDP (Fukumoto, Kaibuchi et al. 1990; Ueda, Kikuchi et al. 1990). Rho GDI was found to be active on Cdc42 and Rac as well (Abo, Pick et al. 1991; Leonard, Hart et al. 1992). Further studies demonstrated that Rho GDI also associated weakly with the GTP-bound form of Rho, Rac, and Cdc42 (Hart, Maru et al. 1992; Chuang, Xu et al. 1993), leading to an inhibition of the intrinsic and GAP-stimulated GTPase activity of the Rho GTPases. Therefore, Rho GDI appears to be a molecule capable of blocking both the GDP/GTP exchange step and the GTP hydrolytic step. It was also reported that the Rho GDIs play a crucial role in the translocation of the Rho GTPases between membranes and the cytoplasm. In resting cells, the Rho proteins are found in the cytosol as a complex with Rho GDIs, which inhibit their

GTP/GDP exchange ratio, but are released from the GDI and translocated to the membranes during the course of cell activation (Takai, Sasaki et al. 1995).

3.2 Effectors of the Rho GTPases

The Rho GTPases have been implicated in a wide varity of cellular processes, including cytoskeletal organization, cell adhesion to the substratum, cell polarity, and transcriptional activation. Several lines of evidence indicate that Rho GTPases link plasma membrane receptors to the assembly and organization of the actin cytoskeleton. Rho GTPases control individual aspects of the actin cytoskeleton through distinct effector proteins. In fact, over 60 targets of the three common Rho GTPases (Rho, Rac, Cdc42) have been found (Fig. 2).

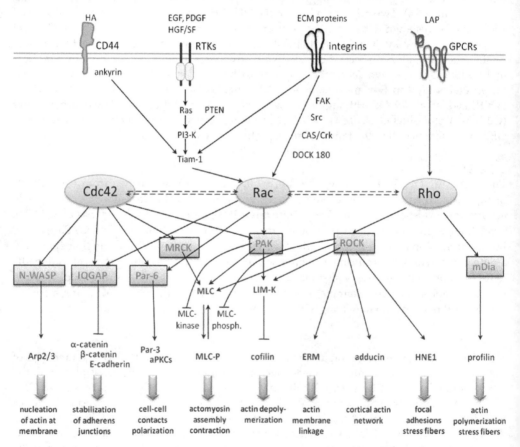

Fig. 2. Regulators and mammalian targets of the Rho family GTPases.

Transmembrane receptors activate Rho GTPases through GEFs such as Tiam-1 or adaptor proteins. Activated Rho GTPases bind to and activate protein kinases, including these of the MRCK, PAK and ROCK families. The effector proteins then interact with several proteins with distinct effects on the actin cytoskeleton and cellular morphology. See text for details.

3.2.1 Rho signaling

Rho was originally studied for its role in regulate the formation of stress fibers and focal adhesion (FA) complexes (Nobes and Hall 1995) which precursors actomyosin assembly and contractile potential, both of which are required for the cellular movement. Rho is also involved in cell-cell adhesion. In particular, inactivation of RhoA by C3 transferase disrupts the organization of actin filaments at cell-cell contact, leading to the inhibition of the proper formation of both adherens junctions (AJs) and tight junctions (TJs) (Braga, Machesky et al. 1997; Takaishi, Sasaki et al. 1997). For example, in normal mammary epithelial cells, MCF10 cells, E-cadherin cytoskeletal links in AJs was disrupted by C3 transferase. In addition, inhibition of Rho blocks the formation of new AJs in MCF10 cells (Zhong, Kinch et al. 1997). It has been suggested that the function of Rho can be either promoted or antagonized by Rac and Cdc42, depending on different variables, such as cellular context, stimulus, and extracellular matrix (ECM) (Zhang, Nie et al. ; Narumiya and Morii 1993; Nobes and Hall 1995). In Swiss 3T3 fibroblasts, the Rho GTPases have been placed in a hierarchical order where Cdc42 activates Rac, and Rac activates Rho (Nobes and Hall 1995); however, in N1E-115 neuroblastoma and Madine-Darby canine kidney (MDCK) cells, constitutively activated Rac down-regulates Rho (Leeuwen, Kain et al. 1997; Michiels and Collard 1999).

Rho is widely studied for its involvement in the acquisition of migratory, invasive, and metastatic phenotypes. Expression of a dominant negative form of RhoA led to the attenuation of membrane ruffling, lamellipodia formation and migration (O'Connor, Nguyen et al. 2000). In addition, RhoA localization to lamellipodia was blocked by inhibiting phosphodiesterase activity while enhanced by inhibiting cAMP-dependent protein kinase activity (O'Connor, Nguyen et al. 2000). Furthermore, activation of Rho either by LPA treatment or by stimulating the actomyosin system has been associated with the migratory ability of tumor cells. For example, in an experimental metastasis model, NIH3T3 fibroblasts expressing a constitutively active form of RhoA were injected into the tail vein of nude mice and formed increased number metastasis nodules in the lung (del Peso, Hernandez-Alcoceba et al. 1997). Moreover, in the absence of serum, activated RhoA is capable of promoting invasion of cultured rat MM1 hepatoma cells through a mesothelial cell monolayer (Yoshioka, Matsumura et al. 1998). Although these are not oncogenes by themselves, RhoA and RhoC are frequently found to be overexpressed in clinical cancers (Sahai and Marshall 2002), and RhoC has been repeatedly associated with metastasis. For example, the expression of RhoA, RhoB and RhoC in 33 pancreatic ductal adnocarcinoma cases were examined in a study (Suwa, Ohshio et al. 1998), it was found that the expression level of RhoC was higher in tumors than in non-malignant tissues, higher in metastatic lesions than in primary tumors, and correlated with perineural invasion and lymph node metastasis as well as poorer prognosis. Although early studies showed that RhoB has a positive role in cell growth, more recent studies suggested that RhoB is down-regulated in human tumors, and its expression inversely correlates with tumor aggressiveness. For example, RhoB protein is found expressed in normal lung tissue and is lost progressively throughout lung cancer progression (Mazieres, Antonia et al. 2004). In line with this, higher expression of RhoB is associated with favorable prognosis in bladder cancer (Kamai, Tsujii et al. 2003). It has been suggested that RhoB can act as a tumor suppressor, since it is activated in response to several stress stimuli, such as DNA damage and hypoxia, inhibits tumor growth, cell migration, and invasion, and has proapoptotic functions in cells (Huang and Prendergast 2006).

3.2.2 Effectors of Rho

There are two major effectors that are downstream of Rho: Rho associated coiled-coil forming kinase (ROCK/Rho kinase/ROK) (Leung, Manser et al. 1995; Ishizaki, Maekawa et al. 1996) and mammalian homolog of Drosophila diaphanous (mDia) (Watanabe, Madaule et al. 1997; Wasserman 1998). While mDia is a formin molecule that can catalyze actin nucleation, polymerization,and produce long, straight actin filaments (Goode and Eck 2007), ROCK is a serine/threonine kinase that phosphorylates a number of substrates (Riento and Ridley 2003). The actions of ROCK and mDia on actin and myosin are believed to work together to induce actomyosin bundles in cells. Expression of an active form of mDia induces stress fibers in cultured cells, and treatment of these cells with a specific ROCK inhibitor, Y-27632 (Narumiya, Ishizaki et al. 2000), causes dissolution of the bundles, leaving the cells with diffusely distributed actin filaments (Watanabe, Kato et al. 1999). It has also been reported that ROCK and mDia are required in contractile ring formations (Kosako, Yoshida et al. 2000; Watanabe, Ando et al. 2008).

At least six substrates of ROCK are known to play roles in actin cytoskeletal reorganization, including myosin light chain (MLC), myosin-binding subunit of MLC phosphatase, LIM-kinase, adducin, ezrin/radixin/moesin (ERM) family of proteins, and Na^+/H^+ exchange protein (NHE1). Among the six substrates, MLC-phosphatase, MLC, and LIM-kinase, are the three best studied ROCK effectors and have been found to play important roles in driving ROCK's physiological function on the actin cytoskeleton. ROCK inactivates myosin-binding subunit of MLC-phosphatase by phosphorylation (Kimura, Ito et al. 1996; Uehata, Ishizaki et al. 1997). ROCK is also able to phosphorylate myosin light chain directly (Maekawa, Ishizaki et al. 1999). These two actions of ROCK increase the myosin light chain phosphorylation, stimulate cross-linking of actin by myosin and enhance actomyosin contractility. ROCK also phosphorylates and activates LIM-kinase, which in turn phosphorylates and inactivates actin-depolymerizing and severing factor, cofilin (Amano, Ito et al. 1996). The later action of ROCK results in stabilization of existing actin filaments and increase in their content.

The ROCK effectors adducin and the ERM family of proteins regulate actin cytoskeleton in a more direct way. ROCK has been shown to phosphorylate adducin (Kimura, Fukata et al. 1998; Fukata, Oshiro et al. 1999), which, together with spectrin, is an important component of the cortical actin network underlying the plasma membrane (Gardner and Bennett 1987). ROCK-phosphorylated adducin interacts with filamentous-actin (F-actin), and its localization suggests a role in regulating cellular migration. In HGF/SF-stimulated MDCK cells, phosphoadducin localizes to membrane ruffles, and ROCK-phosphorylated adducin localizes to the leading edge of migrating NRK49F fibroblasts in wound healing assays (Fukata, Oshiro et al. 1999); while the introduction of nonphosphorylatable adducin into MDCK and NRK49F cells inhibited membrane ruffling and migration, as did a dominant negative ROCK mutant (Fukata, Oshiro et al. 1999). ROCK can also phosphorylate the ERM proteins that are important for linking actin filaments to the plasma membrane (Matsui, Maeda et al. 1998). Interestingly, it has been demonstrated that the TSC1 tumor suppressor hamartin regulates cell adhesion to cell substrates through the ERM family of actin-binding proteins and RhoA (Lamb, Roy et al. 2000). Finally, NHE1 is well known as a ubiquitous Na^+/H^+ exchange protein that enables stress fiber formation (Tominaga, Ishizaki et al. 1998).

3.2.3 Rac and Cdc42 signaling

In classical Swiss 3T3 fibroblast model, activation of Cdc42 leads to filopodia formation, Rac results in lamellipodia formation and membrane ruffling, and Rho results in stress fibers formation (Nobes and Hall 1995). The cytoskeletal rearrangements caused by Rho GTPases activation play a key role in cell motility. In addition to their effects on the actin cytoskeleton and motility, Rac and Cdc42 also play a role in cell-cell adhesion in epithelial cells. Expression of a constitutively active form of Rac in MDCK cells or keratinocytes leads to an increase in E-cadherin complex members and F-actin at cell-cell contacts, while a dominant negative mutant was found to disrupt cell-cell adhesions (Braga, Machesky et al. 1997; Takaishi, Sasaki et al. 1997; Jou and Nelson 1998). A number of studies have suggested that Cdc42 plays an important role in establishing the initial polarization of epithelial cells, which is required for the proper formation of cell-cell adhesions. For example, transfection of a dominant negative form of Cdc42 in MDCK cells results in the selective depolarization of basolateral membrane proteins due to inhibition of membrane transport (Kroschewski, Hall et al. 1999). Expression of a constitutively active form of Cdc42 in MDCK cells increased AJs and blocked cellular migration induced by HGF/SF (Kodama, Takaishi et al. 1999).

Given the importance of Rac and Cdc42 in the regulation of cell cytoskeletal, adhesion and motility, it has been widely considered that they play important roles in cellular processes related to invasion and metastasis. The first evidence of Rac's role in invasion was obtained when Rac-specific GEF T-lymphoma invasion and metastasis (Tiam-1) was identified in a retroviral insertional mutagenesis screen. Virus-infected T-lymphoma cells were repeatedly selected for *in vitro* invasion through a layer of fibroblasts and the proviral insertions in invasive clones were used to identify the Tiam-1 gene (Habets, Scholtes et al. 1994). Subsequently, Rac, and later Cdc42, were shown to also confer an invasive potential to these T-lymphoma cells (Michiels, Habets et al. 1995; Stam, Michiels et al. 1998). More evidence for Rac and Cdc42's involvement in invasion and metastasis has been provided since then. Expression of the laminin-receptor α6β4 integrin in the melanoma cell line MDA-MB-435 promotes invasiveness in a Rac and PI3-kinase-dependent manner (Shaw, Rabinovitz et al. 1997). In addition, constitutively active forms of Rac and Cdc42 in breast carcinoma cell line T47D promote invasion through a collagen matrix. However, this invasion can be blocked by PI3-Kinase inhibitors, indicating that PI3-kinase acts downstream of Rac and Cdc42 (Keely, Westwick et al. 1997).

3.2.4 Effectors of Rac and Cdc42

A number of Rac and Cdc42 effectors have been identified. Some of these have been found to specifically mediate cell motility, whereas others play a more prominent role in mediating cell adhesion. It is well established that WASP and MRCKs are Cdc42 specific effectors that regulate actin organization and filopodia formation which promotes a more motile phenotype (Aspenstrom, Lindberg et al. 1996; Miki, Miura et al. 1996). In addition, members of the p21-activated kinase family (PAK), downstream of Rac and Cdc42, play important roles in cytoskeletal-mediated changes that affect motility (Manser, Leung et al. 1994). The scallfold proteins IQGAP and Par-6, both of which can be activated by Cdc42 and rac, promote cell polarization and contribute to cell-cell adhesion.

The scaffold protein N-WASP binds to Arp2/3 complexes that are crucial for the assembly of within filopodia (Kolluri, Tolias et al. 1996). It has been shown that both N-WASP and Arp2/3 complexes are required for Cdc42 to trigger actin filament assembly (Welch, DePace et al. 1997; Miki, Sasaki et al. 1998). Therefore, N-WASP may promote cellular motility through proper filopodia formation. MRCKs α and β are Cdc42 specific effectors that can phosphorylate MLC via a ROCK-like kinase domain (Leung, Chen et al. 1998). It is well accepted that phosphorylation of MLC is required for actomyosin complex assembly and contraction. Overexpression of MRCKα and Cdc42 synergizes to promote filopodia formation, while a MRCKα kinase-deficient mutant inhibits the formation of Cdc42-induced filopodia (Leung, Chen et al. 1998). Therefore, MRCDs are believed to play important roles in cytoskeletal organization and contraction, and contribute to migration. PAK, a protein kinase downstream of Rac and Cdc42, plays a crucial role in actin dynamics and adhesion (Manser, Leung et al. 1994). PAK has been demonstrated to phosphorylate and inactivate MLCK, subsequently causing a decrease in MLC phosphorylation (Sanders, Matsumura et al. 1999). Thus, inactivation of MLCK leads to stress fiber and focal adhesion disassembly. Moreover, PAK controls the actin cytoskeletion through the phosphorylation and subsequent activation of LIM-kinase. Phosphor-LIM-kinsae can further phosphorylate and inactivate the actin-depolymerizing protein cofilin, thus inhibiting actin depolymerization when Rac is activated and causing extreme membrane ruffling (Arber, Barbayannis et al. 1998; Yang, Higuchi et al. 1998). The IQGAP1 and IQGAP2 scaffolding effectors of Cdc42 and Rac regulate cell-cell adhesion through actin polymerization and sequestration of β-catenin (Kuroda, Fukata et al. 1996; Erickson, Cerione et al. 1997). *In vitro*, IQGAP oligomerizes and cross-links F-catin it has also been found to complex with Cdc42 and F-actin *in vivo* (Fukata, Kuroda et al. 1997). In addition, one study has shown that the IQGAP protein also competes with α-catenin for binding to β-catenin, thus preventing E-cadherin/α-catenin/β-catenin complex from attaching to the actin cytoskeleton, and thereby disrupting cell-cell contacts (Erickson, Cerione et al. 1997). Another scaffolding protein, Par-6, was identified using activated Cdc42 and TC10 mutants as baits in yeast two-hybrid screens (Joberty, Petersen et al. 2000; Qiu, Abo et al. 2000). It is known that Par-6 binds to a second scaffolding protein, Par-3, and both Par-6 and Par-3 bind independently to atypical protein kinase C (aPKC) isoforms (Lin, Edwards et al. 2000). In addition, endogenous Par-3 localizes to TJs in MDCK cells, overexpression of Par-6 or the N-terminal portion of Par-3 (the Par-6-interaction responsible region) disrupts TJ formation (Joberty, Petersen et al. 2000).

4. Expression of Rho GTPases in breast tumors

Aberrant Rho signalling resulting from alterations in Rho GTPase protein level, changes in activation status, and abnormal quantity of effector proteins are found in a large variety of human tumors. of GTPases: the Rho family (RhoA, RhoB and RhoC), the Rac family (Rac1, Rac2 and Rac3) and the Cdc42 family, in order to avoid repetitions.

4.1 Rho GTPases in breast tumors

Overexpression of RhoC has been found in inflammatory breast cancer (IBC), an aggressive form of breast cancer that is highly infiltrative and metastatic with poor prognosis for the patients, using in situ hybridization (van Golen, Davies et al. 1999). Compared to normal untransformed parental cells, RhoC-transformed cells produce and secrete high levels of proangiogenic factors such as vascular endothelial growth factor (VEGF), basic fibroblast growth factor (bFGF), interleukin-6 (IL-6), and interleukin-8 (IL-8). when compared to normal untransformed parental cells (van Golen, Wu et al. 2000). In addition, microarray analysis has shown that MCF10A breast cells stably transfected with wild type RhoC or a constitutively active mutant of RhoC overexpress genes associated with invasion and metastasis (Wu, Wu et al. 2004). Other RhoGTPases are also involved in breast tumors. RhoA is found overexpressed in breast tumor tissues but not in the normal tissue (Fritz, Brachetti et al. 2002). The expression of dominant negative RhoA in rat mammary adenocarcinoma cells affects tumor cell growth *in vivo* and reduces intravasation into the peripheral blood, resulting in decrease in lung colonization ability (Fritz, Just et al. 1999). Other studies have indirectly shown an important role of RhoA in breast carcinogenesis. For example, highly metastatic MDA-MB-231 cells that were treated with HMG-CoA reductase inhibitor, namely cerivastain, showed reduced proliferation and invasion through Matrigel, in a RhoA- but not Ras-dependent manner (Denoyelle, Vasse et al. 2001). However, poorly metastatic breast cancer cells such as MCF-7 are less sensitive to cerivastain treatment, indicating that RhoA might be more significantly overexpressed in late stages of breast cancer as with other tumors.

Rho proteins are also important players in breast tumor progression and metastasis exerted by the CD44 hyaluronan receptor (Bourguignon 2001). CD44 is expressed in human breast tumors and promotes cell growth and metastasis in tumor cells. Studies have found that RhoA and CD44 directly interact with each other *in vivo* in highly metastatic human breast cancer cell lines. Accordingly, inhibition of Rho signaling results in the abrogation of the metastatic phenotype elicited by CD44 (Bourguignon, Zhu et al. 1999). RhoA has also been found to be involved in insulin signaling via Shc in human breast cancer (Finlayson, Chappell et al. 2003). Overexpression of insulin receptors correlates with development, progression and outcome of breast cancer, and insulin signaling involves hyperphosphorylation of Shc. Hence, Shc leads to the activation of geranyl transferases, which results in an increased amount of prenylated RhoA in the tumor tissue compared with normal mammary tissue (Finlayson, Chappell et al. 2003). Furthermore, RhoA has been reported to increase the metastatic potential of tumor cells via its ability to promote tumor angiogenesis through the downregulation of thrombospodin-1 (Tsp-1) (Watnick, Cheng et al. 2003). Rho pathway is part of the downstream signaling cascade that is activated by PI3K and leads to ROCK stimulation, Myc phosphorylation and Tsp-1 repression.

4.2 Rac GTPases in breast tumors

The involvement of Rac GTPases in breast cancer was first reported in rodents (Bouzahzah, Albanese et al. 2001). Expression of a dominant negative Rac1 mutant indicated that Rac1 affects tumor cell growth and metastasis *in vivo*. Deregulation of Rac3, closely related to Rac1, has also been detected in breast cancer (Mira, Benard et al. 2000). Rac3 maps to chromosome band 17q25.3, a region known to contain candidate tumor suppressor genes both in breast and ovarian cancers (Morris, Haataja et al. 2000). Highly proliferative breast cancer cells, T47D and MCF-7, but not normal breast cell lines, contain constitutively active Rac3 in a Ras-independent manner (Morris, Haataja et al. 2000). It has also been shown that expression of a dominant negative mutant Rac3 (N17) leads to inhibition of S-phase entry and cellular proliferation in breast tumor cells, which indicate that Rac3 may promote cell growth (Leung, Nagy et al. 2003). Further, the Rac-PAK signaling pathway is essential for receptor tyrosine kinase ErbB2-mediated transformation of human breast epithelial cancer cells (Mazieres, Antonia et al. 2004). Activation of Rac-PAK1 pathway by ErbB2 homodimers can induce growth factor-independent proliferation and promote disruptions to the three-dimensional (3D) mammary acinar-like structures, via activation of the Erk and

Akt pathways (Mazieres, Antonia et al. 2004). Moreover, Rac1 enhances estrogen receptor α (ERα) transcriptional activity, resulting in increased proliferation in breast cancer cells (Rosenblatt, Garcia et al. ; Folkman 1972).

4.3 Cdc42 family in breast tumors

Cdc42 is overexpressed in some breast cancers and there is accumulating evidence that activated Cdc42 contributes to the accumulation of ErbB1 in cells through the regulation of c-Cbl function (Abraham, Kuriakose et al. 2001; Marionnet, Lalou et al. 2003). The view that Cdc42 is involved in human breast carcinogenesis is supported by a rodents model of breast carcinoma where the expression of a dominant negative mutant of Cdc42 reduced the number of focal contacts, inhibited colony formation in soft agar and affected cell growth *in vivo* (Fritz, Just et al. 1999). The dominant negative Cdc42 also reduced intravasation of tumor cells into peripheral blood and ability to form lung metastasis. In addition, through the activation of Cdc42, transforming growth factor α (TGF-α) mediates the invasion of MDA-MB-231 cells into 3-D collagen matrices by initiating the formation of protrusions into collagen. (Kamai, Tsujii et al. 2003; Fisher, Sacharidou et al. 2009). Further, another study has shown that membrane-type-1 matrix metalloproteinase (MT1-MMP) and Cdc42 are fundamental components of a co-associated invasion-signaling complex that controls directed single-cell invasion of 3D collagen matrices (Fisher, Sacharidou et al. 2009).

5. Multiple functions mediated by Rho GTPases in breast cancer

Rho GTPases mediate housekeeping aspects of cell biology including cell growth, cell polarity, cell adhesion, membrane trafficking and motility. They function as signaling switches that regulate lipid metabolism, microtubules- and actin-based structures, epithelial cell-junctions, cell cycle and apoptosis regulatory proteins, and transcription factors.

5.1 Rho GTPases and cytoskeleton organization

Eukaryotic cellular morphology and attachment to the substratum in response to extracellular signals are largely dependent on rearrangements of the actin cytoskeleton. Cell motility, cytokinesis and phagocytosis all rely on coordinated regulation of the actin cytoskeleton (Small 1994; Zigmond 1996). Filamentous actin can be organized into several discrete structures: (a) filopodia, finger-like protrusions that contain a tight bundle of long actin filaments in the direction of the protrusion. These are found primarily in motile cells and neuronal growth cones. (b) lamellipodia, thin protrusive actin sheets that dominate the edges of cultured fibroblasts and many other motile cells. Membrane ruffles observed at the leading edge of the cell result from lamellipodia that lift up off the substrate and fold backward. (c) actin stress fibers, bundles of actin filaments that traverse the cell and are linked to the ECM through focal adhesion (Van Aelst and D'Souza-Schorey 1997). The actin polymerization is tightly regulated by Rho GTPases.

Rho activation in fibroblasts is known to stimulate the assembly of contractile actin/myosin filaments, the formation of stress fibers, and the clustering of integrins involved in the formation of focal adhesion complexes. Activation of Rac facilitates actin polymerization at the cell periphery to generate protrusive actin-rich lamellipodia and membrane ruffling. And activation of Cdc42 results in actin polymerization to form peripheral actin microspikes and filopidia. As described previously, a number of proteins have been identified as targets of Rho, Rac and Cdc42 (Fig. 3). Most of them are involved in Rho GTPases mediated cytoskeletal rearrangements (Tang, Olufemi et al. 2008).

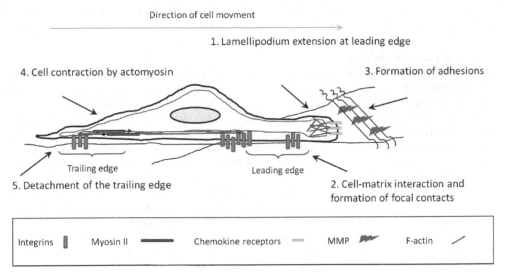

Fig. 3. A model of the cellular migratory process. See text for detailed explanation of motility phases.

5.2 Rho GTPases in cell migration

Cell migration is a multistep process involving polarization, sequential cell protrusion and adhesion formation in the direction of migration, cells body contraction, and tail detachment (Pinner and Sahai 2008). During the migration process, cells move with extending protrusions at the front and a retracting tail at the rear, both regulated by members of the Rho GTPases family (Ridley, Schwartz et al. 2003). The idea that Rho family GTPases could regulate cell migration derives from observations that they mediate the formation of specific actin containing structures. In addition, Rho proteins regulate several other processes that are relevant to cell migration, including cell-substrate adhesion, cell-cell adhesion, protein secretion, vesicle trafficking, and transcription.

5.2.1 Cell polarization and lamellipodium extension at the leading edge

An asymmetrical organization of intracellular activities is required for a cell to move, that means the molecular processes at the leading and trailing edges of a moving cell must be different. Establishing and maintaining cell polarity in response to extracellular stimuli appear to be mediated by Rho family GTPases.

Cdc42 is well accepted as a master regulator of cell polarity in eukaryotic organisms ranging from yeast to human.Cdc42 was first studied in a budding yeast model for its involvement in cell polarity. During the cell cycle, yeast cells adopt alternative states of growth to non-focused isotropic growth. In the absence of Cdc42, *Saccharomyces cerevisiae* fail to establish focused apical growth and, cells expand isotropically (Pruyne and Bretscher 2000). Cdc42 regulates cell polarity by deciding the location of lamellipodia formation (Srinivasan, Wang et al. 2003). In addition, Cdc42 directs the localization of the microtubule-organizing center

(MTOC) and Golgi apparatus to the front of the nucleus, oriented toward the direction of movement. MTOC orientation at the leading edge then facilitates the delivery of Golgi derived vesicles to the leading edge and microtubule growth into the lamellipodium (Rodriguez, Schaefer et al. 2003). It has been further studied that Cdc42 exerts its effect on MTOC through its downstream effector, PAK1 (Li, Hannigan et al. 2003).

5.2.2 Protrusion formation
Inherent polarity drives the formation of membrane protrusions, and the organization of filaments depends on the type of protrusion. Actin filaments form a branching dendritic network in lamellipodia, but form long parallel bundles in filopodia (Pollard, Blanchoin et al. 2000). The dendritic organization of lamelipodia that provides a tight brush-like structure, formed via the actin-nucleating activity of the actin-related proteins 2/3 (Arp2/3) protein complex (Urban, Jacob et al.). Rac stimulates new actin polymerization by acting on Arp2/3 complexes, which binds to pre-existing filaments (Campellone and Welch). Activation of Arp2/3 complexes by Rac is carried out through its target IRSp53. Upon activation, IRSp53 interacts with WAVE through its SH3 domain, it then binds to and activates Arp2/3 complexes (Chesarone and Goode 2009). It has also been reported that IRSp53 binds to Cdc42 through a separate domain (Miki, Yamaguchi et al. 2000). So, IRSp53 can serve as a direct link between Cdc42 and Rac, which explains how Cdc42 induces Rac involvement in lamellipodium formation. Furthermore, IRSp53 can bind to a Rho target, Dia1, which might underlie the capability of Rho to facilitate lamellipodium extension (Cox and Huttenlocher 1998; Fujiwara, Mammoto et al. 2000).

5.2.3 Cell-substrate adhesions
Newly formed focal adhesion complexes are localized in the lamellipodia of most migrating cells. Once the lamellipodium attach to the ECM, integrins come into contact with ECM ligands and cluster in the cell membrane where they interact with FAK, α-actin, and talin (Cox and Huttenlocher 1998). All these proteins can bind to adaptor proteins through Src-homologous domain 2 and 3 (SH2, SH3) as well as proline rich domains to more actin binding proteins (vinculin, paxillin and α-actin) and regulatory molecules PI3K to focal complexes (Zamir and Geiger 2001). Rac is required for focal complex assembly, and Rac itself can be activated by cell-substrate ECM adhesion (Rottner, Hall et al. 1999). It is suggested that the adhesion assemblies in migrating cells begin with small-scale clustering and the speed of the cell migration is dependent on ECM composition, which determines the relative activated levels of Rho, Rac and Cdc42 (Price, Leng et al. 1998). Therefore, interactions between ECM and integrins at the leading edge of cells play an important role in maintaining the level of active Rac. This indicates the existence of a positive feedback loop that allows continuous crosstalk between integrins and Rac, and allows cells to respond to changing ECM composition.

5.2.4 Cell body contraction by actomyosin complexes
Cell body contraction is driven by actomyosin contractility and the force transmitted to sites of adhesion derives from myosin II. Myosin II, which is predominantly induced by Rho and its downstream effector ROCK, controls stress fiber assembly and contraction. Rho acts via ROCKs to affect MLC phosphorylation by inhibiting MLC phosphatase or the MLC phosphorylation. MLC phosphorylation is also regulated by MLCK, which is controlled by both intracellular calcium concentration and ERK MAPKs (Fukata, Amano et al. 2001).

ROCKs and MLCK have been suggested to act in concert to regulate different aspects of cell contractility, since ROCK appears to be required for MLC phosphorylation which are associated with actin filaments in the cell body, and MLCK is required at the cell periphery (Totsukawa, Yamakita et al. 2000).

5.2.5 Adhesion disassembly and tail detachment
Tail detachment occurs when cell-substrate linkages are preferentially disrupted at the rear of a migrating cell, while the leading edge remains attached to the ECM and continues to elongate (Palecek, Huttenlocher et al. 1998). Mechanisms underlying the focal complex disassembly and tail detachment depend on the type of cell and strength of adhesion to the extracellular matrix at the trailing edge (Wear, Schafer et al. 2000). In slow moving cells, tail detachment depend on the action of a calcium-dependent, non-lysosomal cysteine protease calpain that cleaves focal complex components like talin and cytoplasmic tail of $\beta 1$ and $\beta 3$ integrins along the trailing edge (Potter, Tirnauer et al. 1998). Strong tension forces exerted across the cells at the rear adhesions is required to break the physical link between integrin and the actin cytoskeleton. Rho and myosin II are involved in this event. Furthermore, Rho plays important roles in reducing adhesion and promoting tail detachment in fibroblasts, which have relatively large focal adhesion complexes (Cox and Huttenlocher 1998).

5.3 Rho GTPases and transcriptional activation
A number of studies have suggested that Rho family GTPases are involved in the regulation of nuclear signaling. Rac and Cdc42, but not Rho, have been demonstrated to regulate the activation of JNK and reactivate kinase p38RK in certain cell types (Seger and Krebs 1995). Expression of constitutively active forms of Rac and Cdc42 in HeLa, NIH-3T3, and Cos cells stimulates JNK and p38 activity (Coso, Chiariello et al. 1995). Furthermore, these same effects were observed with oncogenic GEFs for these Rho proteins (Minden, Lin et al. 1995). However in human kidney 293 T cells, Cdc42 and the Rho protein, but not Rac, induces the activation of JNK (Teramoto, Crespo et al. 1996). Upon activation, JNKs and p38 translocate to the nucleus where they phosphorylate transcription factors, including c-Jun, ATF2, and Elk (Derijard, Hibi et al. 1994; Gille, Strahl et al. 1995). Further, Rac has been shown to activate PEA3, a member of the Ets family, in a JNK-dependent manner (O'Hagan, Tozer et al. 1996). Activated p38 phosphorylates ATF2, Elk, Max, and the cAMP response element binding protein.

PAKs are the farthest known upstream kinases that connect Rho GTPases to JNK and p38 through GTP-dependent bindings to Rac and Cdc42 *in vitro* and are activated after binding to activated Rac and Cdc42. (Manser, Chong et al. 1995). In addition, certain constitutively active forms of PAK can activate JNK and p38 (Zhang, Han et al. 1995). Further, a mutant effector of Rac that cannot bind to PAK remains a potent JNK activator (Westwick, Lambert et al. 1997). These observations suggest that other kinases, in addition to PAK, participate in the signalling from Rho GTPases to JNK. Supporting this, MLK3 and MEKK4 are found to be regulated by Cdc42 and Rac, and selectively activate the JNK pathway (Gerwins, Blank et al. 1997). It has also been reported that Cdc42/Rac can bind to MLK3 both *in vitro* and *in vivo* and that the coexpression of activated Cdc42/Rac mutants elevates the enzymatic activity of MLK3 in Cos-7 cells (Teramoto, Coso et al. 1996; Gerwins, Blank et al. 1997). In addition, Rho, Rac and Cdc42 stimulate the activation of the serum responsive factor (SRF) (Hill, Wynne et al. 1995). SRF forms a complex with TCF/Elk proteins to stimulate transcription with serum response elements (SREs) at their promoter enhancer regions, for example the Fos promoter (Treisman 1990).

5.4 Rho GTPases and cell growth control

Several lines of evidence have suggested that Rho family members play important roles in several aspects of cell growth. The Rho proteins have been shown to increase expression of cyclin D1, a cell cycle regulator that controls the transition from G_1 phase to S phase, in Swiss 3T3 fibroblasts (Yamamoto, Marui et al. 1993; Olson, Ashworth et al. 1995) and in mammary epithelial cells (Liberto, Cobrinik et al. 2002). Overexpression of RhoE inhibits cell cycle progression by inhibiting translation of cyclin D1 mRNA (Villalonga, Guasch et al. 2004). In fibroblasts, RhoA is involved in ERK activation and subsequent cyclin D1 expression (Roovers and Assoian 2003). RhoA also downregulates cdk inhibitors p21 and p27 during the G1 phase of the cell cycle (Weber, Hu et al. 1997). Rac 1 is capable of regulating the cell cyle through the activation of a number of distinct intra-cellular pathways, including the NFκB pathway. In contrast to other Rho proteins, Rac1 can directly activate cyclin D1 expression (Page, Li et al. 1999).

Furthermore, Rho, Rac, and Cdc42 have been demonstrated to possess transforming and oncogenic potential in some cell lines. For example, cells with constitutively active forms of Rac and Rho display enhanced anchorage independent growth ability, and initiate tumor formation when inoculated into nude mice (Khosravi-Far, Solski et al. 1995). The observation that Tiam, a Rac GEF, can transform NIH-3T3 cells suggests a role for Rac in transformation (van Leeuwen, van der Kammen et al. 1995). While expression of constitutively activated Rac is sufficient to cause malignant transformation of rodent fibroblasts (Qiu, Chen et al. 1995), this is not the case with Rho (Qiu, Chen et al. 1995), suggesting that the growth-promoting effects of the Rho GTPases are specific to cell type. Evidence of Cdc42's role in cell growth has been provided in fibroblasts. The constitutively active mutant of Cdc42 stimulates anchorage independent growth and proliferation in nude mice (Qiu, Abo et al. 1997). Using a Cdc42 mutant, Cdc42(F28L), that can undergo GTP-GDP exchange in the absence of GEF, one study demonstrated that cells stably tranfected with Cdc42(F28L) exhibited not only anchorage-independent growth but also lower dependence on serum for growth (Lin, Bagrodia et al. 1997). A role for Cdc42 in Ras transformation has also been established in Rat 1 fibroblasts. Coexpression of a dominant negative form of Cdc42, Cdc42N17, with oncogenic Ras results in inhibition of RasV12-induced focus formation and anchorage-independent growth, and reversed the change in morphology in RasV12-transformed cells (Qiu, Abo et al. 1997).

5.5 Rho GTPases and angiogenesis

Beside their roles in multiple processes of cellular control, tumor growth, progression and metastasis, the Rho proteins have also been shown to be involved in angiogenesis, a process Where new blood vessels arise from existing mature vessels. This process is controlled by a number of pro-angiogenic and anti-angiogenic factors at different stages (Folkman 1972). The major pro-angiogenic factors are comprised of vascular endothelial growth factor (VEGF), fibroblast growth factors (FGF), platelet derived growth factor-β (PDGFβ), angiopoietins 1 and 2 (Ang-1 and 2), tumor necrosis factor (TNF), interleukin 6 and 8 (IL-6 and 8), and epidermal growth factor (EGF). The main anti-angiogenic foctors include the thrombospondins (TSPs), angiostatin, and endostain (Merajver and Usmani 2005). The Rho proteins are believed to be capable of altering the expression and activity of pro-angiogenic and anti-angiogenic factors during angiogenesis.

5.5.1 Regulation of VEGF and hypoxia inducible factor-1 (HIF1)

It has been reported that hypoxia increases the expression and activity of Cdc42, Rac1 and RhoA in renal cell carcinoma cell lines and a human microvascular endothelial cell line (Turcotte, Desrosiers et al. 2003). This study demonstrated that reactive oxygen species (ROS) are responsible for the upregulation of Rho proteins and that RhoA is required for the accumulation of HIF-1α (Turcotte, Desrosiers et al. 2003), a transcription factor induced by hypoxia that plays important roles in the process of angiogenesis by inducing the transcription of crucial mediators, including VEGF, PDGFβ and Ang-2 (Gleadle and Ratcliffe 1998). In contrast, Rac1 is shown to be involved in hypoxia-induced PI3K activation of HIF-1α through a different mechanism (Hirota and Semenza 2001). Hypoxia-induced expression of Rac1 also contributes to the upregulation of HIF-1α and, subsequently, VEGF in gastric and hepatocellular cancer cells (Xue, Bi et al. 2004). VEGF has been reported to increase RhoA activity and localization to the cell membrane, and the RhoA /ROCK pathway has been implicated in the VEGF-mediated angiogenesis (van Nieuw Amerongen, Koolwijk et al. 2003). In addition, RhoA activation also increases tyrosine phosphorylation of the primary VEGF receptor, VEGFR-2 (Gingras, Lamy et al. 2000).

Overexpression of RhoC in human mammary epithelial cells (HME) and a highly aggressive breast cancer cell line, SUM-149, increases VEGF expression (van Golen, Wu et al. 2000). Similar finding were found in the MCF10A cells (Wu, Wu et al. 2004), further suggesting that RhoC plays a role in, further suggesting that RhoC plays a role in increasing VEGF in mammary neoplasis.

5.5.2 IL-6 and IL-8 expression

IL-6 is a multifunctional cytokine that is involved in many different biological process, including immunological and inflammatory processes, tumor growth and angiogenesis (Hirano, Akira et al. 1990; Mateo, Reichner et al. 1994). IL-8 is another important cytokine that acts as a pro-angiogenic factor. Both of these cytokines can be induced by hypoxia (Yan, Tritto et al. 1995; Mizukami, Jo et al. 2005) and have been shown to upregulate VEGF mRNA expression (Cohen, Nahari et al. 1996). Studies indicate that active Rho proteins upregulate the expression of NFκB components in NIH-3T3 cells (Perona, Montaner et al. 1997; Montaner, Perona et al. 1998). Consistent with Rho-mediated activation of NFκB, HKG-CoA reductase inhibitors had been reported to reduce IL-6 expression by inhibiting Rho proteins (Ito, Ikeda et al. 2002). Rac1 has been shown to mediate the activation of a potential oncogen, STAT3, through NFκB regulated IL-6 signaling (Faruqi, Gomez et al. 2001).

IL-8 expression has also been found to be regulated by Rho proteins. In human endothelial cells, it has been shown that inhibition of RhoA, Rac1 and Cdc42 decreases NFκB activation and, therefore, decreases IL-8 mRNA and IL-8 protein expression (Hippenstiel, Soeth et al. 2000; Warny, Keates et al. 2000). In addition, RhoC has been shown to increase IL-6 and IL-8 expression in aggressive breast cancer cell lines (Xue, Bi et al. 2004). These evidences suggest that different Rho proteins modulate IL-6 and IL-8 through distinct signaling pathways.

5.5.3 FGF activation

FGF1 and FGF2 are the two earliest characterized members of the FGF family of growth factors. FGF is an angiogenic factor that is frequently overexpressed in breast and prostate cancers. Rac1 and Cdc42 have been reported to increase FGF1 expression by stimulating the FGF1 gene promoter region (Chotani, Touhalisky et al. 2000). One study demonstrated that Rac1 activity is required for FGF2-induced activation of Ras/MAPK signaling in human breast cell line MCF7 (Liu, Chevet et al. 1999). In addition, medium collected from RhoC stably transfected HME and SUM149 cells present higher level of FGF2, in comparison to those collected from control transfected HME cells (van Golen, Wu et al. 2000). However, how Rho proteins regulate FGF expression remains unclear.

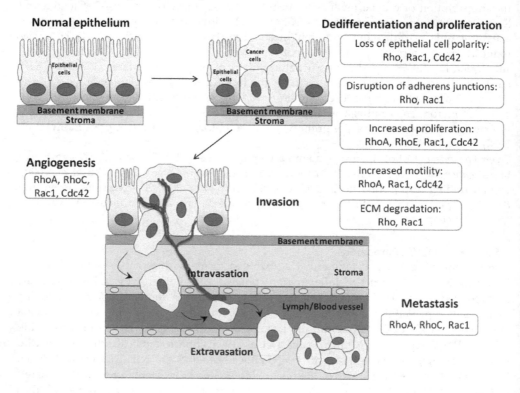

Fig. 4. Rho family GTPases are involved in different stages of breast cancer progression: dedifferentiation and upregulation of uncontrolled proliferation, angiogenesis, invasion and metastasis.

5.5.4 Repression of Tsp-1

The anti-angiogenic molecule Tsp-1 is capable of inhibiting metalloproteinase-9 (MMP9) from releasing the VEGF sequestered in ECM. The oncoprotein Ras has been reported to increase VEGF expression and inhibit Tsp-1 expression. One study showed that the inhibitory function of Ras on Tsp-1 via PI3K pathway also involve RhoA and RhoC in human embryonic kidney cell lines, human mammary cell lines, and breast cancer cell lines

(Watnick, Cheng et al. 2003). And the suppression of Tsp-1 always correlates with promotion of angiogenesis.

6. Conclusion

It is apparent that individual members of Rho GTPases play specific roles in different aspects in breast cancer development (Fig. 4). Aberrant expression and activity of Rho proteins contribute to the transformation from normal epithelial phenotype, increases in proliferation, the promotion of angiogenesis, elevated motility, and metastasis to distant organs. RhoA, RhoC and Rac1 are frequently overexpressed in metastatic breast cancers. Manipulating the Rho GTPases' regulatory proteins and their effectors can induce activation of Rho proteins, , leading to aberrant transcription factor activation, including that of NFκB, that contribute to invasive phenotypes. All this evidence suggests that Rho GTPases could be targets in cancer therapy. Therefore, better knowledge of the the regulation mechanisms of Rho GTPases in breast cancer may be critical for a more in-depth understanding of tumor biology, facilitating development of novel approaches for cancer treatment.

7. References

Abo, A., E. Pick, et al. (1991). "Activation of the NADPH oxidase involves the small GTP-binding protein p21rac1." Nature 353(6345): 668-70.

Abraham, M. T., M. A. Kuriakose, et al. (2001). "Motility-related proteins as markers for head and neck squamous cell cancer." Laryngoscope 111(7): 1285-9.

Amano, M., M. Ito, et al. (1996). "Phosphorylation and activation of myosin by Rho-associated kinase (Rho-kinase)." J Biol Chem 271(34): 20246-9.

Arber, S., F. A. Barbayannis, et al. (1998). "Regulation of actin dynamics through phosphorylation of cofilin by LIM-kinase." Nature 393(6687): 805-9.

Aspenstrom, P., U. Lindberg, et al. (1996). "Two GTPases, Cdc42 and Rac, bind directly to a protein implicated in the immunodeficiency disorder Wiskott-Aldrich syndrome." Curr Biol 6(1): 70-5.

Bourguignon, L. Y. (2001). "CD44-mediated oncogenic signaling and cytoskeleton activation during mammary tumor progression." J Mammary Gland Biol Neoplasia 6(3): 287-97.

Bourguignon, L. Y., H. Zhu, et al. (1999). "Rho-kinase (ROK) promotes CD44v(3,8-10)-ankyrin interaction and tumor cell migration in metastatic breast cancer cells." Cell Motil Cytoskeleton 43(4): 269-87.

Bouzahzah, B., C. Albanese, et al. (2001). "Rho family GTPases regulate mammary epithelium cell growth and metastasis through distinguishable pathways." Mol Med 7(12): 816-30.

Braga, V. M., L. M. Machesky, et al. (1997). "The small GTPases Rho and Rac are required for the establishment of cadherin-dependent cell-cell contacts." J Cell Biol 137(6): 1421-31.

Campellone, K. G. and M. D. Welch "A nucleator arms race: cellular control of actin assembly." Nat Rev Mol Cell Biol 11(4): 237-51.

Cerione, R. A. and Y. Zheng (1996). "The Dbl family of oncogenes." Curr Opin Cell Biol 8(2): 216-22.

Chang, J. H., S. Gill, et al. (1995). "c-Src regulates the simultaneous rearrangement of actin cytoskeleton, p190RhoGAP, and p120RasGAP following epidermal growth factor stimulation." J Cell Biol 130(2): 355-68.

Chesarone, M. A. and B. L. Goode (2009). "Actin nucleation and elongation factors: mechanisms and interplay." Curr Opin Cell Biol 21(1): 28-37.

Chotani, M. A., K. Touhalisky, et al. (2000). "The small GTPases Ras, Rac, and Cdc42 transcriptionally regulate expression of human fibroblast growth factor 1." J Biol Chem 275(39): 30432-8.

Chuang, T. H., X. Xu, et al. (1993). "GDP dissociation inhibitor prevents intrinsic and GTPase activating protein-stimulated GTP hydrolysis by the Rac GTP-binding protein." J Biol Chem 268(2): 775-8.

Cohen, T., D. Nahari, et al. (1996). "Interleukin 6 induces the expression of vascular endothelial growth factor." J Biol Chem 271(2): 736-41.

Coso, O. A., M. Chiariello, et al. (1995). "The small GTP-binding proteins Rac1 and Cdc42 regulate the activity of the JNK/SAPK signaling pathway." Cell 81(7): 1137-46.

Cox, E. A. and A. Huttenlocher (1998). "Regulation of integrin-mediated adhesion during cell migration." Microsc Res Tech 43(5): 412-9.

Crespo, P., K. E. Schuebel, et al. (1997). "Phosphotyrosine-dependent activation of Rac-1 GDP/GTP exchange by the vav proto-oncogene product." Nature 385(6612): 169-72.

del Peso, L., R. Hernandez-Alcoceba, et al. (1997). "Rho proteins induce metastatic properties in vivo." Oncogene 15(25): 3047-57.

Denoyelle, C., M. Vasse, et al. (2001). "Cerivastatin, an inhibitor of HMG-CoA reductase, inhibits the signaling pathways involved in the invasiveness and metastatic properties of highly invasive breast cancer cell lines: an in vitro study." Carcinogenesis 22(8): 1139-48.

Derijard, B., M. Hibi, et al. (1994). "JNK1: a protein kinase stimulated by UV light and Ha-Ras that binds and phosphorylates the c-Jun activation domain." Cell 76(6): 1025-37.

DerMardirossian, C. and G. M. Bokoch (2001). "Regulation of cell function by Rho GTPases." Drug News Perspect 14(7): 389-95.

Erickson, J. W., R. A. Cerione, et al. (1997). "Identification of an actin cytoskeletal complex that includes IQGAP and the Cdc42 GTPase." J Biol Chem 272(39): 24443-7.

Eva, A. and S. A. Aaronson (1985). "Isolation of a new human oncogene from a diffuse B-cell lymphoma." Nature 316(6025): 273-5.

Faruqi, T. R., D. Gomez, et al. (2001). "Rac1 mediates STAT3 activation by autocrine IL-6." Proc Natl Acad Sci U S A 98(16): 9014-9.

Finlayson, C. A., J. Chappell, et al. (2003). "Enhanced insulin signaling via Shc in human breast cancer." Metabolism 52(12): 1606-11.

Fisher, K. E., A. Sacharidou, et al. (2009). "MT1-MMP- and Cdc42-dependent signaling co-regulate cell invasion and tunnel formation in 3D collagen matrices." J Cell Sci 122(Pt 24): 4558-69.

Folkman, J. (1972). "Anti-angiogenesis: new concept for therapy of solid tumors." Ann Surg 175(3): 409-16.

Fritz, G., C. Brachetti, et al. (2002). "Rho GTPases in human breast tumours: expression and mutation analyses and correlation with clinical parameters." Br J Cancer 87(6): 635-44.

Fritz, G., I. Just, et al. (1999). "Rho GTPases are over-expressed in human tumors." Int J Cancer 81(5): 682-7.

Fujiwara, T., A. Mammoto, et al. (2000). "Rho small G-protein-dependent binding of mDia to an Src homology 3 domain-containing IRSp53/BAIAP2." Biochem Biophys Res Commun 271(3): 626-9.

Fukata, M., S. Kuroda, et al. (1997). "Regulation of cross-linking of actin filament by IQGAP1, a target for Cdc42." J Biol Chem 272(47): 29579-83.

Fukata, Y., M. Amano, et al. (2001). "Rho-Rho-kinase pathway in smooth muscle contraction and cytoskeletal reorganization of non-muscle cells." Trends Pharmacol Sci 22(1): 32-9.

Fukata, Y., N. Oshiro, et al. (1999). "Phosphorylation of adducin by Rho-kinase plays a crucial role in cell motility." J Cell Biol 145(2): 347-61.

Fukumoto, Y., K. Kaibuchi, et al. (1990). "Molecular cloning and characterization of a novel type of regulatory protein (GDI) for the rho proteins, ras p21-like small GTP-binding proteins." Oncogene 5(9): 1321-8.

Gardner, K. and V. Bennett (1987). "Modulation of spectrin-actin assembly by erythrocyte adducin." Nature 328(6128): 359-62.

Gerwins, P., J. L. Blank, et al. (1997). "Cloning of a novel mitogen-activated protein kinase kinase kinase, MEKK4, that selectively regulates the c-Jun amino terminal kinase pathway." J Biol Chem 272(13): 8288-95.

Gille, H., T. Strahl, et al. (1995). "Activation of ternary complex factor Elk-1 by stress-activated protein kinases." Curr Biol 5(10): 1191-200.

Gingras, D., S. Lamy, et al. (2000). "Tyrosine phosphorylation of the vascular endothelial-growth-factor receptor-2 (VEGFR-2) is modulated by Rho proteins." Biochem J 348 Pt 2: 273-80.

Glaven, J. A., I. P. Whitehead, et al. (1996). "Lfc and Lsc oncoproteins represent two new guanine nucleotide exchange factors for the Rho GTP-binding protein." J Biol Chem 271(44): 27374-81.

Gleadle, J. M. and P. J. Ratcliffe (1998). "Hypoxia and the regulation of gene expression." Mol Med Today 4(3): 122-9.

Goode, B. L. and M. J. Eck (2007). "Mechanism and function of formins in the control of actin assembly." Annu Rev Biochem 76: 593-627.

Gulbins, E., K. M. Coggeshall, et al. (1993). "Tyrosine kinase-stimulated guanine nucleotide exchange activity of Vav in T cell activation." Science 260(5109): 822-5.

Habets, G. G., E. H. Scholtes, et al. (1994). "Identification of an invasion-inducing gene, Tiam-1, that encodes a protein with homology to GDP-GTP exchangers for Rho-like proteins." Cell 77(4): 537-49.

Hall, A. (1990). "ras and GAP--who's controlling whom?" Cell 61(6): 921-3.

Han, J., B. Das, et al. (1997). "Lck regulates Vav activation of members of the Rho family of GTPases." Mol Cell Biol 17(3): 1346-53.

Hart, M. J., Y. Maru, et al. (1992). "A GDP dissociation inhibitor that serves as a GTPase inhibitor for the Ras-like protein CDC42Hs." Science 258(5083): 812-5.

Hill, C. S., J. Wynne, et al. (1995). "The Rho family GTPases RhoA, Rac1, and CDC42Hs regulate transcriptional activation by SRF." Cell 81(7): 1159-70.

Hippenstiel, S., S. Soeth, et al. (2000). "Rho proteins and the p38-MAPK pathway are important mediators for LPS-induced interleukin-8 expression in human endothelial cells." Blood 95(10): 3044-51.

Hirano, T., S. Akira, et al. (1990). "Biological and clinical aspects of interleukin 6." Immunol Today 11(12): 443-9.

Hirota, K. and G. L. Semenza (2001). "Rac1 activity is required for the activation of hypoxia-inducible factor 1." J Biol Chem 276(24): 21166-72.

Huang, M. and G. C. Prendergast (2006). "RhoB in cancer suppression." Histol Histopathol 21(2): 213-8.

Ishizaki, T., M. Maekawa, et al. (1996). "The small GTP-binding protein Rho binds to and activates a 160 kDa Ser/Thr protein kinase homologous to myotonic dystrophy kinase." EMBO J 15(8): 1885-93.

Ito, T., U. Ikeda, et al. (2002). "HMG-CoA reductase inhibitors reduce interleukin-6 synthesis in human vascular smooth muscle cells." Cardiovasc Drugs Ther 16(2): 121-6.

Joberty, G., C. Petersen, et al. (2000). "The cell-polarity protein Par6 links Par3 and atypical protein kinase C to Cdc42." Nat Cell Biol 2(8): 531-9.

Jou, T. S. and W. J. Nelson (1998). "Effects of regulated expression of mutant RhoA and Rac1 small GTPases on the development of epithelial (MDCK) cell polarity." J Cell Biol 142(1): 85-100.

Kamai, T., T. Tsujii, et al. (2003). "Significant association of Rho/ROCK pathway with invasion and metastasis of bladder cancer." Clin Cancer Res 9(7): 2632-41.

Keely, P. J., J. K. Westwick, et al. (1997). "Cdc42 and Rac1 induce integrin-mediated cell motility and invasiveness through PI(3)K." Nature 390(6660): 632-6.

Khosravi-Far, R., P. A. Solski, et al. (1995). "Activation of Rac1, RhoA, and mitogen-activated protein kinases is required for Ras transformation." Mol Cell Biol 15(11): 6443-53.

Kimura, K., Y. Fukata, et al. (1998). "Regulation of the association of adducin with actin filaments by Rho-associated kinase (Rho-kinase) and myosin phosphatase." J Biol Chem 273(10): 5542-8.

Kimura, K., M. Ito, et al. (1996). "Regulation of myosin phosphatase by Rho and Rho-associated kinase (Rho-kinase)." Science 273(5272): 245-8.

Kodama, A., K. Takaishi, et al. (1999). "Involvement of Cdc42 small G protein in cell-cell adhesion, migration and morphology of MDCK cells." Oncogene 18(27): 3996-4006.

Kolluri, R., K. F. Tolias, et al. (1996). "Direct interaction of the Wiskott-Aldrich syndrome protein with the GTPase Cdc42." Proc Natl Acad Sci U S A 93(11): 5615-8.

Kosako, H., T. Yoshida, et al. (2000). "Rho-kinase/ROCK is involved in cytokinesis through the phosphorylation of myosin light chain and not ezrin/radixin/moesin proteins at the cleavage furrow." Oncogene 19(52): 6059-64.

Kroschewski, R., A. Hall, et al. (1999). "Cdc42 controls secretory and endocytic transport to the basolateral plasma membrane of MDCK cells." Nat Cell Biol 1(1): 8-13.

Kuroda, S., M. Fukata, et al. (1996). "Identification of IQGAP as a putative target for the small GTPases, Cdc42 and Rac1." J Biol Chem 271(38): 23363-7.

Lamb, R. F., C. Roy, et al. (2000). "The TSC1 tumour suppressor hamartin regulates cell adhesion through ERM proteins and the GTPase Rho." Nat Cell Biol 2(5): 281-7.

Lancaster, C. A., P. M. Taylor-Harris, et al. (1994). "Characterization of rhoGAP. A GTPase-activating protein for rho-related small GTPases." J Biol Chem 269(2): 1137-42.

Leeuwen, F. N., H. E. Kain, et al. (1997). "The guanine nucleotide exchange factor Tiam1 affects neuronal morphology; opposing roles for the small GTPases Rac and Rho." J Cell Biol 139(3): 797-807.

Leonard, D., M. J. Hart, et al. (1992). "The identification and characterization of a GDP-dissociation inhibitor (GDI) for the CDC42Hs protein." J Biol Chem 267(32): 22860-8.

Leung, K., A. Nagy, et al. (2003). "Targeted expression of activated Rac3 in mammary epithelium leads to defective postlactational involution and benign mammary gland lesions." Cells Tissues Organs 175(2): 72-83.

Leung, T., X. Q. Chen, et al. (1998). "Myotonic dystrophy kinase-related Cdc42-binding kinase acts as a Cdc42 effector in promoting cytoskeletal reorganization." Mol Cell Biol 18(1): 130-40.

Leung, T., E. Manser, et al. (1995). "A novel serine/threonine kinase binding the Ras-related RhoA GTPase which translocates the kinase to peripheral membranes." J Biol Chem 270(49): 29051-4.

Li, Z., M. Hannigan, et al. (2003). "Directional sensing requires G beta gamma-mediated PAK1 and PIX alpha-dependent activation of Cdc42." Cell 114(2): 215-27.

Liberto, M., D. Cobrinik, et al. (2002). "Rho regulates p21(CIP1), cyclin D1, and checkpoint control in mammary epithelial cells." Oncogene 21(10): 1590-9.

Lin, D., A. S. Edwards, et al. (2000). "A mammalian PAR-3-PAR-6 complex implicated in Cdc42/Rac1 and aPKC signalling and cell polarity." Nat Cell Biol 2(8): 540-7.

Lin, R., S. Bagrodia, et al. (1997). "A novel Cdc42Hs mutant induces cellular transformation." Curr Biol 7(10): 794-7.

Liu, J. F., E. Chevet, et al. (1999). "Functional Rac-1 and Nck signaling networks are required for FGF-2-induced DNA synthesis in MCF-7 cells." Oncogene 18(47): 6425-33.

Maekawa, M., T. Ishizaki, et al. (1999). "Signaling from Rho to the actin cytoskeleton through protein kinases ROCK and LIM-kinase." Science 285(5429): 895-8.

Manser, E., C. Chong, et al. (1995). "Molecular cloning of a new member of the p21-Cdc42/Rac-activated kinase (PAK) family." J Biol Chem 270(42): 25070-8.

Manser, E., T. Leung, et al. (1994). "A brain serine/threonine protein kinase activated by Cdc42 and Rac1." Nature 367(6458): 40-6.

Marionnet, C., C. Lalou, et al. (2003). "Differential molecular profiling between skin carcinomas reveals four newly reported genes potentially implicated in squamous cell carcinoma development." Oncogene 22(22): 3500-5.

Mateo, R. B., J. S. Reichner, et al. (1994). "Interleukin-6 activity in wounds." Am J Physiol 266(6 Pt 2): R1840-4.

Matsui, T., M. Maeda, et al. (1998). "Rho-kinase phosphorylates COOH-terminal threonines of ezrin/radixin/moesin (ERM) proteins and regulates their head-to-tail association." J Cell Biol 140(3): 647-57.

Mazieres, J., T. Antonia, et al. (2004). "Loss of RhoB expression in human lung cancer progression." Clin Cancer Res 10(8): 2742-50.

Merajver, S. D. and S. Z. Usmani (2005). "Multifaceted role of Rho proteins in angiogenesis." J Mammary Gland Biol Neoplasia 10(4): 291-8.

Michiels, F. and J. G. Collard (1999). "Rho-like GTPases: their role in cell adhesion and invasion." Biochem Soc Symp 65: 125-46.

Michiels, F., G. G. Habets, et al. (1995). "A role for Rac in Tiam1-induced membrane ruffling and invasion." Nature 375(6529): 338-40.

Miki, H., K. Miura, et al. (1996). "N-WASP, a novel actin-depolymerizing protein, regulates the cortical cytoskeletal rearrangement in a PIP2-dependent manner downstream of tyrosine kinases." EMBO J 15(19): 5326-35.

Miki, H., T. Sasaki, et al. (1998). "Induction of filopodium formation by a WASP-related actin-depolymerizing protein N-WASP." Nature 391(6662): 93-6.

Miki, H., H. Yamaguchi, et al. (2000). "IRSp53 is an essential intermediate between Rac and WAVE in the regulation of membrane ruffling." Nature 408(6813): 732-5.

Minden, A., A. Lin, et al. (1995). "Selective activation of the JNK signaling cascade and c-Jun transcriptional activity by the small GTPases Rac and Cdc42Hs." Cell 81(7): 1147-57.

Mira, J. P., V. Benard, et al. (2000). "Endogenous, hyperactive Rac3 controls proliferation of breast cancer cells by a p21-activated kinase-dependent pathway." Proc Natl Acad Sci U S A 97(1): 185-9.

Mizukami, Y., W. S. Jo, et al. (2005). "Induction of interleukin-8 preserves the angiogenic response in HIF-1alpha-deficient colon cancer cells." Nat Med 11(9): 992-7.

Montaner, S., R. Perona, et al. (1998). "Multiple signalling pathways lead to the activation of the nuclear factor kappaB by the Rho family of GTPases." J Biol Chem 273(21): 12779-85.

Morris, C. M., L. Haataja, et al. (2000). "The small GTPase RAC3 gene is located within chromosome band 17q25.3 outside and telomeric of a region commonly deleted in breast and ovarian tumours." Cytogenet Cell Genet 89(1-2): 18-23.

Narumiya, S., T. Ishizaki, et al. (2000). "Use and properties of ROCK-specific inhibitor Y-27632." Methods Enzymol 325: 273-84.

Narumiya, S. and N. Morii (1993). "rho gene products, botulinum C3 exoenzyme and cell adhesion." Cell Signal 5(1): 9-19.

Nobes, C. D. and A. Hall (1995). "Rho, rac and cdc42 GTPases: regulators of actin structures, cell adhesion and motility." Biochem Soc Trans 23(3): 456-9.

Nobes, C. D. and A. Hall (1995). "Rho, rac, and cdc42 GTPases regulate the assembly of multimolecular focal complexes associated with actin stress fibers, lamellipodia, and filopodia." Cell 81(1): 53-62.

O'Connor, K. L., B. K. Nguyen, et al. (2000). "RhoA function in lamellae formation and migration is regulated by the alpha6beta4 integrin and cAMP metabolism." J Cell Biol 148(2): 253-8.

O'Hagan, R. C., R. G. Tozer, et al. (1996). "The activity of the Ets transcription factor PEA3 is regulated by two distinct MAPK cascades." Oncogene 13(6): 1323-33.

Olofsson, B. (1999). "Rho guanine dissociation inhibitors: pivotal molecules in cellular signalling." Cell Signal 11(8): 545-54.

Olson, M. F., A. Ashworth, et al. (1995). "An essential role for Rho, Rac, and Cdc42 GTPases in cell cycle progression through G1." Science 269(5228): 1270-2.

Page, K., J. Li, et al. (1999). "Characterization of a Rac1 signaling pathway to cyclin D(1) expression in airway smooth muscle cells." J Biol Chem 274(31): 22065-71.

Palecek, S. P., A. Huttenlocher, et al. (1998). "Physical and biochemical regulation of integrin release during rear detachment of migrating cells." J Cell Sci 111 (Pt 7): 929-40.

Pasteris, N. G., A. Cadle, et al. (1994). "Isolation and characterization of the faciogenital dysplasia (Aarskog-Scott syndrome) gene: a putative Rho/Rac guanine nucleotide exchange factor." Cell 79(4): 669-78.

Perona, R., S. Montaner, et al. (1997). "Activation of the nuclear factor-kappaB by Rho, CDC42, and Rac-1 proteins." Genes Dev 11(4): 463-75.

Pinner, S. and E. Sahai (2008). "PDK1 regulates cancer cell motility by antagonising inhibition of ROCK1 by RhoE." Nat Cell Biol 10(2): 127-37.

Pollard, T. D., L. Blanchoin, et al. (2000). "Molecular mechanisms controlling actin filament dynamics in nonmuscle cells." Annu Rev Biophys Biomol Struct 29: 545-76.

Potter, D. A., J. S. Tirnauer, et al. (1998). "Calpain regulates actin remodeling during cell spreading." J Cell Biol 141(3): 647-62.

Price, L. S., J. Leng, et al. (1998). "Activation of Rac and Cdc42 by integrins mediates cell spreading." Mol Biol Cell 9(7): 1863-71.

Pruyne, D. and A. Bretscher (2000). "Polarization of cell growth in yeast. I. Establishment and maintenance of polarity states." J Cell Sci 113 (Pt 3): 365-75.

Qiu, R. G., A. Abo, et al. (1997). "Cdc42 regulates anchorage-independent growth and is necessary for Ras transformation." Mol Cell Biol 17(6): 3449-58.

Qiu, R. G., A. Abo, et al. (2000). "A human homolog of the C. elegans polarity determinant Par-6 links Rac and Cdc42 to PKCzeta signaling and cell transformation." Curr Biol 10(12): 697-707.

Qiu, R. G., J. Chen, et al. (1995). "An essential role for Rac in Ras transformation." Nature 374(6521): 457-9.

Qiu, R. G., J. Chen, et al. (1995). "A role for Rho in Ras transformation." Proc Natl Acad Sci U S A 92(25): 11781-5.

Ridley, A. J., H. F. Paterson, et al. (1992). "The small GTP-binding protein rac regulates growth factor-induced membrane ruffling." Cell 70(3): 401-10.

Ridley, A. J., M. A. Schwartz, et al. (2003). "Cell migration: integrating signals from front to back." Science 302(5651): 1704-9.

Riento, K. and A. J. Ridley (2003). "Rocks: multifunctional kinases in cell behaviour." Nat Rev Mol Cell Biol 4(6): 446-56.

Rodriguez, O. C., A. W. Schaefer, et al. (2003). "Conserved microtubule-actin interactions in cell movement and morphogenesis." Nat Cell Biol 5(7): 599-609.

Ron, D., M. Zannini, et al. (1991). "A region of proto-dbl essential for its transforming activity shows sequence similarity to a yeast cell cycle gene, CDC24, and the human breakpoint cluster gene, bcr." New Biol 3(4): 372-9.

Roovers, K. and R. K. Assoian (2003). "Effects of rho kinase and actin stress fibers on sustained extracellular signal-regulated kinase activity and activation of G(1) phase cyclin-dependent kinases." Mol Cell Biol 23(12): 4283-94.

Rosenblatt, A. E., M. I. Garcia, et al. "Inhibition of the Rho GTPase, Rac1, decreases estrogen receptor levels and is a novel therapeutic strategy in breast cancer." Endocr Relat Cancer 18(2): 207-19.

Rottner, K., A. Hall, et al. (1999). "Interplay between Rac and Rho in the control of substrate contact dynamics." Curr Biol 9(12): 640-8.

Sahai, E. and C. J. Marshall (2002). "RHO-GTPases and cancer." Nat Rev Cancer 2(2): 133-42.

Sanders, L. C., F. Matsumura, et al. (1999). "Inhibition of myosin light chain kinase by p21-activated kinase." Science 283(5410): 2083-5.

Scheffzek, K. and M. R. Ahmadian (2005). "GTPase activating proteins: structural and functional insights 18 years after discovery." Cell Mol Life Sci 62(24): 3014-38.

Seger, R. and E. G. Krebs (1995). "The MAPK signaling cascade." FASEB J 9(9): 726-35.

Shaw, L. M., I. Rabinovitz, et al. (1997). "Activation of phosphoinositide 3-OH kinase by the alpha6beta4 integrin promotes carcinoma invasion." Cell 91(7): 949-60.

Small, J. V. (1994). "Lamellipodia architecture: actin filament turnover and the lateral flow of actin filaments during motility." Semin Cell Biol 5(3): 157-63.

Srinivasan, S., F. Wang, et al. (2003). "Rac and Cdc42 play distinct roles in regulating PI(3,4,5)P3 and polarity during neutrophil chemotaxis." J Cell Biol 160(3): 375-85.

Stam, J. C., F. Michiels, et al. (1998). "Invasion of T-lymphoma cells: cooperation between Rho family GTPases and lysophospholipid receptor signaling." EMBO J 17(14): 4066-74.

Suwa, H., G. Ohshio, et al. (1998). "Overexpression of the rhoC gene correlates with progression of ductal adenocarcinoma of the pancreas." Br J Cancer 77(1): 147-52.

Takai, Y., T. Sasaki, et al. (1995). "Rho as a regulator of the cytoskeleton." Trends Biochem Sci 20(6): 227-31.

Takaishi, K., T. Sasaki, et al. (1997). "Regulation of cell-cell adhesion by rac and rho small G proteins in MDCK cells." J Cell Biol 139(4): 1047-59.

Tang, Y., L. Olufemi, et al. (2008). "Role of Rho GTPases in breast cancer." Front Biosci 13: 759-76.

Tarakhovsky, A., M. Turner, et al. (1995). "Defective antigen receptor-mediated proliferation of B and T cells in the absence of Vav." Nature 374(6521): 467-70.

Teramoto, H., O. A. Coso, et al. (1996). "Signaling from the small GTP-binding proteins Rac1 and Cdc42 to the c-Jun N-terminal kinase/stress-activated protein kinase pathway. A role for mixed lineage kinase 3/protein-tyrosine kinase 1, a novel member of the mixed lineage kinase family." J Biol Chem 271(44): 27225-8.

Teramoto, H., P. Crespo, et al. (1996). "The small GTP-binding protein rho activates c-Jun N-terminal kinases/stress-activated protein kinases in human kidney 293T cells. Evidence for a Pak-independent signaling pathway." J Biol Chem 271(42): 25731-4.

Tominaga, T., T. Ishizaki, et al. (1998). "p160ROCK mediates RhoA activation of Na-H exchange." EMBO J 17(16): 4712-22.

Totsukawa, G., Y. Yamakita, et al. (2000). "Distinct roles of ROCK (Rho-kinase) and MLCK in spatial regulation of MLC phosphorylation for assembly of stress fibers and focal adhesions in 3T3 fibroblasts." J Cell Biol 150(4): 797-806.

Treisman, R. (1990). "The SRE: a growth factor responsive transcriptional regulator." Semin Cancer Biol 1(1): 47-58.

Turcotte, S., R. R. Desrosiers, et al. (2003). "HIF-1alpha mRNA and protein upregulation involves Rho GTPase expression during hypoxia in renal cell carcinoma." J Cell Sci 116(Pt 11): 2247-60.

Ueda, T., A. Kikuchi, et al. (1990). "Purification and characterization from bovine brain cytosol of a novel regulatory protein inhibiting the dissociation of GDP from and the subsequent binding of GTP to rhoB p20, a ras p21-like GTP-binding protein." J Biol Chem 265(16): 9373-80.

Uehata, M., T. Ishizaki, et al. (1997). "Calcium sensitization of smooth muscle mediated by a Rho-associated protein kinase in hypertension." Nature 389(6654): 990-4.

Urban, E., S. Jacob, et al. "Electron tomography reveals unbranched networks of actin filaments in lamellipodia." Nat Cell Biol 12(5): 429-35.

Van Aelst, L. and C. D'Souza-Schorey (1997). "Rho GTPases and signaling networks." Genes Dev 11(18): 2295-322.

van Golen, K. L., S. Davies, et al. (1999). "A novel putative low-affinity insulin-like growth factor-binding protein, LIBC (lost in inflammatory breast cancer), and RhoC GTPase correlate with the inflammatory breast cancer phenotype." Clin Cancer Res 5(9): 2511-9.

van Golen, K. L., Z. F. Wu, et al. (2000). "RhoC GTPase overexpression modulates induction of angiogenic factors in breast cells." Neoplasia 2(5): 418-25.

van Leeuwen, F. N., R. A. van der Kammen, et al. (1995). "Oncogenic activity of Tiam1 and Rac1 in NIH3T3 cells." Oncogene 11(11): 2215-21.

van Nieuw Amerongen, G. P., P. Koolwijk, et al. (2003). "Involvement of RhoA/Rho kinase signaling in VEGF-induced endothelial cell migration and angiogenesis in vitro." Arterioscler Thromb Vasc Biol 23(2): 211-7.

Villalonga, P., R. M. Guasch, et al. (2004). "RhoE inhibits cell cycle progression and Ras-induced transformation." Mol Cell Biol 24(18): 7829-40.

Warny, M., A. C. Keates, et al. (2000). "p38 MAP kinase activation by Clostridium difficile toxin A mediates monocyte necrosis, IL-8 production, and enteritis." J Clin Invest 105(8): 1147-56.

Wasserman, S. (1998). "FH proteins as cytoskeletal organizers." Trends Cell Biol 8(3): 111-5.

Watanabe, N., T. Kato, et al. (1999). "Cooperation between mDia1 and ROCK in Rho-induced actin reorganization." Nat Cell Biol 1(3): 136-43.

Watanabe, N., P. Madaule, et al. (1997). "p140mDia, a mammalian homolog of Drosophila diaphanous, is a target protein for Rho small GTPase and is a ligand for profilin." EMBO J 16(11): 3044-56.

Watanabe, S., Y. Ando, et al. (2008). "mDia2 induces the actin scaffold for the contractile ring and stabilizes its position during cytokinesis in NIH 3T3 cells." Mol Biol Cell 19(5): 2328-38.

Watnick, R. S., Y. N. Cheng, et al. (2003). "Ras modulates Myc activity to repress thrombospondin-1 expression and increase tumor angiogenesis." Cancer Cell 3(3): 219-31.

Wear, M. A., D. A. Schafer, et al. (2000). "Actin dynamics: assembly and disassembly of actin networks." Curr Biol 10(24): R891-5.

Weber, J. D., W. Hu, et al. (1997). "Ras-stimulated extracellular signal-related kinase 1 and RhoA activities coordinate platelet-derived growth factor-induced G1 progression through the independent regulation of cyclin D1 and p27." J Biol Chem 272(52): 32966-71.

Welch, M. D., A. H. DePace, et al. (1997). "The human Arp2/3 complex is composed of evolutionarily conserved subunits and is localized to cellular regions of dynamic actin filament assembly." J Cell Biol 138(2): 375-84.

Wennerberg, K. and C. J. Der (2004). "Rho-family GTPases: it's not only Rac and Rho (and I like it)." J Cell Sci 117(Pt 8): 1301-12.

Westwick, J. K., Q. T. Lambert, et al. (1997). "Rac regulation of transformation, gene expression, and actin organization by multiple, PAK-independent pathways." Mol Cell Biol 17(3): 1324-35.

Wu, M., Z. F. Wu, et al. (2004). "RhoC induces differential expression of genes involved in invasion and metastasis in MCF10A breast cells." Breast Cancer Res Treat 84(1): 3-12.

Xue, Y., F. Bi, et al. (2004). "[Expressions and activities of Rho GTPases in hypoxia and its relationship with tumor angiogenesis]." Zhonghua Zhong Liu Za Zhi 26(9): 517-20.

Yamamoto, M., N. Marui, et al. (1993). "ADP-ribosylation of the rhoA gene product by botulinum C3 exoenzyme causes Swiss 3T3 cells to accumulate in the G1 phase of the cell cycle." Oncogene 8(6): 1449-55.

Yan, S. F., I. Tritto, et al. (1995). "Induction of interleukin 6 (IL-6) by hypoxia in vascular cells. Central role of the binding site for nuclear factor-IL-6." J Biol Chem 270(19): 11463-71.

Yang, N., O. Higuchi, et al. (1998). "Cofilin phosphorylation by LIM-kinase 1 and its role in Rac-mediated actin reorganization." Nature 393(6687): 809-12.

Yoshioka, K., F. Matsumura, et al. (1998). "Small GTP-binding protein Rho stimulates the actomyosin system, leading to invasion of tumor cells." J Biol Chem 273(9): 5146-54.

Zamir, E. and B. Geiger (2001). "Molecular complexity and dynamics of cell-matrix adhesions." J Cell Sci 114(Pt 20): 3583-90.

Zhang, S., J. Han, et al. (1995). "Rho family GTPases regulate p38 mitogen-activated protein kinase through the downstream mediator Pak1." J Biol Chem 270(41): 23934-6.

Zhang, X., D. Nie, et al. "Growth factors in tumor microenvironment." Front Biosci 15: 151-65.

Zheng, Y., D. Zangrilli, et al. (1996). "The pleckstrin homology domain mediates transformation by oncogenic dbl through specific intracellular targeting." J Biol Chem 271(32): 19017-20.

Zhong, C., M. S. Kinch, et al. (1997). "Rho-stimulated contractility contributes to the fibroblastic phenotype of Ras-transformed epithelial cells." Mol Biol Cell 8(11): 2329-44.

Zigmond, S. H. (1996). "Signal transduction and actin filament organization." Curr Opin Cell Biol 8(1): 66-73.

Permissions

The contributors of this book come from diverse backgrounds, making this book a truly international effort. This book will bring forth new frontiers with its revolutionizing research information and detailed analysis of the nascent developments around the world.

We would like to thank Prof. Dr. Mehmet Gunduz, for lending his expertise to make the book truly unique. He has played a crucial role in the development of this book. Without his invaluable contribution this book wouldn't have been possible. He has made vital efforts to compile up to date information on the varied aspects of this subject to make this book a valuable addition to the collection of many professionals and students.

This book was conceptualized with the vision of imparting up-to-date information and advanced data in this field. To ensure the same, a matchless editorial board was set up. Every individual on the board went through rigorous rounds of assessment to prove their worth. After which they invested a large part of their time researching and compiling the most relevant data for our readers. Conferences and sessions were held from time to time between the editorial board and the contributing authors to present the data in the most comprehensible form. The editorial team has worked tirelessly to provide valuable and valid information to help people across the globe.

Every chapter published in this book has been scrutinized by our experts. Their significance has been extensively debated. The topics covered herein carry significant findings which will fuel the growth of the discipline. They may even be implemented as practical applications or may be referred to as a beginning point for another development. Chapters in this book were first published by InTech; hereby published with permission under the Creative Commons Attribution License or equivalent.

The editorial board has been involved in producing this book since its inception. They have spent rigorous hours researching and exploring the diverse topics which have resulted in the successful publishing of this book. They have passed on their knowledge of decades through this book. To expedite this challenging task, the publisher supported the team at every step. A small team of assistant editors was also appointed to further simplify the editing procedure and attain best results for the readers.

Our editorial team has been hand-picked from every corner of the world. Their multi-ethnicity adds dynamic inputs to the discussions which result in innovative outcomes. These outcomes are then further discussed with the researchers and contributors who give their valuable feedback and opinion regarding the same. The feedback is then collaborated with the researches and they are edited in a comprehensive manner to aid the understanding of the subject.

Apart from the editorial board, the designing team has also invested a significant amount of their time in understanding the subject and creating the most relevant covers. They scrutinized every image to scout for the most suitable representation of the subject and create an appropriate cover for the book.

The publishing team has been involved in this book since its early stages. They were actively engaged in every process, be it collecting the data, connecting with the contributors or procuring relevant information. The team has been an ardent support to the editorial, designing and production team. Their endless efforts to recruit the best for this project, has resulted in the accomplishment of this book. They are a veteran in the field of academics and their pool of knowledge is as vast as their experience in printing. Their expertise and guidance has proved useful at every step. Their uncompromising quality standards have made this book an exceptional effort. Their encouragement from time to time has been an inspiration for everyone.

The publisher and the editorial board hope that this book will prove to be a valuable piece of knowledge for researchers, students, practitioners and scholars across the globe.

List of Contributors

Xue-Gang Luo, Shu Guo, Yu Guo and Chun-Ling Zhang
Tianjin University of Science and Technology, P. R. China

Majed Saleh Alokail
Department of Biochemistry, College of Science, King Saud University, Saudi Arabia

Fatemeh Kalalinia, Fatemeh Mosaffa and Javad Behravan
Biotechnology Research Center and Department of Pharmaceutical Biotechnology, Mashhad University of Medical Sciences, Mashhad, Iran

Tilen Koklic and Rok Podlipec
Jozef Stefan Institute, Ljubljana, Slovenia
Center of Excellence NAMASTE, Ljubljana, Slovenia

Maja Garvas and Marjeta Šentjurc
Jozef Stefan Institute, Ljubljana, Slovenia

Janez Mravljak
Faculty of Pharmacy, University of Ljubljana, Ljubljana, Slovenia

Reiner Zeisig
Max-Delbrück-Centre for Molecular Medicine, Berlin-Buch, Germany

Shao-Wen Hung, Chiao-Li Chu, Yu-Ching Chang and Shu-Mei Liang
Agricultural Biotechnology Research Center, Academia Sinica, Taipei, Taiwan

Ann Marie Kieber-Emmons, Fariba Jousheghany and Behjatolah Monzavi-Karbassi
Department of Pathology and Winthrop P. Rockefeller Cancer institute, University of Arkansas for Medical Sciences, Little Rock, USA

Khoo Boon Yin
Institute for Research in Molecular Medicine (INFORMM), University Sains Malaysia, Penang, Malaysia

P. Di Stefano, M. del P. Camacho Leal, B. Bisaro, G. Tornillo, D. Repetto, A. Pincini, N. Sharma, S. Grasso, E. Turco, S. Cabodi and P. Defilippi
Molecular Biotechnology Center, Università di Torino, Torino, Italy

Sanaa Al Saleh and Yunus A. Luqmani
Faculty of Pharmacy, Kuwait University, Kuwait

Anthony Magliocco and Cay Egan
University of Calgary, Canada

Jenna E. Fong and Svetlana V. Komarova
Faculty of Dentistry, McGill University, Montreal, Canada

Gozie Offiah, Kieran Brennan and Ann M. Hopkins
Royal College of Surgeons in Ireland, Beaumont Hospital, Dublin, Ireland

Xuejing Zhang and Daotai Nie
Department of Medical Microbiology, Immunology, and Cell Biology Southern Illinois, University School of Medicine and Simmons Cancer Institute, Springfield, USA

Printed in the USA
CPSIA information can be obtained
at www.ICGtesting.com
JSHW011503221024
72173JS00005B/1185

9 781632 410665